New

Dimensions

in Women's

Health

AIDS II Smartbook, Kopec

Aquatic Exercise, Sova

Aquatics: The Complete Reference Guide for Aquatic Fitness Professionals, Sova

Aquatics Activities Handbook, Sova

An Athlete's Guide to Agents, Ruxin

Basic Law for the Allied Health Professions, Cowdrey

The Biology of AIDS, Third Edition, Fan, et al.

The Birth Control Book, Belcastro

Bloodborne Pathogens, National Safety Council

A Challenge for Living: A Comprehensive View of Dying, Death, and Bereavement, Corless, et al.

CPR Manual, National Safety Council

Contemporary Health Issues, Banister, et al.

Dawn Brown's Complete Guide to Step Aerobics, Brown

Drugs and Society, Third Edition, Witters, et al.

Essential Medical Terminology, Stanfield

Dying, Death, and Bereavement: Theoretical Perspectives and Other Ways of Knowing, Corless, et al.

Emergency Encounters: EMTs and Their Work, Mannon

Ethics Consultation: A Practical Guide, LaPuma/Schiedermayer

First Aid, National Safety Council

First Aid and CPR, Second Edition, National Safety Council

First Aid and CPR, Infants and Children, National Safety Council

Fitness and Health: Life-Style Strategies, Thygerson

Fostering Emotional Well-Being in the Classroom, Page/Page

Golf: Your Turn for Success, Fisher/Geertsen

Health and Wellness, Fourth Edition, Edlin/Golanty

Healthy Children 2000, U.S. Department of Health and Human Services

Healthy People 2000, U.S. Department of Health and Human Services

Healthy People 2000—Summary Report, U.S. Department of Health and Human Services

Human Aging and Chronic Disease, Kart, et al.

Human Anatomy and Physiology Coloring Workbook and Study Guide, Anderson

Interviewing and Helping Skills for Health Professionals, Cormier, et al.

Introduction to Human Disease, Third Edition, Crowley

Introduction to Human Immunology, Huffer, et al.

Introduction to the Health Professions, Stanfield

Medical Terminology, Stanfield

The Nation's Health, Fourth Edition, Lee/Estes

Omaha Orange: A Popular History of EMS in America, Post

Personal Health Choices, Smith/Smith

Safety, Second Edition, Thygerson

Sexuality Today, Nass/Fisher

Skill-Building Activities for Alcohol and Drug Education, Bates/Wigtil

Sports Equipment Management, Walker/Seidler

Sports Injury Care, Abdenour/Thygerson

Teaching Elementary Health Science, Third Edition, Bender/Sorochan

Weight Management the Fitness Way, Dusek

Weight Training for Strength and Fitness, Silvester

Writing a Successful Grant Application, Reif-Lehrer

New Dimensions in Women's Health

Linda Lewis Alexander, PhD, RN,C

Department of Health Education
University of Maryland
College Park, Maryland

Director of Women's Health
American Social Health Association
Research Triangle Park, North Carolina

Judith H. LaRosa, PhD, RN

Deputy Director
Office of Research on Women's Health
National Institutes of Health
Bethesda, Maryland

JONES AND BARTLETT PUBLISHERS
Boston　　　　　London

Editorial, Sales, and Customer Service Offices
Jones and Bartlett Publishers
One Exeter Plaza
Boston, MA 02116
617-859-3900
800-832-0034

Jones and Bartlett Publishers International
PO Box 1498
London W6 7RS
England

Library of Congress Cataloging-in-Publication Data
Alexander, Linda Lewis.
    New dimensions in women's health / Linda Lewis Alexander, Judith H. LaRosa.
      p. cm.
    Includes bibliographical references and index.
    ISBN 0-86720-777-9
    1. Women—Health and hygiene.   2. Women—Health and hygiene—Social aspects. I. La Rosa, Judith H. II. Title.
    [DNLM: 1. Women's Health.   WA 300 A376n 1994]
  RA778.A438   1994
  613′ .0424—dc20
  DNLM/DLC
  for Library of Congress   93-50822
                                               CIP

Acquisitions Editor Joseph E. Burns
Production Editor Judy Songdahl
Manufacturing Buyer Dana L. Cerrito
Editorial Production Service Michael Bass & Associates
Text Design Joy Dickinson / Editorial Design
Typesetting Modern Graphics
Cover Design Beth Santos Design
Printing and Binding Courier
Cover Printing Henry N. Sawyer

Printed in the United States of America
98 97 96 95 94 10 9 8 7 6 5 4 3 2 1

This book is dedicated to women everywhere— Witness our complexity and celebrate the strength in our diversity.

Contents

PART II

Personal and Sexual Dimensions of Women's Health

10. *Reproductive Tract Infections* 292

PART III

Chronic Conditions and Aging Dimensions of Women's Health

11. Cardiovascular Disease

Preface

In the last half of the twentieth century women have gained acceptance as complete human beings, and have come to be regarded as more than extensions of their families, more than (e.g.,) wives, mothers, or daughters. They are multi-faceted individuals who are artists, scientists, generals, clergy members, and housewives. Similarly, it has been realized that understanding a woman's health means more than understanding her gynecological or reproductive health. The traditional concept of a woman's gynecological health of the early twentieth century has evolved into a more accurate, sensitive, and enlightened one.

The feminist movement and social activism of the 1960s and '70s became the foundation for the new understanding and actions in the '90s. The concept of women's health has changed from the view that "raging hormones" rule a woman's life during her three critical periods of menarche, pregnancy, and menopause to one that appreciates the full spectrum of factors that constitute illness or well-being.

Another result of this change in thinking was that women began taking control of their health and well-being rather than being passive recipients of illness-driven health care. Women began entering into decision-making partnerships with health care providers and demanding investigation and understanding of the diseases, disorders, and conditions that affect them. In the '90s, women began demanding redress from research neglect. The biomedical research agencies of the federal government had to ensure that gaps in knowledge on women's health issues were addressed, that women as a group be included in study populations, and that gender differences in conditions be discerned whenever possible. Thus, the '90s approach to women's health has evolved into one that melds the traditional medical model with enlightened self-interest and advocacy for scientifically valid research that discerns the similarities and differences between genders. The result of these efforts is improved personal and public health for women.

Like the times, the book is neither traditional nor feminist in tone or scope, but an amalgam of both with a focus on personal decision making in all dimensions of women's health. Each chapter comprehensively reviews an important dimension and examines the contributing epidemiological, historical, psycho-social, cultural/ethnic, legal, political, and economic influences. Special populations of women—adolescents, minorities, lesbians, and others—are recognized in terms of their particular needs or unique factors that influence their well-being. Information boxes and self-assessments are distributed throughout each chapter highlighting and summarizing significant concepts.

New Dimensions in Women's Health is organized for the time constraints of a single academic semester. It is intended to provide a comprehensive overview of critical, contemporary women's health topics and a framework for informed personal decision making. The explosion of contemporary interest in women's health makes this book ideally suited as a core textbook for courses in women's health, women's studies, health education, and nursing. It is also appropriate as a supplemental reading or background text for studies in sociology, psychology, anthropology, public health, health behavior, medicine, and allied health.

This work has benefited greatly from the support and guidance of our families and friends. We are indebted to them for their patience, understanding, and encouragement. Special people at Jones and Bartlett deserve an extra thank you for their help and support in the production of this book. Mr. Joseph Burns, Vice President, and Amina Sharma, Editorial Assistant, have been continuous sources of guidance and assistance. Special thanks also to Judy Songdahl, Production Administrator; Michael Bass and Debbie Frank of Michael Bass & Associates; and Maxine Effenson Chuck of B. Czar Productions, Inc., for sharing their insights, experiences, and support.

We would also like to thank the reviewers whose critical judgment and editorial suggestions helped strengthen and improve the final draft of this text. I am very grateful for the comments and wise counsel of Denise Amschler, Ball State University; Nancy Ellis, Indiana University; Kathy Fischer, Western Illinois University; and Roberta Ogletree and Eileen Zunich, both of Southern Illinois University.

New

Dimensions

in Women's

Health

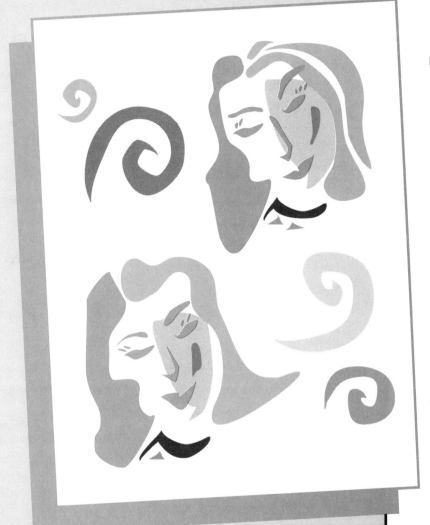

Lifestyle and Social Dimensions in Women's Health

CHAPTER 1

Nutrition

CHAPTER OBJECTIVES

On completion of this chapter, the student should be able to discuss:

1. How nutritional issues for women represent a complex spectrum of subjects.

2. The basic building blocks of nutrition.

3. How to select a fortified food.

4. The significance of the food pyramid.

5. Differences between saturated and unsaturated fats; monounsaturated and polyunsaturated fats; low-density lipoproteins and high-density lipoproteins.

6. How to calculate daily fat intake.

7. Differences between water-soluble and fat-soluble vitamins.

8. Why calcium is of special dietary significance to women.

9. Which groups of women are at risk for iron deficiency.

10. Significance of beta-carotene in the diet.

11. Differences between crude and dietary fiber.

12. How sugar is detrimental to health.

13. Why dieting is an ineffective way to lose weight.

14. What is the position of the antidiet movement.

15. What is a safe weight loss rate.

16. What is yo-yo dieting and how it contributes to future difficulty in losing weight.

17. The risks associated with obesity.

18. How to calculate body mass index.

19. Significance of basal metabolic rate with dieting.

20. Why exercise is the best way to increase basal metabolic rate.

21. How body image has changed with time.

22. Concerns with "apple" versus "pear" shape for women.

Introduction

Nutritional issues for women represent a complex spectrum of subjects from dietary guidelines to sociological phenomena. Contemporary society is weight conscious, fashion conscious, diet conscious, and not very tolerant of perceived physical imperfection. Society sends a message suggesting that thin women are somehow smarter than, luckier than, more interesting than, and generally superior to those who aren't thin. The resultant female obsession with dieting and weight loss is also primarily an American phenomenon. Compared with women worldwide, studies show that girls and women in the United States diet more and are less satisfied and more self-conscious about their bodies than women in other countries.[1] This obsession begins early, with inappropriate eating habits and high anxiety about obesity prevalent among adolescent girls. More than half of the underweight adolescent participants in one study were found to be extremely fearful of being overweight.[2] Another interesting finding regarding nutrition and adolescent girls is that a high-fat, low-fiber diet appears to expedite sexual development. Specifically a study found that breast development was delayed the longest in those girls who consumed the most fruits, vegetables, and whole grains.[3] Clearly the spectrum of nutritional issues is complex and begins early with women, lasting throughout the lifetime.

A woman informed about lifetime nutrition needs to understand what is meant by healthy eating, how body image influences women and their eating (or dieting) decisions, issues in weight control, and how women are especially vulnerable to an array of possible eating disorders.

Healthful Eating

Nutrition

Nutrition is the science that explores the need for and the effects of food on organisms. Nutritional jargon refers to the terminology used to describe nutritional issues and concepts (Information Box 1.1). The fundamental building blocks of the body include protein, carbohydrates, and fats. **Protein** provides the framework for muscles, bones, blood, hair, and fingernails. The National Academy of Science recommends that women have 50 gm of protein a day.[4] Most Americans actually ingest nearly twice as much as that daily. Only 12 to 15 percent of daily calories should come from protein sources. Extra protein, like other excess calories,

Nutritional Jargon

Enriched: Replacing nutrients in a product that may have been lost during processing. For example, bread may be enriched with iron, niacin, thiamine, and riboflavin.

Fortified: The addition of vitamins and minerals to a food product that were not originally present. For example, orange juice may be fortified with calcium.

Light or lite: A relatively meaningless descriptor that may refer to reduced calories, low sodium, taste, reduced alcohol, or fluffy texture.

Low-calorie: Means that a food has less than 40 calories per serving *and* less than 0.4 calories per gram.

Natural: A relatively meaningless descriptor that may refer to minimal processing or a product that is free of artificial ingredients. Many foods labeled as natural are highly processed, high in fat or sugar, or loaded with preservatives.

RDA: Recommended Dietary Allowance, the estimated amount of various nutrients needed each day to maintain good health. The guidelines were developed to address population-based dietary needs such as pregnant women; individual needs may vary owing to genetic, personal, and demographic factors.

Reduced-calorie: Foods labeled as reduced calorie must have at least one-third fewer calories than regular preparations. The nutritional comparison must be displayed on the product label.

Sugarless and sugar-free: Another misleading descriptor because current FDA definition of "sugar" means sucrose but does not include other forms of sugar such as glucose, fructose, or sorbitol, which contain as many calories as sucrose.

---

is stored as fat. **Carbohydrates** provide the basic fuel for the body and are present in two forms: **simple carbohydrates** (sugars) and **complex carbohydrates** (starches). Sugars provide little more than a quick spurt of energy, whereas starches are rich in vitamins, minerals, and other nutrients. Complex carbohydrates should provide the major supply of calories in diets. There is no recommended allowance for **fats,** although fats perform many important bodily functions, such as storing energy, maintaining healthy hair and skin, carrying fat-soluble vitamins, supplying essential fatty acids, affecting levels of blood cholesterol, and promoting satiety. According to the US Department of Agriculture (USDA) and the US Health and Human Services Joint Nutrition Committee, the principal nutrition-related problems in the United States today arise from overconsumption of fat, saturated fatty acids, cholesterol, and sodium.[5]

Fortified Foods

Food fortification is an important contemporary nutritional issue. **Fortification** is defined as any addition of a nutrient to a food. The addition of vitamin D to milk to prevent rickets and niacin to flour to fight pellagra are classic examples of fortification. Today many processed foods, such as ready-to-eat cereals, fruit drinks, and frozen items, are fortified without regulation. Vitamins, minerals, and fiber are added to these products in varying amounts. Consumers are often confused about how much and what type of fortification is really necessary for healthy eating. Fortified foods should be part of a healthy eating plan for women, *not* a substitute for one. Fortified foods should be carefully chosen. A cereal fortified to 100 percent of the recommended dietary allowance (RDA) can add badly needed iron to a woman's diet, but it can also present a problem if the woman is tempted by high-fat fast foods later on with the mistaken perception that she is "nutritionally sound" for the day based on the morning bowl of fortified cereal. When selecting fortified foods, a woman should first determine, "is this food itself nutritious?" There is no value in eating a fortified cookie or snack bar. Fortified foods should derive less than 30 percent of their calories from fat (3 to 4 gm per 100-calorie serving), and the food itself should be a "real" food, that is 100 percent fruit products, milk products, and breads and whole-grain mixtures, fortified to less than 50 percent of the RDA for nutrients often found in inadequate amounts in women's diets: iron, calcium, magnesium, zinc, vitamin B_6 and folacin.[6]

Dietary Guidelines

Several publications have highlighted the significance of diet on health. In 1988, the *Surgeon General's Report on Nutrition and Health* identified the reduction of fat intake as the primary dietary priority for public health action.[7] This report led to the 1992 revision of the USDA dietary guidelines (Figure 1.1) with an

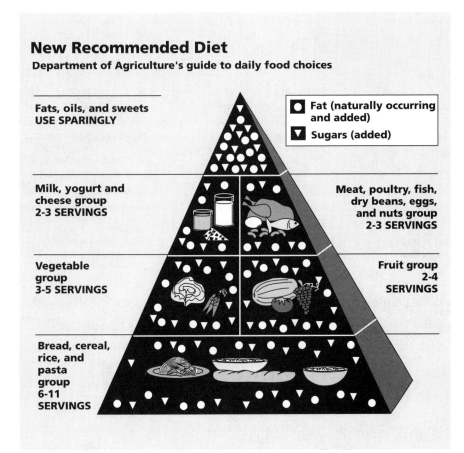

FIGURE 1.1

USDA recommended diet—food pyramid.
SOURCE: USDA, 1992.

emphasis on promoting less fat and sugar and more fruits, vegetables, and grains. The schematic format for the guidelines is a pyramid, which replaced the traditional food-wheel pie. The pie had equal representations of the traditional four major food groups: fruits and vegetables; dairy products; breads and other grains; and meat, poultry, eggs, and fish. The pyramid emphasizes the importance of eating in moderation and what nutritionists call "proportionality"—eating different amounts of food daily from the basic food

---

INFORMATION BOX 1.2

Dietary Guidelines to Reduce Risk of Cancer

Substance	Major Dietary Sources	Suspected Role in Cancer	Comment
Possible protectors			
Beta carotene (transformed into vitamin A by the body)	Yellow, orange, and green leafy vegetables and fruit, such as carrots, cantaloupe, broccoli, yams, spinach	Deficiency may increase risk of lung, stomach, cervical, bladder, and other cancers	This antioxidant is thought to be more anticarcinogenic than dietary vitamin A. Extra carotene is stored in most tissue for future use. Not toxic
Vitamin A	Liver, butter, milk, cheese, egg yolk, fish oil	Deficiency may cause abnormal cell growth, possibly leading to cancerous tumors	Much of its protectiveness is due to beta carotene (above). Avoid vitamin A supplements—megadoses can be toxic
Vitamin C	Citrus fruits, tomatoes, broccoli, strawberries, potatoes, peppers, kale (C is destroyed by improper storage or long cooking)	Deficiency of this antioxidant may increase risk of cancer of stomach and esophagus. May block conversion of nitrites and nitrates to cancer-causing agents	Adult RDA is 60 mg, supplied by 4 oz of fresh orange juice. Unused C is excreted. Megadoses (over 1 gm daily) can cause diarrhea and may result in kidney stones
Vitamin E	Nuts, vegetable oils, liver, margarine, whole grains, wheat germ, dried beans	An antioxidant. Shown to protect laboratory animals against some cancers	Adult RDA is supplied by 1 tablespoon of margarine
Selenium	Seafood, liver, meats, grains, egg yolks, tomatoes	An antioxidant. Shown to protect laboratory animals against some cancers	No RDA. Plentiful in most diets. Supplements can be extremely dangerous
Fiber	Found only in plant foods, such as fruits, vegetables, whole grains	Promotes healthy bowel function. May lower risk of colon and rectal cancer	Choose whole-grain breads and cereals. Eat fruit and vegetables with skins when possible
Cruciferous vegetables	Vegetables of the cabbage family, e.g., broccoli, kale, Brussels sprouts, cauliflower	Contain antioxidants that may block production of potential cancer-causing agents in laboratory animals	Eat at least 2–3 servings each week. Excellent sources of fiber, minerals, and vitamins

groups. The pyramid conveys at a glance that fruit and vegetables and grains should make up the bulk of the diet. Eating the proper foods in moderation and proportionately maximizes nutritional benefit. Diet plays a major role in the development of cardiovascular disease and is believed to play a significant role in cancer development as well. Based on current research, nutritional guidelines have been developed by the National Cancer Institute to maximize the possible benefits from a healthy diet (Information Box 1.2). It is estimated

Substance	Major Dietary Sources	Suspected Role in Cancer	Comment
Possible villains			
Fats	Meats, poultry skin, whole milk and milk products, vegetable oils	Excess consumption of fats may contribute to cancers of the digestive and reproductive systems and to obesity, another risk factor for cancer	Choose low-fat dairy products and lean meats; trim all visible fat and discard poultry skin; don't fry meats. Eat fish. Avoid high-fat processed foods
Alcohol	Beer, wine, liquor	Heavy drinking, especially combined with smoking, contributes to cancers of the mouth, throat, liver, and bladder. May also be a factor in breast cancer	Drink only in moderation, if at all: no more than 2 drinks a day
Nitrites	Used to preserve cured meats, such as bacon, hot dogs, sausages, ham	Promotes cancers of stomach and esophagus in laboratory animals	Avoid eating cured meats habitually. Use low-temperature cooking methods. Microwaved bacon, e.g., is lower in carcinogens, especially if you drain the fat
Aflatoxins	Poisons formed in moldy peanuts, peanut butter, seeds, corn, and other crops	If eaten in large amounts, can cause liver cancer, a rare disease in the US	Discard moldy, shriveled, discolored peanuts. Refrigerate freshly ground peanut butter; discard entire jar if moldy
Browned foods	Meats grilled, barbecued, or fried at high temperatures	These cooking methods create cancer-causing agents. Most dangerous when cooking fatty meat over a heat source	As often as possible, choose other cooking methods—steam, bake, roast, or microwave. Scrape off charred material

SOURCE: American Cancer Society, 1992.

Fat Content of Selected Foods

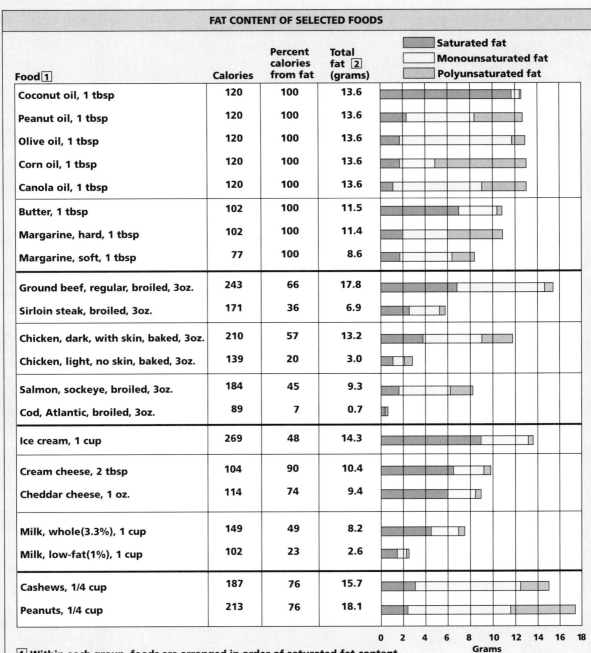

FAT CONTENT OF SELECTED FOODS

Food [1]	Calories	Percent calories from fat	Total fat [2] (grams)
Coconut oil, 1 tbsp	120	100	13.6
Peanut oil, 1 tbsp	120	100	13.6
Olive oil, 1 tbsp	120	100	13.6
Corn oil, 1 tbsp	120	100	13.6
Canola oil, 1 tbsp	120	100	13.6
Butter, 1 tbsp	102	100	11.5
Margarine, hard, 1 tbsp	102	100	11.4
Margarine, soft, 1 tbsp	77	100	8.6
Ground beef, regular, broiled, 3oz.	243	66	17.8
Sirloin steak, broiled, 3oz.	171	36	6.9
Chicken, dark, with skin, baked, 3oz.	210	57	13.2
Chicken, light, no skin, baked, 3oz.	139	20	3.0
Salmon, sockeye, broiled, 3oz.	184	45	9.3
Cod, Atlantic, broiled, 3oz.	89	7	0.7
Ice cream, 1 cup	269	48	14.3
Cream cheese, 2 tbsp	104	90	10.4
Cheddar cheese, 1 oz.	114	74	9.4
Milk, whole(3.3%), 1 cup	149	49	8.2
Milk, low-fat(1%), 1 cup	102	23	2.6
Cashews, 1/4 cup	187	76	15.7
Peanuts, 1/4 cup	213	76	18.1

Legend: Saturated fat, Monounsaturated fat, Polyunsaturated fat

Grams axis: 0 2 4 6 8 10 12 14 16 18

[1] Within each group, foods are arranged in order of saturated-fat content.
[2] Total fat exceeds the sum of saturated, monounsaturated, and polyunsaturated fats because it also includes other fatty acids.

SOURCE: "Fat Content of Selected Foods." Copyright © 1992 by Consumers Union of U.S., Inc., Yonkers, NY 10703-1057. Reprinted by permission from *Consumer Reports on Health,* June 1992.

that approximately 35 percent of cancers are related to diet. To promote a cancer-reduction diet among Americans, the National Cancer Institute and food industry have launched the largest public-private sponsored nutrition education program ever undertaken to encourage the public to eat five servings of fruits and vegetables every day.

Cholesterol

The body normally produces **cholesterol,** which is a necessary component of various body cells. Cholesterol is a vital constituent of cell membranes and nerve fibers and serves as a building block for certain hormones. Too much cholesterol, however, is dangerous, especially to the cardiovascular system. The connection between diet and elevated blood cholesterol is evident: generally the lower the blood cholesterol level, the better. Diet has been identified as one of the major modifiable risk factors for coronary heart disease (atherosclerosis), along with smoking, high blood pressure, obesity, and physical inactivity. Cholesterol is found only in foods from animal sources, such as eggs, meats, and dairy products. Fats are classified as **saturated,** which come primarily from animal sources, and **unsaturated,** which come from plants and include most vegetable oils. Saturated fats are loaded with all the hydrogen atoms they can carry. Unsaturated fats, which have proportionately fewer hydrogen atoms, include **polyunsaturated** fats, such as those in safflower and sunflower oil, and **monounsaturated** fats, such as those in olive and canola oil. Information Box 1.3 demonstrates the relationship of saturated and unsaturated fats among popular food items. The way cholesterol is distributed in the body is complex and not fully understood. Both fats, known as **triglycerides,** and cholesterol are transported in the bloodstream in protein packages called **lipoproteins,** which are assembled in the intestinal tract and liver. Polyunsaturated fats have demonstrated effectiveness in not only lowering cholesterol levels, but also **low-density lipoproteins** (LDL)—the "bad" cholesterol—and **high-density lipoproteins** (HDL)—the "good" cholesterol. Monounsaturated fats have been shown to lower only LDL. Research also suggests that monounsaturated fats may also benefit the heart by reducing blood pressure and blood sugar levels.[8] In general terms, LDL carry the cholesterol through the system, dropping it off where it is needed for cell building and leaving any excess in arterial walls and other tissue. Other molecular packages, HDL, pick up these cholesterol deposits and bring them to the liver for reprocessing or excretion. This is why LDL has been called "bad cholesterol" and HDL "good cholesterol."

A panel of experts from the National Heart, Lung, and Blood Institute recommends that less than 10 percent of total calories come from saturated fatty acids and an average of not more than 30 percent of total calories come from all fat. Self-Assessment 1.1 reviews the method for calculating daily fat intake. Very few American women currently are meeting this standard (Figure 1.2). In addition, diet should provide adequate energy (calorie) levels to maintain desirable weight and contain less than 300 mg of cholesterol per day.[9] These

---

SELF-ASSESSMENT 1.1

Calculating Daily Fat Limits

To determine the maximum number of daily grams of fat:

1. Calculate approximately how many calories are consumed on a daily basis: _____

2. Multiply the answer in (1) by 0.30: _____

3. Divide the result of (2) by 9: _____

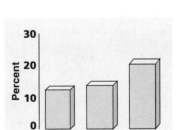

FIGURE 1.2

Percentage of women aged 19 to 50 meeting dietary guidelines for fat (≤30%), by race, 1985–86.

SOURCE: Adapted from Thompson, F.E., Sowers, M.F., Frongillo, E.A., and Parpia, B.J. (1992). Sources of fiber and fat in diets of U.S. women aged 19 to 50: Implications for nutrition education and policy. *American Journal of Public Health, 82*(5), 695–702.

guidelines parallel the guidelines released by other federal agencies and emphasize the importance of careful eating patterns for women from early childhood to old age.

Vitamins

Vitamins, organic substances needed by the body in very small amounts that perform a variety of functions in metabolism and nutrition, are often misunderstood and misused substances. When a woman consumes a nutritious diet, there is no need for vitamin supplements. Despite all the advertising claims, scientific evidence offers *no* indication that extra vitamins prolong life, enhance sexual pleasures, or enhance athletic performance. Vitamins are often viewed as a lazy way or a shortcut to good nutrition. Vitamins work well with other nutrients in food. They cannot replace food or turn a junk-food meal into a healthy one. Vitamins are essential for life, promoting good vision, forming normal blood cells, creating strong bones and teeth, and ensuring proper functioning of the heart and nervous system. Although vitamins do not supply any energy, they do aid in the efficient conversion of foods into energy. Scientific consensus is that there are 13 essential vitamins: A, C, D, E, K, and the eight vitamins of the B complex. Vitamins are classified as **fat-soluble** (A, D, E, and K), which are stored in the liver for relatively long periods of time, and as **water-soluble,** which are stored for very short periods of time. Each vitamin carries out specific functions. The body generally cannot manufacture vitamins; they must be derived from food sources. A particular disease usually results if a certain vitamin is lacking or is improperly used by the body. Information Box 1.4 provides a summary of the facts and myths of each of the essential vitamins.

Minerals

Minerals are inorganic substances essential to a variety of vital body functions, from basic bone formation (calcium) and enzyme synthesis (iron) to the regulation of the heart muscle (potassium) and normal functioning of the digestive process. Minerals are basic constituents of the earth's surface. Carried into the soil, groundwater, and sea by erosion, they are taken up by plants and consumed by animals and humans. As components of the body, minerals are present in small amounts. Although there are more than 60 different minerals, 6 of them (calcium, chloride, magnesium, phosphorus, potassium, and sodium) are generally designated as **macrominerals,** or major minerals. From a women's health perspective, calcium and iron are especially important minerals. Because of the complex interactions between minerals and the dangers of overdosing, self-administration of mineral supplements in doses greater than RDAs should be avoided. Megadoses of certain minerals may do serious harm. The best way to ensure an adequate supply of minerals is to eat a varied, balanced diet.

Facts and Myths about Vitamins

Vitamin	Adult RDA*	Sources	What It Does	Myths
A	800–1,000 mcg	Liver, eggs, fortified milk, carrots, tomatoes, apricots, cantaloupe, fish	Promotes good vision; helps form and maintain healthy skin and mucous membranes; may protect against some cancers	Cures cancer; enhances normal vision; promotes smooth, youthful skin
C	50–60 mg	Citrus fruits, strawberries, tomatoes	Promotes healthy gums, capillaries, and teeth; aids iron absorption; may block production of nitrosamines; maintains normal connective tissue; aids in healing wounds	Prevents or cures the common cold; cures cancer; reduces cholesterol and protects against heart disease; prevents allergies; prevents or cures poisoning; cures a wide range of infections; cures arthritis
D	5–10 mcg (200–400 IU)	Fortified milk, fish; also produced by the body in response to sunlight	Promotes strong bones and teeth; necessary for absorption of calcium	Cures arthritis
E	8–10 mg	Nuts, vegetable oils, whole grains, olives, asparagus, spinach	Protects tissue against oxidation; important in formation of red blood cells; helps body use vitamin K	Prevents or alleviates coronary heart disease; enhances sexual performance; improves muscle strength and stamina; heals burns and wounds; slows aging
K	70–140 mcg†	Body produces about half of daily needs; cauliflower, broccoli, cabbage, spinach, cereals, soybeans, beef liver	Aids in clotting of blood	
B₁ (Thiamine)	1–1.5 mg	Whole grains, dried beans, lean meats (especially pork), fish	Helps release energy from carbohydrates; necessary for healthy brain and nerve cells and for functioning of heart	Prevents fatigue; cures depression
B₂ (Riboflavin)	1.2–1.7 mg	Nuts, dairy products, liver	Aids in release of energy from foods; interacts with other B vitamins	Cures baldness; improves vision
B₃ (Niacin)	13–19 mg	Nuts, dairy products, liver	Aids in release of energy from foods; involved in synthesis of DNA; maintains normal functioning of skin, nerves, and digestive system	Fights heart disease; alleviates schizophrenia; cures depression
B₅ (Pantothenic acid)	4–7 mg†	Whole grains, dried beans, eggs, nuts	Aids in release of energy from foods; essential for synthesis of numerous body materials	Cures allergies; helps you cope with stress; restores gray hair to normal color

(continued)

Facts and Myths about Vitamins

Vitamin	Adult RDA*	Sources	What It Does	Myths
B_6 (Pyridoxine)	1.8–2.2 mg	Whole grains, dried beans, eggs, nuts	Important in chemical reactions of proteins and amino acids; involved in normal functioning of brain and formation of red blood cells	Helps arthritis; cures migraines; relieves nausea; acts as a tranquilizer; relieves nervous and muscle disorders; prevents tooth decay; lowers blood cholesterol
B_{12}	3 mcg	Liver, beef, eggs, milk, shellfish	Necessary for development of red blood cells; maintains normal functioning of nervous system	Helps nervous disorders
Folacin	400 mcg	Liver, wheat bran, leafy green vegetables, beans, grains	Important in the synthesis of DNA; acts together with B_{12} in the production of hemoglobin	Alleviates mental illness; cures anemia
Biotin	100–200 mcg†	Yeast, eggs, liver, milk	Important in formation of fatty acids; helps metabolize amino acids and carbohydrates	Cures baldness; alleviates muscle pain; cures dermatitis

*These figures are not applicable to pregnant women, who need additional vitamins.
†Although there is no RDA for this vitamin, the Food and Nutrition Board recommends this range of intakes.
SOURCE: Excerpted from the University of California at Berkeley Wellness Letter, © Health Letter Associates, 1986.

Information Box 1.5 provides a summary of the facts and myths of each of the essential minerals.

Calcium

Calcium is a mineral of special concern to women. Calcium is an integral component of bones and teeth and also plays a role in regulating heartbeat, blood clotting, muscle contraction, and nerve conduction. Evidence also suggests that this essential mineral helps prevent high blood pressure and may play a role in preventing colon cancer. Calcium deficiency is one of the strongest contributors to osteoporosis. When calcium levels in the blood are too low, the body draws the mineral from bones to meet its needs. This accelerates the gradual bone loss that occurs most dramatically in postmenopausal women. The daily RDA for women is 800 mg except for adolescents and young adults (aged 11 to 24) and pregnant or lactating women, who are advised to consume

INFORMATION BOX 1.5

Facts and Myths about Minerals

Mineral	Adult RDA or Estimated Intake	Food Sources	What It Does	Myths
Calcium	800 mg* (1,200–1,500 mg for older women, according to an NIH consensus report) 1 quart milk = 1,250 mg	Milk and milk products, sardines and salmon eaten with bones, dark green leafy vegetables, shellfish, hard water	Builds bones and teeth and maintains bone density and strength; helps prevent osteoporosis in older population; plays a role in regulating heartbeat, blood clotting, muscle contraction, and nerve conduction; may help prevent hypertension	Helps prevent insomnia and anxiety
Chloride	1,900–5,000 mg†	Table salt, fish, pickled and smoked foods	Maintains normal fluid shifts; balances pH of the blood; forms hydrochloric acid to aid digestion	
Magnesium	300 mg (women), 350 mg (men)* 1 cup spinach = 160 mg	Wheat bran, whole grains, raw leafy green vegetables, nuts (especially almonds and cashews), soybeans, bananas, apricots, hard water, spices	Aids in bone growth; aids function of nerves and muscles, including regulation of normal heart rhythm	Cures alcoholism, prostate problems, kidney stones, and heart disease
Phosphorus	800 mg* 1 cup milk = 993 mg; 1 serving chicken = 231 mg	Meats, poultry, fish, cheese, egg yolks, dried peas and beans, milk and milk products, soft drinks, nuts; present in almost all foods	Aids bone growth and strengthening of teeth; important in energy metabolism	Reduces stress; accelerates growth in children; helps reduce arthritis
Potassium	1,500–6,000 mg† 1 cup raisins = 524 mg; 1 banana = 400 mg; 1 small potato = 400 mg	Oranges and orange juice, bananas, dried fruits, peanut butter, dried peas and beans, potatoes, coffee, tea, cocoa, yogurt, molasses, meat	Promotes regular heartbeat; active in muscle contraction; regulates transfer of nutrients to cells; controls water balance in body tissues and cells; contributes to regulation of blood pressure	Cures acne, alcoholism, allergies, burns, and heart disease
Sodium	2,000–3,300 mg† 1 frozen pot pie = 1,600 mg	All from salt	Helps regulate water balance in body; plays a role in maintaining blood pressure	Lowers fevers; prevents heat stroke
Chromium	0.05–0.20 mg†	Meat, cheese, whole grains, dried peas and beans, peanuts, brewer's yeast	Important for glucose metabolism; may be a cofactor for insulin	Relieves atherosclerosis, diabetes, and hypoglycemia

(continued)

Facts and Myths about Minerals

Mineral	Adult RDA or Estimated Intake	Food Sources	What It Does	Myths
Copper	2.0–3.0 mg†	Shellfish (especially oysters), nuts, beef and pork liver, cocoa powder, chocolate, kidneys, dried beans, raisins, corn oil margarine	Formation of red blood cells; cofactor in absorbing iron into blood cells; assists in production of several enzymes involved in respiration; interacts with zinc	Stimulates hair growth in bald men; relieves anemia
Fluorine (fluoride)	1.5–4.0 mg†	Fluoridated water; foods grown with or cooked in fluoridated water; fish, tea, gelatin	Contributes to solid bone and tooth formation; may help prevent osteoporosis in older people	Causes cancer
Iodine	0.15 mg*	Primarily from iodized salt, but also seafood, seaweed food products, vegetables grown in iodine-rich areas, vegetable oil	Necessary for normal function of the thyroid gland; essential for normal cell function; keeps skin, hair, and nails healthy; prevents goiter	Cures anemia
Iron	10 mg (male), 18 mg (female, during childbearing years, expected to be lowered to 16 mg)* 4 oz calf's liver = 12 mg	Liver (especially pork liver), kidneys, red meats, egg yolks, peas, beans, nuts, dried fruits, green leafy vegetables, enriched grain products, blackstrap molasses	Essential to formation of hemoglobin, the oxygen-carrying factor in the blood; part of several enzymes and proteins in the body	Controls alcoholism and menstrual discomfort
Manganese	2.5–5.0 mg† ½ cup peanut butter = 2 mg	Nuts, whole grains, vegetables, fruits, instant coffee, tea, cocoa powder, beets, egg yolks	Required for normal bone growth and development, normal reproduction, and cell function	Helps asthma, diabetes, sterility, fatigue, and myasthenia gravis
Molybdenum	0.15–0.50 mg†	Peas, beans, cereal grains, organ meats, some dark green vegetables	Important for normal cell function	
Selenium	0.05–0.20 mg† 4 oz fish = 0.038 mg	Fish, shellfish, red meat, egg yolks, chicken, garlic, tuna, tomatoes	Complements vitamin E to fight cell damage by oxygen	Cures cancer and arthritis

*These figures are not applicable to pregnant women, who need additional vitamins.
†Although there is no RDA for this vitamin, the Food and Nutrition Board recommends this range of intakes.
SOURCE: Excerpted from the University of California at Berkeley Wellness Letter, © Health Letter Associates, 1985.

1,200 mg daily. Most experts now recommend that postmenopausal women consume at least that much, too. The typical American woman consumes less than 600 mg of calcium daily. Three to five cups of milk or servings of other calcium-rich foods such as cheese, broccoli, or sardines supply the 1,000 to 1,500 mg of essential daily calcium. The vitamin D added to milk and the lactose in milk and dairy products are believed also to aid in the body's absorption of calcium. Information Box 1.6 shows the amount of calcium present in some food products. Calcium may be a difficult nutrient for women who do not like or cannot tolerate milk and other dairy products. The calcium shortfall has led to promotion of calcium supplementation and additional questions about their effectiveness. Proponents of calcium fortification compare it with other forms of nutritional fortification, such as iodine in table salt, which virtually eliminated goiter in the United States. The link between calcium and osteoporosis, however, is not nearly as clear-cut. There may be detrimental effects of calcium supplements. Women susceptible to kidney stones should avoid supplements and calcium-fortified foods. Although large amounts of calcium may not be toxic for healthy women, no one has documented how much calcium specifically constitutes an overdose. It is known, however, that large doses of calcium can interfere with the absorption of other nutrients, such as iron and zinc.

Iron

Women with diets chronically deficient in iron are at serious risk for anemia. Anemia is characterized by a lack of **hemoglobin,** a key component of red blood cells and the oxygen-carrying protein that gives blood its red color. When hemoglobin is not produced, the body becomes fatigued and weak. In severe cases, anemia can lead to heart failure. Iron deficiency anemia is one of the most common nutritional shortfalls in the United States today, with up to 15 percent of women of childbearing age experiencing some form of iron deficiency. Iron is stored in the liver, spleen, bone marrow, and other tissues. An iron deficit is not necessarily due to poor eating habits. An otherwise balanced diet may not supply adequate iron with the following special groups of women:

1. *Menstruating women* have a higher RDA for iron as a result of monthly blood losses. Women who bleed heavily should pay special attention to their iron intake.
2. *Dieters* are another special group. The average balanced diet offers about 6 mg of iron per 1,000 calories. With reduced caloric consumption, lower levels of iron are ingested. Women consuming less than 1,500 calories daily are not likely to obtain their minimal iron levels.
3. *Pregnant women* have increased dietary needs for iron because of higher blood volume and the increasing demands by the fetus and placenta.
4. *Endurance athletes* have a tendency to have increased iron losses and lower iron absorption rates. This may lead to a higher incidence of

---

INFORMATION BOX 1.6

Calcium Sources

Food	Amount	mg
Yogurt, plain	1 cup	415
Sardines, with bones	3 oz	372
Skimmed milk	1 cup	302
Swiss cheese	1 oz	262
Cheddar cheese	1 oz	213
Salmon, canned with bones	3 oz	167
Collard greens	½ cup	145
Molasses, blackstrap	1 tbsp	137
Spinach, cooked	½ cup	106
Beans, dried and cooked	1 cup	90
Cottage cheese, low fat	½ cup	77
Broccoli, cooked	½ cup	68
Orange	1 medium	54

---

iron depletion, manifested by below-normal iron stores. The physiological significance of these changes is uncertain, and it is not known whether they impair athletic performance.

5. *Vegetarians and women who do not consume red meat* are another group of concern. Although high in saturated fat, beef, pork, and lamb are among the richest sources of iron. The iron in vegetables, grains, and beans is not nearly as well absorbed by the body. Dairy products have negligible amounts of iron.

6. *Adolescents* require high iron intake because of their rapid growth. Menstruating adolescents who are still growing are at high risk, especially if their nutritional status is compromised by junk food or fad diets.

Iron absorption is a complex process that varies with the foods consumed, the combination of foods, and the body's needs. There are several strategies that women can use to increase their dietary intake of iron. Eating lean red meats is an obvious strategy. Liver is one of the best sources of iron, but it should not be eaten more than once a week owing to its high cholesterol content. Chicken and fish usually contain one-third to one-half the iron of red meat. Choosing breads, cereals, and pasta labeled "enriched" or "fortified" and unrefined whole grains, such as whole-wheat bread, supplies a fair amount of iron. Eating foods high in vitamin C helps because it facilitates the body's absorption of iron. For vegetarians, vitamin C with meals is a must. Cooking in cast iron cookware also helps to increase the iron content of foods. The more acidic the food (such as spaghetti sauce) and the longer it cooks, the higher the iron content.

Beta-carotene

The dietary benefits of beta-carotene have been identified. Numerous animal studies have suggested that beta-carotene can defend against tumors and enhance the immune system (see Information Box 1.2). Many studies on humans have found that those who eat few foods rich in beta-carotene have an increased risk of cancer, particularly lung cancer and melanoma. High dietary intake of beta-carotene has also been shown to confer greater protection against ovarian cancer.[10] Beta-carotene appears to protect against heart disease, cataracts, and certain cancers by neutralizing or mopping up toxic particles in the body called **free radicals.** Although there is as yet no official RDA for beta-carotene, nutrition experts recommend 6 mg daily through food sources.[11] The best sources of beta-carotene are yellow-orange fruits and vegetables, such as carrots, sweet potatoes, winter squash, cantaloupe, and apricots, and more of certain green vegetables, such as spinach, kale, asparagus, broccoli, and brussels sprouts.

Fiber

To many women, **fiber** is synonymous with wheat bran or diet supplements. Fiber is not a single substance but rather a large group of widely different chemical substances with varied physical properties. Fiber is an essential dietary component. Formerly called roughage or bulk, fiber was once thought of as a "filler food." Although high-fiber foods tend to be low in fats and calories and usually replace meats and other fatty foods, scientists now recognize that fiber itself may play a role in reducing the risk of leading chronic diseases—heart disease, cancer, and diabetes.[5] Fiber is derived from plants that cannot be digested by enzymes in the human digestive tract. High-fiber diets have been shown to protect against colon and rectal cancer, breast cancer, constipation, diverticulosis, heart disease, diabetes, and obesity.

Fiber can be measured from a **crude** and **dietary** perspective. Crude fiber is the older method, which employed strong chemicals that "digested" the food, and what was left was known as "crude" fiber. Newer methods use milder chemicals and enzymes to analyze "dietary" fiber. Dietary fiber is the more accurate, complete measure, but it has not yet been determined for all foods. These different measures can lead to confusion, and it is important to determine whether a food label is specifying dietary or crude fiber. Fiber can also be classified as **soluble** or **insoluble.** Soluble fiber absorbs water in the digestive tract and is easily fermented by bacteria in the large intestine. Oats, for example, are rich in this type of fiber, which helps lower blood cholesterol and manage blood sugar levels. Most insoluble fiber remains essentially unchanged during the digestive process. Wheat bran and whole-grain breads and cereals are rich in this type of fiber, which tends to increase stool bulk and may be protective against cancer. General strategies for increasing dietary fiber include eating a variety of foods daily, including at least five servings of fruits and vegetables and three to six servings of whole-grain breads, cereals, and legumes. It is better to opt for less-processed food. Whole-wheat flour and brown rice are higher

Ways to Increase Fiber in the Diet

1. Eat whole fresh fruit instead of just drinking the juice.
2. Eat the skins of fruits and vegetables, such as apples and potatoes
3. Eat fruits with edible seeds, such as berries and kiwis.
4. Use whole-grain products.
5. Eat more of the stems when having broccoli or asparagus.
6. Peel citrus fruits and eat the sections with their membranes.
7. Eat more beans and peas.

in fiber than processed varieties, and an apple has twice as much fiber as an equal serving of applesauce. Eating the skin of fruits and vegetables also increases fiber. Also, fiber from food sources provides more nutrients than fiber pills or powders. Information Box 1.7 summarizes specific strategies for getting more fiber in the diet.

Sugar

Sugar is consumed in four forms: sucrose, glucose, fructose, and lactose. Sugar is nearly ubiquitous. This additive is present in products from ice cream to ketchup. A typical 12-ounce soft drink contains the equivalent of 8 teaspoonfuls of sugar, and a typical chocolate bar contains about 3 teaspoonfuls of sugar per ounce. Sugar has been blamed for many conditions in children and adults, but the strongest evidence against sugar relates to its role in tooth decay. Sugar nourishes cavity-causing bacteria. The source of sugar can affect the degree of damage it causes. Sugar in sticky foods, for example, clings to the teeth, encouraging bacterial growth. Liberal use of sugar promotes plaque, the toxin-producing film that forms on teeth and can lead to periodontal (gum) disease, the leading cause of tooth loss among American adults. Although a popular concept among some mothers and teachers, there is no convincing evidence of sugar inducing hyperactivity in children. Research has also not supported the notion that excessive sugar leads to aggressive or criminal behavior.

Although sugar may not be the culprit it has been portrayed to be, it is still not healthy to consume excessive sugar. Foods high in sugar are often high in fat, and research clearly identifies the detrimental consequences of a high-fat diet. Sugar also provides "empty calories"—offering energy to the consumer but no other significant nutritional value. Also, when a sugared product is consumed, as in the case of a soft drink, it is usually in lieu of something else that may be nutritious, such as a glass of skim milk or fruit juice.

Weight Control

Dieting

Dieting appears to be a common phenomenon of contemporary American life. A panel convened by the National Institutes of Health (NIH) in 1992 found that at any given time, 50 percent of American women are on a weight-loss diet. Americans spend more than $30 billion a year on weight control programs and products. Yet the percentage of overweight Americans has been growing during the past 20 years. All these facts have led many to believe that dieting has more negative than positive effects. Dieting is the least effective way to lose weight. For 95 percent of dieters, lost pounds eventually return.[12]

An organized antidiet movement has evolved that says that the lucrative weight-loss industry is a fraud and that chronic dieting is actually an eating disorder, similar to anorexia. These opponents of dieting claim that women are being sold an impossible ideal body image and that people are better off physically and emotionally if they are allowed to eat whatever they want so their bodies "find" their natural weight (see Current Events Box, page 31).

Most medical authorities, including those on the NIH panel, believe that such antidiet proponents go too far and that it is irresponsible to encourage people to remain obese. They agree, however, that being a little overweight is certainly not hazardous and having a flat stomach is not a requisite of good health. Genetic, cultural, and psychological factors are all components of the issue. Experts, however, have revised their guidance on weight loss. In addition to revising the food groups, the US Food and Drug Administration (FDA) and Department of Health and Human Services (DHHS) released Dietary Guidelines for Americans in 1990. Although they still encourage weight loss, the revised guidelines indicate that "safe" weight loss should occur at the level of no more than ½ to 1 pound per week. The guidelines no longer rely on the "desired weight tables" of the Metropolitan Life Insurance Company, which were originally developed in 1959. Instead they have substituted a table recommending "healthy" weights that show weight allowances for people 35 and older, reflecting the fact that people gain weight as they age (Information Box 1.8).

INFORMATION BOX 1.8

Revised Height/Weight Tables*

Height (without shoes)	Weight (without clothes)	
	Age 19 to 34	Age 35 and Up†
5′0″	97–128	108–138
5′1″	101–132	111–143
5′2″	104–137	115–148
5′3″	107–141	119–152
5′4″	111–146	122–157
5′5″	114–150	126–162
5′6″	118–155	130–167
5′7″	121–160	134–172
5′8″	125–164	138–178
5′9″	129–169	142–183
5′10″	132–174	146–188
5′11″	136–179	151–194
6′0″	140–184	155–199
6′1″	144–189	159–205
6′2″	148–195	164–210
6′3″	152–200	168–216
Body Mass Index	**19–25**	**21–27**

*Women or men.
†Based on 1990 *Dietary Guidelines for Americans,* USDHHS.

Yo-yo dieting is a term used to characterize the repeated, chronic pattern of dieting that describes most dieters' behavior. In addition to being frustrating, yo-yo dieting has been found to be hazardous to health. Research confirms that people whose body weight yo-yos often have a higher incidence of coronary heart disease than do people with relatively stable weights and that dieters show a 5-year failure rate of 98 to 99 percent.[13] It has been hypothesized that yo-yo dieters store more and more fat in the abdominal area with each failed diet, and abdominal fat has been shown to be more harmful to health than fat in other places.

Yet despite the health risks of both dieting and cosmetic surgery, many health professionals and most laypeople cling tenaciously to unhealthy myths about body size and weight. The fact is chronic dieting itself, not fatness per se, is actually dangerous to health.

Obesity

Obesity, a medical term meaning the excessive storage of energy in the form of fat, has been identified as a risk for a wide range of disease, including adult-onset diabetes, hypertension, coronary heart disease, certain cancers, gout, gallbladder disease, and certain arthritic conditions.[14] Often referred to as a "disease," obesity is actually a range of disorders from genetic to environmental. Although obesity may be simply an extreme degree of overweight according to ordinary standards, a person can be overweight without being obese. A 150-pound female weightlifter may be overweight according to ordinary standards, but she may actually have a below-average amount of body fat. In contrast, a woman in a normal weight range but with sedentary habits could have a small amount of muscle mass and be storing excess fat and thus be classifiable as obese.

The best way to determine "desirable" weight remains a matter of controversy. The fastest, although not most accurate, is to consult a standard height/weight table. These tables fail to take into account many important factors that affect weight, such as family history, race, or age. Another way to define overweight is to measure the proportion of fat in the body, a difficult task to do accurately, even with professional training. The most pragmatic way to determine healthy body weight effectively is to calculate **body mass index** (Self-Assessment 1.2). This method minimizes the effect of height and provides reasonable guidelines for defining overweight. A value of 25 or greater shows obesity-related health risks.

How Women Can Lose Weight

Women who need to lose weight for health reasons face the dilemma of how to do so. Popular media abound with conflicting guidance on weight loss strategies for women. Information Box 1.9 provides a summary of weight loss strategies that help and do not help women. To lose weight, it is necessary to burn more calories than are ingested. The most important way that the body

---

SELF-ASSESSMENT 1.2

Determining Body Mass Index

Body mass index is determined by dividing weight in kilograms by the square of height in meters:

1. To convert weight to kilograms, divide the number of pounds (without clothes) by 2.2:
   (a) _____

2. To convert to meters, divide height in inches (without shoes) by 39.4 = (b) _____, then square (b) _____

3. Divide (a) by (b²). Body mass = _____

For women, desirable body mass is 21 to 23, overweight begins about 27.5, and seriously overweight is above 31.5.

Helpful and Nonhelpful Weight Loss Strategies for Women

Helpful	Nonhelpful
Plan meals and snacks to include more complex carbohydrates, more fruits and vegetables, and less fat.	Any diet that promotes one particular food such as grapefruit or yogurt.
Limit intake of fat foods, oils, dressings.	Unconventional theories to explain how food combinations add or decrease body weight.
Avoid packaged snack foods.	Diets that omit any one food group.
Develop new interests that don't involve food.	Daily caloric intake less than 1,200 calories unless under medical supervision.
Eat foods slowly.	
Exercise regularly.	Any diet that promotes megadoses of vitamins to make up for nutritional deficits.
Join a support group or share the process with a friend.	Fasting or starvation diets.
Clean pantry—give away foods that are not part of the new healthy eating plan.	Any pill or potion that "melts fat."
	Appetite-suppressant drugs.
	Fiber supplements.
	Giving up all sweets or breads.
	Muscle stimulators.
	Body wraps.

burns calories is through resting metabolism, or **basal metabolic rate** (BMR), the process that maintains body heat and controls automatic activities such as breathing and heartbeat. Nearly 75 percent of calorie use is devoted to these functions. When a woman attempts to lose weight by cutting calories, her body responds as it would to starvation, by actually burning *fewer* calories. Shifting from an intake of about 2,000 calories a day to a 1,200-calorie diet reduces resting metabolism by 5 to 10 percent, and a more stringent 800-calorie diet lowers it by 10 to 20 percent. Even after resuming a more normal calorie consumption, other changes act to keep the metabolic rate low. Much of the weight lost on a low-calorie diet can come from lost muscle tissue, and the muscles may shrink further as the woman stays at the lower weight because they do not have to work as hard to carry the body around. Less muscle tissue means lower metabolic rate. The net effect is simple: The more weight that is lost through dieting, the more the metabolic rate will decline—and the greater the tendency to regain the weight that was lost. Although dieting still has a role in weight control, exercise provides some solution to the metabolic problem.

The key to successful weight loss is increasing the BMR, not counting

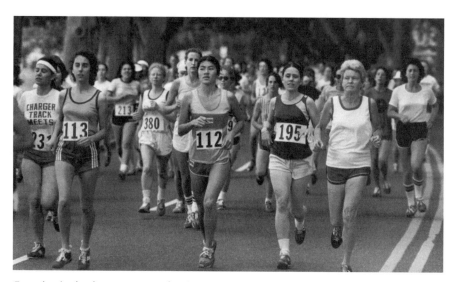

Exercise is the best strategy for increasing BMR.

I have tried every diet in the book. I have had times where I have eaten only grapefruit, only rice, only salads, etc. I have also tried all the gimmicks—pills, liquids, body wraps. You name it, I've tried it. But nothing has really worked. I quickly gain the weight back, sometimes more, within a short time after I lose it. I always swear I won't try another stupid method, but as soon as I read an ad or see a new product, I feel that I have to give it a try.

22-YEAR-OLD WOMAN

calories. Regular exercise is an essential component of any weight control program. Exercise is the best way to increase the BMR. Computerized exercise equipment provides misleading information when it displays the number of calories that the exerciser has burned up. A vigorous 20- to 30-minute workout can easily burn 200 to 300 calories, and even brisk walking can have a significant impact (see Chapter 2). Equally important, exercise helps keep up the metabolic rate by building muscle or by keeping muscle from shrinking as a result of weight loss. Because adding exercise to a diet program helps keep the metabolic rate steady, it makes it easier to keep the weight off. The ways that exercise so dramatically influences metabolism are not totally understood. Exercise does indeed burn up some calories, but the main advantage of exercise is that the metabolism remains higher for several hours afterward, so calories are burned at a higher rate during that period, even during inactivity. Aerobic exercise burns calories faster than weight training, but weight training builds muscle, which is of critical importance in weight loss. A pound of muscle needs 30 to 50 calories a day just for maintenance, whereas fat needs only 2 maintenance calories per day. Substituting muscle for fat not only makes a person trimmer because muscle is more compact than fat, but also it results in an increased daily caloric expenditure. Rather than simply promoting weight loss, exercise may actually affect the body in a more complex, integrated way, bringing appetite and energy expenditure into balance. Exercise can also trim a physical profile even without weight loss. Muscle is denser than fat, so it is possible to become thinner while the weight holds steady if a larger amount of fat is replaced with a smaller amount of muscle. Bathroom scales simply do not measure these changes. Regardless of its direct effects on weight and body fat, exercise serves to improve overall health by lowering blood pressure, improving cholesterol levels, strengthening the cardiovascular system, helping prevent type II diabetes, and reducing stress.

In any weight loss effort, starvation or hunger is not the solution. Food substitution, in which twice as many calories from carbohydrates can be consumed compared with fat, is far better than food restriction. Fat contains 9 calories per gram, whereas protein and carbohydrates have 4 calories per gram. Foods such as pasta, whole-grain bread, and potatoes are nutritious and filling and low in calories as long as they are not smothered in fat products, such as butter, sour cream, mayonnaise, and margarine. Alcohol should also be considered contraindicated in a weight loss effort. The BMR is influenced by a woman's alcohol consumption. Alcohol promotes the storage of body fat. In addition to providing empty calories, alcohol affects the BMR because the body burns fat more slowly in the presence of alcohol.

Before jumping into a weight control program or a fitness center to lose weight, it is important to ascertain if there is a health reason to lose weight or if the goal of losing weight is to conform to an artificial and perhaps impossible image. A medical examination can help rule out any underlying pathology that might be contributing to the weight problem and provide a reliable, realistic professional perspective on the "need" to lose weight. If it is decided that some pounds should be shed, it must be remembered that they did not accumulate overnight and will not disappear overnight. An average weekly loss of 1 pound is a realistic, safe goal for weight loss. The time frame for the loss can be easily calculated with this goal when the desired weight loss is determined. The commitment to lose weight can be reinforced and sustained by joining a group or making a serious arrangement for support with a friend. Keeping a food diary is a help to some women because it enables them to identify eating and exercising patterns. Meals, snacks, and drinks should all be recorded in the diary. After a review of a few days of diary notes, realistic goals can be established that incorporate a change in eating patterns and a focus on healthy foods. Progress can be monitored through the food diary and weekly (not daily) checks with the scale. Once the reasonable desired weight loss is achieved, the focus should be on maintenance, again through sensible eating *and* exercise.

Body Image and Shape

Obsession with Thinness

Women have been socialized to believe that their physical attractiveness determines their social value. Eating disorders, cosmetic and plastic surgery mania, and diet mania have been attributed to modern women's distorted body image. The obsession with thinness has been also blamed on the fitness craze, where not only are women supposed to be thin, but also they are supposed to be fit. This is evidenced by reports indicating that more than one-half of American

I guess when I look in the mirror I see only the things that I feel are wrong. My hair is too limp, and I wish I could look thinner and taller. When I think about it, I realize that there are many things I actually like about myself but I can't seem to focus on them. When I look at other women, I notice their attributes. I wonder why I can't do that with myself?

25-YEAR-OLD WOMAN

girls and women between the ages of 10 and 30 suffer with eating disorders, and 50 percent of adult American wonen are dieting to lose weight and contributing to the $33 billion weight-loss industry. Weight loss dieting is not the only dangerous health strategy women use to alter their bodies in hopes of attaining the "body ideal." Cosmetic surgery, which grossed $300 million in 1988, is expected to grow annually by 10 percent.[15] Sixty-three percent of high school girls are dieting to lose weight. Strategies used by high school girls to lose weight include starvation and fad diets, without any realistic idea of how much weight they ought to lose. A concern with adolescent preoccupation with body image is that the discontent may persist for life. Several surveys of American women find that most are dissatisfied with their bodies.[16]

An irony about body image is that standards for beauty and desirability are not absolute but vary over time and from culture to culture. The twentieth-century trend promoted by Madison Avenue and Hollywood has been an image of emaciation. In former times, big-bellied women were thought of as beautiful. In Greek and Roman representations of Aphrodite and Venus as well as in paintings by Titian, Rubens, and Rembrandt, "ideal" women often had ample thighs, hips, waists, and abdomens. The Venus de Milo, one of the most beautiful of the classical female torsos, is muscular and rounded.

New research findings and growing numbers of activists are seeking to influence the women and girls who are alienated from their bodies and obsessed with dieting. Although the 1990s language of fat liberation has been replaced by the politically milder talk of "size discrimination" and "size acceptance," the goals remain the same: to empower women to accept themselves at their present sizes and to shatter the man-made media image of the body ideal (Figure 1.3). As feminist researcher Rothblum points out:[1]

> There are no objective definitions of obesity.
> Fat is not more prevalent among women than among men.
> Fat people do not consume more calories than thin people.
> Dieting is not an effective way to lose weight.
> Obesity is not related to poor physical health, "fat can be fit."

Body Shape

Women whose body fat distribution favors the upper body ("apples") rather than the hips and thighs ("pears") may be at higher risk of developing breast and endometrial cancer. Distribution of body fat in the upper rather than the lower body predisposes women to diabetes, hypertension, and gallbladder disease, and evidence also links abdominal obesity with breast cancer. Obese women in general are at a slightly higher risk of developing breast cancer, but when the "apples" are isolated, their breast cancer rate is significantly elevated. As the waist-to-hip circumference ratio increases, so does the risk. The relative risk for endometrial cancer also goes up with increasing waist-to-hip circumference ratios or abdomen-to-thigh skin fold ratios.

Eating Disorders

Although eating disorders seem to be modern afflictions, medical history seems to indicate otherwise. A disease similar in description to anorexia was described as early as 1694, and the term "anorexia," meaning loss of appetite or desire, was first used in 1874.[17] Since that time, many other researchers have presented documentation of what is now referred to as **anorexia nervosa. Bulimia,** meaning "appetite like an ox," has also been described in historical writings. Ancient Egyptians believed that purging was a way to prevent disease, and women of the Middle Ages often purged for religious reasons.[18]

Eating disorders know no social or economic barriers. Recent admissions and awareness of eating disorders of prominent public women such as Jane Fonda, Tracey Gold, and Princess Diana have heightened general levels of sensitivity to the issue. Today eating disorders are more prevalent among young Western white females from middle to upper social classes than in other groups, with incidence rates peaking at age 18.[17] Studies indicate that probable causes for eating disorders include biological, emotional, and social factors. Eating disorders are also present in males, although females experience a tenfold prevalence of the conditions. When professionals speak of eating disorders, they generally mean anorexia nervosa or bulimia nervosa. Both are serious problems that can have life-threatening physical consequences. Both disorders reflect an extreme preoccupation with food and body images. Some individuals experience both anorexic and bulimic symptoms. Bulimics often "starve" themselves before a binge and anorexics may purge after consuming even a small amount of food. Once started, eating disorders may become self-perpetuating. Dieting, bingeing, and purging may help a woman cope with strong emotions and feel as if she is in control of her life. At the same time, these behaviors undermine one's health, self-esteem, and sense of competency.

Anorexia Nervosa

Physical symptoms of anorexia nervosa include a huge loss of weight, a refusal to eat, virtually a delusional viewpoint toward food and the body, and a general detachment from family and friends (Information Box 1.10). Psychological symptoms of anorexia nervosa include a distorted body image, a confusion of the self-image, a sense of being incompetent, depression, and withdrawal from others.[19] Individuals also tend to become more socially withdrawn as the disorder progresses. They have been described as follows: a limited range of affective responses, a denial of being fatigued, hyperactive behavior, an indifference to changes in temperature, a negative outlook on life, a disposition to resist authority, stubbornness, unnatural body movements, being unhappy, no sense of humor, and relatively few smiling gestures.[20] Researchers note that the most notable belief shared by anorectics is that weight, shape, or being thin is the predominant reference for establishing personal value or self-worth.[21] Other identified psychological features of the illness include a frustration over becoming overweight, a fear of losing

I look in the mirror and see myself as grotesquely fat— a real blimp. My legs and arms are really fat and I can't stand what I see. I know that others say I am too thin, but I can see myself and I have to deal with this my way.

100-POUND-ANORECTIC GIRL

INFORMATION BOX 1.10

Symptoms of Anorexia Nervosa

Loss of at least 15 percent of body weight.

Intense fear of weight gain.

Distorted body image (feeling fat even when too thin).

Absence of three consecutive menstrual periods.

Insistence on keeping weight below a healthy minimum.

FIGURE 1.3

Measurements are only statistics.

Reprinted with permission of NIKE, Inc. and the Roger Richman Agency, Inc.

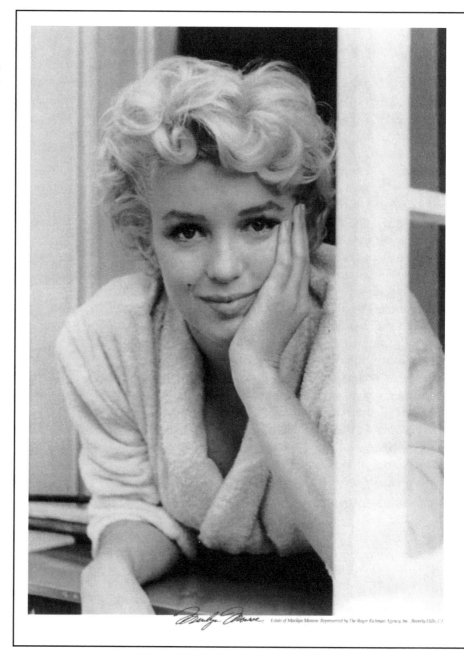

control over eating, a loss of judgment relative to the requirement of food as a basic need for the body, and an unrealistic sense of body image.

Identified psychodynamic problems of the individual with anorexia nervosa include poor self-esteem, a confused identity, and fear of becoming an independent individual.[22] A general characteristic of the anorectic personality is a feeling of overall ineffectiveness as a person. The typical individual is highly critical of herself and believes that she is quite inadequate in most areas of personal

A WOMAN IS OFTEN MEA-
SURED BY THE THINGS SHE CANNOT
CONTROL. SHE IS MEASURED BY THE WAY
HER BODY CURVES OR DOESN'T CURVE, BY
WHERE SHE IS FLAT OR STRAIGHT OR ROUND.
SHE IS MEASURED BY 36-24-36 AND INCHES
AND AGES AND NUMBERS, BY ALL THE OUT-
SIDE THINGS THAT DON'T EVER ADD UP TO
WHO SHE IS ON THE INSIDE. AND SO IF A
WOMAN IS TO BE MEASURED, LET HER BE
MEASURED BY THE THINGS SHE CAN
CONTROL, BY WHO SHE IS AND WHO SHE IS
TRYING TO BECOME. BECAUSE AS EVERY
WOMAN KNOWS, MEASUREMENTS ARE ONLY
STATISTICS. AND STATISTICS LIE.

and social functioning.[21] Extremely malnourished individuals with anorexia may display denial and suppress negative emotions. Symptoms of depression, with large mood swings, are commonly seen in individuals with the disorder. Just as the individual with the disorder ignores hunger pains and resists or rejects food, she also tends to reject compliments and nurturance.

The prototype of the young girl with anorexia nervosa has been described as:

- Obessional in character makeup.
- Introverted and often socially uncertain.
- Self-denying.
- Respectful of others.
- Extremely compliant.
- Somewhat self-abashing with limited spontaneity and little self-directed autonomy.
- Thinking that is stereotyped despite being structured, industrious, and competent intellectually.

Bulimia Nervosa

Bulimia is a disorder characterized by cyclic binge eating followed by purging (Information Box 1.11). It was first identified in 1873, and by the 1940s it was considered symptomatic of anorexia nervosa—self-imposed starvation. In 1976, the term "bulimarexia" was coined and the symptom was determined to be a separate disorder from anorexia. Prevalence rates for bulimia range from 1 to 16 percent, with the highest rates occurring in adolescents and young adults.[18] Currently bulimia nervosa is classified in the American Psychological Association Diagnostic and Statistical Manual (DSM-III-R) as an eating disorder associated with five factors:

1. Recurrent episodes of binge eating.
2. Feeling of lack of control over eating behavior during the binge.
3. Regular engagement in purges.
4. Minimum average of two episodes a week for at least 3 months.
5. Persistent overconcern with body shape and weight.

Bulimia is a progressive disorder that usually begins with extreme hunger as a result of long periods of food deprivation from fasting or dieting and subsequent attempts at eating while still trying to control weight. Some bulimics have reported that in their preadolescent years, they gained feelings of self-control and power through this self-denial. The situation progresses to out-of-control binge/purges because the artificial elimination methods have relieved the feeling of being "stufffed," and the bulimic believes it is a good way to lose weight. Binges often occur when bulimics feel that they have passed a self-imposed limit on acceptable food intake. Consequently they feel defeated and generally gorge until they are interrupted or the food runs out. During such binges, the caloric intake can be as high as 60,000 calories and generally lasts for less than 2 hours but has been reported to last as long as 8 hours. The binge foods of choice are usually high-calorie, easily ingested "junk" food that requires little preparation and can be obtained while keeping the binge secret from others. Bulimics have been known to use several modes of purging, including emetics,

INFORMATION BOX 1.11

Symptoms of Bulimia Nervosa

Repeated (usually secretive) episodes of bingeing and vomiting.

Feeling out of control during a binge.

Purging after a binge (vomiting, use of laxatives or diuretics, excessive exercise).

Frequent dieting.

Extreme concern with body weight and shape.

diuretics, laxatives, fasts, enemas, diet pills, chewing for hours and then spitting out the food, regurgitation by placing fingers or other objects down the throat, and excessive exercise. The number of different methods of purging is a stronger severity index than is the frequency of use of any one type.

The binge-purge cycle may occur anywhere from once a day to 12 or more per week. The psychological components of the cycle vary from person to person; however, there are certain similarities. The cycle begins in response to a strong emotion, either positive or negative; this can be food craving, stress, sleeplessness, anxiety, joy, excitement, physical or emotional pain, helplessness, hopelessness, loneliness, or sadness. After the binge, some say they initially feel unique, relaxed, soothed, but then these feelings turn to shame, guilt, self-hatred, and then to the need to purge to relieve the fear of weight gain and because of a desire to regain control and purity. After the purge, bulimics may feel relieved that they have controlled their weight but guilty and negative about succumbing to the cycle again. These guilt feelings invariably lead the bulimic to perpetuate the behavior.

Bulimia has characteristically afflicted adolescent to young adult females from middle-class backgrounds but exists in members of other groups as well. Many women trace their cyclical behaviors to transition points in their lives when they were changing their dependent status, such as when they were going to college or getting married. In the past several decades, the media has promoted unreasonable thinness as the epitome of beauty. Bulimic women have often been socialized to attain this ideal. The victims often appear to be independent high achievers and are of normal weight. They are invariably poised, pleasant, and intelligent. However, these young women are often perfectionistic, obsessive-compulsive, depressed, intense, insecure, sensitive to rejection, anxious to please, dependent on others, and nonassertive. They tend to have rigid thinking and suppress their feelings, particularly anger. They are socially isolated, often as a result of their all-consuming preoccupation with food and weight and their struggle to hide their eating behavior, and because of their strong negative self-concept, they fear rejection. The majority of them are aware that their eating habits are abnormal, but some may feel that they have the ultimate weight control secret of being able to "have their cake and eat it too."

In addition to the pychological problems, bulimia nervosa can cause a myriad of physical problems (Information Boxes 1.12 and 1.13).

Theories about Eating Disorders

There is no single explanation for an eating disorder. There are certain medical conditions that result in weight loss, and those can be ruled out with a medical examination. Most likely, eating disorders arise from a combination of long-standing emotional, psychological, and social conditions. Poor self-image, depression, anxiety, loneliness, and certain family and personal relationships may contribute to the development of an eating disorder. The stresses associated with adult life can also precipitate anorexia or bulimia. Our culture, with its unrelenting idealization of thinness and "the perfect body," is also partly to

---

INFORMATION BOX 1.12

Binge Eating

Binge eating is known to cause:

Hypoglycemia, a sugar deficiency that may cause dizziness, headaches, fatigue, irritability, numbness, anxiety, and depression.

Neurological abnormalities.

Lethargy, inactivity, lowered metabolism.

Purging

Purging is known to cause:

Spontaneous regurgitation ("reverse peristalsis" after about 5 years of persistent vomiting).

Dental erosion on the palatal (inner) surface of the teeth as a result of the continual exposure to stomach acids in vomitus. This erosion is compounded by high sugar intake; excessive citric juices, which are taken to quench continuous thirst; and decreased saliva. Eventually erosion may lead to cavities, tooth loss, faulty bite, and gum disease.

Abscesses and sores in the mouth.

Bleeding in the esophagus.

Choking feelings from stomach protrusion into the diaphragm—known as a hiatal hernia.

Salivary gland infection and swelling.

Hypokalemia—a deficiency of potassium because of impairment in the uptake of minerals in the alimentary canal—leads to muscle fatigue, numbness, erratic heartbeats, kidney damage, and paralysis depending on the duration of the disorder.

Sodium and potassium—mineral deficiencies that cause electrolyte imbalances, dehydration, kidney malfunction, seizures, and muscle spasm depending on the severity of the illness. Sodium deficiency leads to loss of skin elasticity, dry tongue, and low blood pressure.

Substance abuse of laxatives and diuretics, which leads to or is concurrent with abuse of and addiction to appetite suppressants, including cocaine, and amphetamine/diet pills.

Constipation for laxative users. Intestinal distress similar to inflammatory bowel disease for irritant (castor oil, cascara) users.

---

blame. Although research has been conducted on eating disorders, it is fairly limited in scope, and findings are often contradictory.

Treatment of Eating Disorders

The treatment of eating disorders usually involves weight restoration through nutrition and medical support in conjunction with individual, behavioral, or dynamic psychotherapy or family therapy. Most experts agree that a realistic body image concept is a precondition for recovery from an eating disorder. Treatment and prevention strategies often emphasize the importance of body acceptance and development of positive self-esteem. There is some evidence of successful treatment of anorexia nervosa,[23] but most evaluations are not as encouraging.

Several approaches are usually used to treat both disorders, including motivating the patient, enlisting family support, and providing nutrition counseling and psychotherapy. Behavior modification therapy and drug therapy may be used as well. Hospitalizations may be required for those with life-threatening complications or extreme psychological problems. If the patient's life is not in danger, treatment may be provided on an outpatient basis and may last for a year or longer. Psychotherapy may be in many forms. In individual sessions, the victim is encouraged to explore her attitudes about weight, food, and body image. Then, as she becomes more aware of her problems in relating to others and dealing with situational stress, the focus changes to her self-esteem, guilt, anxiety, depression, or helplessness. Constructive, nonjudgmental feedback is given to promote growth and independence. In behavior modification therapy, the focus is on eliminating self-defeating behaviors. Family therapy is usually encouraged to improve overall family functioning. Group therapy may help to reduce feelings of isolation and secrecy and may be especially important for bulimics. Self-help groups are usually an adjunct to primary treatment. Through sharing of experiences, members provide mutual emotional support, exchange information, and diminish feelings of isolation.

I really was confused about this cholesterol thing. I wanted to eat well. I knew that nutrition really influences how I feel, but I didn't really understand what I should eat or why. Finally I decided that was really foolish. I am an educated and knowledgeable person in so many other areas. So I sat down and read everything that I could and I asked lots of questions. Now I am confident about my diet, and I am working to eat wholesome foods that are good for me.

24-YEAR-OLD COLLEGE STUDENT

Summary

The nutritional dimensions of women's health include a complex spectrum of topics. Dietary guidelines have been revised and will continue to change as scientists unlock the mysteries of diet and its relationship with health and illness. Weight control is a topic that has both wellness and psychosocial dimensions. A woman's body image is also determined by another myriad of issues that influence her sense of worth and personal confidence. The prevalence and personal destruction of eating disorders among women dramatically underscore the need to better understand, manage, treat, and most importantly prevent these devastating conditions. It is every woman's personal responsibility to maintain a high level of awareness of all nutritional issues and to execute informed nutritional decision making on a daily basis.

CURRENT EVENTS

"The Government Weighs the Claims of Diets"

Washington Post
May 31, 1992

The Federal Trade Commission (FTC) is expected to soon complete a two-year probe of advertising and marketing practices by more than a dozen diet-center operators, such as Weight Watchers International, Diet Center, Inc, Nutri/System, Inc, and Jenny Craig. Another probe is on going as well that is targeting the marketing of diet food products. Behind both FTC investigations is a common set of suspicions that diet companies exaggerate the ease and effectiveness of their services or products, that claims of dramatic weight loss aren't substantiated and that advertising doesn't adequately disclose potential health risks. The industry is essentially unregulated with current legislation. Diet marketers generated $17 billion in revenues in 1991 through weight-loss centers, hospital-run programs, and sales of over-the-counter pills and foods. The stakes for consumers are high with estimates of 100 million Americans who are trying to lose weight. Nearly 8 million people signed up for these structured weight loss programs in 1991. Advertising by the industry has been accused of contributing to the distorted body images of women, the most frequent dieters. Another advertising concern is that commercial dieting programs often work, but the results are almost always temporary, a fact that is rarely disclosed with advertising.

Philosophical Dimensions–Nutrition

1. Should the food industry be regulated regarding the fortification of foods? Why not develop a "superfortified Twinkie"?

2. If a young adolescent female has more body weight than her peers, should she be advised about her weight? If so, how? If not, why not?

References

1. Rothblum, E. (1990). Women and weight: Fad and fiction. *Journal of Psychology, 124* (Jan), 5–24.

2. Moses, N., Banilivy, M., and Lifshitz, F. (1989). Fear of obesity among adolescent girls. *Pediatrics, 83*(3), 393–398.

3. De Ridder, C.M., Thijssen, J.H.H., Van 't Veer, P., van Duuren, R., Bruning, P.F., Zonderland, M.L., and Erich, W.B.M. (1991). Dietary habits, sexual maturation, and plasma hormones in pubertal girls: a longitudinal study. (1991). *American Journal of Clinical Nutrition, 54,* 805–813.

4. National Academy of Sciences, National Research Council Committee on Diet and health (1989). *Diet and health: Implications for reducing chronic disease risk.* Washington, D.C.: National Academy Press.

5. U.S. Department of Agriculture/U.S. Department of Health and Human Services (1989). *Nutrition monitoring in the United States: An update report on nutrition monitoring* (DHHS Publication No. (PHS) 89-1255). Washington, DC: U.S. Government Printing Office.

6. Zigouras, S. (1989). Food fortification, the good, the bad, and the hype. *Women's Health and Fitness News, 4*(4), 1–2.

7. U.S. Department of Health and Human Services (1988). *The Surgeon General's Report on Nutrition and Health: Summary and Recommendations, 1988.* Washington, DC: U.S. Government Printing Office.

8. American Medical Association Council on Scientific Affairs (1990). Saturated fatty acids in vegetable oils. *Journal of the American Medical Association, 263*(5).

9. National Heart, Lung, and Blood Institute (1990). *Report of the Expert Panel on Population Strategies for Blood Cholesterol Reduction.* National Cholesterol Education Program. (NIH Publication No. 91-2732). Washington, DC: U.S. Government Printing Office.

10. Slattery, M.L., Schuman, K.L., and West, D.W. (1989). Nutrient intake and ovarian cancer. *American Journal of Epidemiology, 130*(3), 497–502.

11. Beta-carotene: Recipes for good health. (1992). *University of Texas Lifetime Health Letter, 4*(6), 6.

12. Weight control: Give up dieting so you can lose weight. (1991). *University of Texas Lifetime Health Letter, 3*(6), 4–5.

13. Lissner, L., Odell, P.M., D'Agostino R.B., Stokes, J. III, Kreger, B.E., Belanger, A.J., & Brownell, K.D. (1991). Variability of body weight and health outcomes in the Framingham population. *New England Journal of Medicine, 324*(26), 1837–1844.

14. National Institutes of Health (1985). *Health implications of obesity.* Bethesda, MD: Consensus Development Conference Statement, *5*(9).

15. Wolf, N. (1991). *The beauty myth: How images of beauty are used against women.* New York: William Morrow.

16. Berkman, S. (1990). Body image: Larger than life? *Women's Health and Fitness News, 4*(8), 1–2.

17. Hsu, L.K.G., (1990). *Eating Disorders.* Guilford Press: New York.

18. Crowther, J.H., Tennenbaum, D.L., Hobfoll, S.E., and Paris-Stephens, M.A. (1992). *The etiology of bulimia nervosa.* Washington, D.C.: Hemisphere Publishers.

19. Kalliopuska, M. (1982). Body-image disturbance in patients with anorexia nervosa. *Psychological Reports, 51*:715.

20. Bruch, H. (1973). *Eating disorders: Obesity, anorexia nervosa, and the person within.* New York: Basic Books.

21. Garner, D.M., and Bemis, J.R. (1984). Cognitive therapy for anorexia nervosa. In D.M. Garner and P.E. Garfinkel (Eds.), *Anorexia nervosa and bulimia* (pp. 84–133). New York: Guilford Press.

22. Maloney, M.T., and Farrell, M.K. (1981). Treatment of severe weight loss in anorexia nervosa with hyperalimentation and psychotherapy. *American Journal of Psychiatry, 137,* 310.

23. Kreipe, R.E., Churchhill, B.H., and Strauss, J. (1989). Long-term outcome of adolescents with anorexia nervosa. *American Journal of Diseases in Children, 143*(11), 1322–1327.

Resources

A-HELP, THE ASSOCIATION FOR THE HEALTH ENHANCEMENT OF LARGE PERSONS

800-368-3468

Multidisciplinary group of health professionals who reject dieting and weight loss as crucial for healthy living. Promote the development of healthy living and self-accepting patterns and messages. Focus on promoting the physical and emotional well-being of large people.

AMERICAN ANOREXIA/ BULIMIA ASSOCIATION

418 E. 76th Street
New York, NY 10021
212-734-1114

ANOREXIC/BULIMIC ANONYMOUS

PO Box 112214
San Diego, CA 92111
619-277-3737

Helps in starting groups.

ANOREXIA NERVOSA AND RELATED EATING DISORDERS (ANRED)

PO Box 5102
Eugene, OR 97405
503-344-1144

BULIMIA/ANOREXIA SELF-HELP (BASH)

6125 Clayton Avenue Suite 215
St. Louis, MO 63139
800-277-4785

Information on national self-help groups.

GLENBEIGH FOOD ADDICTION HOTLINE

800-4A BINGE

Crisis hotline for prompt support and help.

HUMAN NUTRITION INFORMATION SERVICE (NHIS)

Department of Agriculture
6505 Belcrest Road
Hyattsville, MD 20782
301-436-8617

Publications on research on food consumption, food composition, and dietary guidance in both technical and public publications.

NATIONAL ANOREXIC AID SOCIETY

5796 Karl Road
Columbus, OH 43229
614-436-1112

NATIONAL ASSOCIATION FOR THE ADVANCEMENT OF FAT ACCEPTANCE (NAAFA)

PO Box 188620
Sacramento, CA 95818
916-443-0303

Social, educational, and human rights network of fat people and their allies who work for the acceptance of fat people. They are active in fighting size discrimination and promoting self-acceptance of all sizes.

NATIONAL ASSOCIATION OF ANOREXIA NERVOSA AND ASSOCIATED DISORDERS (ANAD)

PO Box 7
Highland Park, IL 60035
708-831-3438

Oldest organization; helps in forming self-help groups and holds conferences in addition to its information services.

NATIONAL HEART, LUNG, AND BLOOD INSTITUTE (NHLBI) INFORMATION CENTER

PO Box 30105
Bethesda, MD 20824-0105
301-951-3260

Nutrition, lifestyle, and chronic disease information.

NATIONAL INSTITUTE OF MENTAL HEALTH EATING DISORDERS UNIT

Bldg. 10, Room 35231
900 Rockville Pike
Bethesda, MD 20892
301-496-1891

Average stay 2 months; ages 18–40; research setting; services are free.

OFFICE OF DISEASE PREVENTION AND HEALTH PROMOTION (ODPHP)

National Health Information Center
PO Box 1133
Washington, DC 20013-1133
800-336-4797, 301-565-4167

Assists the public and health professionals locate health information through the identification of health information resources, an information and referral system, and publications.

OFFICE OF MINORITY HEALTH RESOURCES (OMH-RC)

PO Box 37337
Washington, DC 20013
800-444-6472

Information on minority health organizations, publications on minority health, and health statistics.

THE COUNCIL ON SIZE AND WEIGHT DISCRIMINATION

PO Box 238
Columbia, MD 21045

Council that works to influence public policy and public opinion to end fat discrimination.

These organizations offer weight control and general nutrition information:

AMERICAN DIETETIC ASSOCIATION

216 West Jackson Blvd., Suite 800
Chicago, IL 60606-6995

CENTER FOR SCIENCE IN THE PUBLIC INTEREST (CSPI)

1501 16th Street NW
Washington, DC 20036
202-332-9110

CENTERS FOR DISEASE
CONTROL
CENTER FOR DISEASE
PREVENTION AND
HEALTH PROMOTION
NUTRITION DIVISION

5B17 CDC-3
1600 Clifton Road NE
Atlanta, GA 30333
404-639-3107

FOOD AND NUTRITION
INFORMATION CENTER
U.S. DEPARTMENT OF
AGRICULTURE

National Agricultural
    Building
Room 304
Beltsville, MD 20705
301-344-3719

INSTITUTE OF MEDICINE
NATIONAL ACADEMY OF
SCIENCE

Office of Communications
2101 Constitution Avenue
Washington, DC 20418
202-344-2352

SOCIETY FOR NUTRITION
EDUCATION

1700 Broadway Suite 300
Oakland, CA 94612
415-444-7133

CHAPTER 2

$\mathscr{2}$

Exercise and Fitness

CHAPTER OBJECTIVES

On completion of this chapter, the student should be able to discuss:

1. The concept of physical fitness and how it relates to health.
2. The physiological benefits of physical fitness.
3. The psychological benefits of physical fitness.
4. The six major components of physical fitness.
5. What is meant by aerobic exercise.
6. The difference between muscular strength and muscular endurance.
7. How flexibility protects the body.
8. How body composition is affected by exercise.
9. How psycho-social-cultural dimensions contribute to the overall physical fitness status of women.
10. Biological differences between men and women that affect physical performance levels.
11. How pelvic floor fitness contributes to a woman's well-being.
12. The major exercise myths often held by women.
13. The major components of Total Fitness.
14. The benefits of strength training.
15. The three major variables of exercise capacity.
16. Maximum and target range heart rate.
17. Significance of a warm-up and cool-down.
18. Why walking may be the best exercise.
19. How exercise counters some of the natural conditions of the aging process.
20. Athletic amenorrhea.
21. Physical and psychological side effects of anabolic steroid use.

Introduction

The 1980s witnessed the emergence of a renewed national interest in physical fitness and exercise. Scientific research documented that exercise extends life. Specifically physical fitness greatly reduces the risk of dying of heart disease, cancer, and other chronic illnesses.[1] In addition to increasing the quantity of life by slowing natural aging processes, exercise enhances the quality of life by promoting psychological well-being and controlling body fat and fat distribution. This chapter examines the concepts of physical fitness and exercise, identifying the critical components and issues of each. The concepts of total fitness, aerobic exercise, and strength training are examined and discussed from a women's health perspective. The maintenance of a personal fitness program, exercise and aging issues, and exercise abuse are also explored.

Physical Fitness

Physical fitness is an elusive term that is difficult to define. It means different things to different people; for example, "fitness" to a dancer is a different concept than "fitness" to a long-distance swimmer. Fitness is also relative—a woman may be "more fit" this year than she was last year, and there is no clear end point at which fitness occurs. Fitness can also be defined as the ability to meet routine physical demands with a reserve to meet sudden challenges. The point is that with fitness as a goal, exercise is the means to get there. Fitness provides both short-term and long-term benefits. A low physical fitness level is a strong, consistent factor for early death from all causes in otherwise healthy adults (Fig. 2.1). Increasing fitness level through moderate exercise, such as a brisk 30- to 60-minute walk daily, may reduce an unfit woman's risk of early death by nearly 50 percent.[1]

Benefits of Physical Fitness

Regular physical activity, recreational or work-related, contributes to overall health and well-being. Specific physical benefits of exercise include the utilization of calories; reduction in body fat; improved cardiovascular status; lowered blood pressure; and decreased risk of developing diabetes, osteoporosis, and certain forms of cancer.[2,3] Physical activity also protects against premature death. Women with an almost completely sedentary lifestyle have the highest risk of death from all causes (see Fig. 2.1). Physiological benefits are not the only positive outcome of exercise. Psychological benefits are also a result of physical activity. Although most individuals who exercise regularly report that they "feel better" when they exercise, until recently, the scientific community has not been able to measure this phenomenon objectively. One review of studies on exercise and mental health found that exercise serves as a coping strategy or "inoculator" against stress. Because exercise itself stresses the body, repeated exercise sessions ("inoculations") may increase the exerciser's capacity for dealing with stress in all forms.[4]

FIGURE 2.1

Women's fitness level and risk of death.

SOURCE: Blair, S.N., Kohl, H.W., Paffenberger, R.S., Clark, D.G., Cooper, K.H., and Gibbons, L.W. (1989). Physical fitness and all-cause mortality. *Journal of the American Medical Association. 262,* 2395–2401. Copyright 1989, American Medical Association.

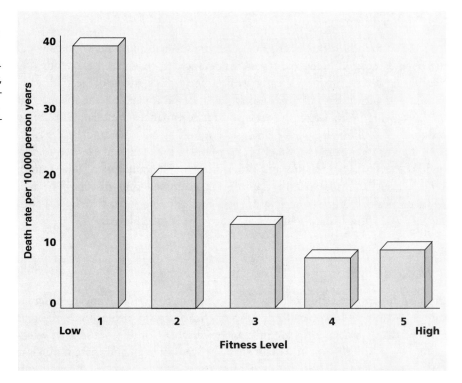

Components of Physical Fitness

Exercise physiologists usually define fitness in six major areas: (1) cardiovascular endurance, (2) muscular strength and endurance, (3) flexibility, (4) balance, (5) coordination and agility, and (6) body composition that falls within the normal range of body weight and percent body fat. Modern lifestyles do not require much physical movement, and few American women are naturally fit as a result of day-to-day living activity. For most women, contemporary life requires a commitment of time and energy to achieve fitness in these six areas.

1. *Cardiovascular endurance,* the ability to carry on a vigorous physical activity for an extended period of time, is the most vital element of fitness. **Cardiovascular fitness** is the ability of the heart to pump blood through the body efficiently. The development of cardiovascular fitness begins with the enhancement of the ability of the heart, blood vessels, and blood to deliver oxygen to the body's cells and then remove waste products. Although muscles are able to draw on quick sources of energy for short-term exertion, when exercise lasts more than a minute or two, the muscles must derive their energy from a process that requires oxygen from the blood. Because blood-derived oxygen is used in this process, it is called **aerobic exercise.** With repeated regular exercise, the heart becomes able to pump more blood and deliver more oxygen with greater efficiency. In

addition, the muscles' capacity to use this oxygen becomes enhanced. The two coupled events are referred to as the "training effect." The heart rate, both at rest and exertion, decreases as a result of this regular exercise, and the heart acquires the ability to recover from the stress of exercise more quickly.

2. *Muscular strength* is the total force muscle groups produce in one effort, such as a lift, jump, or heave. Working out with weights is the best way to increase muscle strength. Strength gains come most quickly from heavy resistance and few repetitions. *Muscular endurance* refers to the ability to perform repeated muscular contractions in quick succession. Although muscle endurance requires strength, it is not a single all-out effort. The key to increasing endurance is repetition, working at a moderate level, and building up to a specified goal. Free weights and weight machines can also be used to build endurance.

3. *Flexibility* refers to the ability of the joints to move through their full range of motion. Flexibility is best improved through the use of static exercises that apply steady pressure at the extreme range of motion without undue bouncing. Flexibility varies from person to person and from joint to joint. Women tend to be more flexible than men because of differences in their skeletons, muscle mass, and body composition. Good flexibility is thought to protect the muscles against pulls and tears because short, tight muscles may be more likely to be overstretched. Flexibility and calisthenic exercises must be selected carefully, however, because some movements may actually cause injury to the lower back and knees. Some women find that stretching certain muscle groups helps relieve or prevent pain. For example, stretching hamstring and lower back muscles may alleviate lower back pain, and calf stretches may help prevent leg cramps. Other examples of flexibility exercises are described in Information Box 2.1.

4. *Balance* can be significantly improved with exercise. Balance "skills" are frequently neglected and can be maintained only through regular use. Problems with balance are responsible for a major portion of falls and other accidents among the elderly. Exercise activities that can improve balance include dancing, some calisthenics, yoga, and skipping rope.

5. *Coordination and agility* are both enhanced with regular exercise. **Coordination** is the ability to organize physical activities involving all parts of the body in a skillful manner and to coordinate different actions with each other and with the eyes. **Agility** is the ability to coordinate such movements and change directions quickly and safely. Racket sports are particularly helpful in promoting coordination and agility.

6. *Body composition* can be dramatically affected by exercise, which can help prevent and control obesity by reducing excess body weight and fat. Calories are burned not only during the period of physical exercise (Information Box 2.2), but also for several hours after the exercise. This process is

Flexibility Exercises

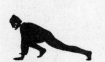

Ski stretch
Hold 30 seconds.

Hurdle stretch
Keep knee straight.
Hold 30 seconds.

Trunk circling
Take 5 seconds to circle clockwise, relax. Repeat in counter-clockwise direction. Do each direction at least twice.

Cobra posture
Lie face down with hands under shoulders. With forehead on floor, slowly raise forehead, then nose, then chin, then shoulders, upper and middle back. Take 10 seconds to complete extension; hold extension 5 seconds. Relax.

Hamstring stretch I
Slowly raise one leg to an angle of 90°, keeping the knee as straight as possible. Grasp the raised ankle with both hands and gently increase the stretch. Hold 5 seconds; relax. Repeat for other leg. Do each leg twice.

Hamstring stretch II
Bend at the waist holding onto toes or ankles. Attempt to place head on knees, hold 30 or 60 seconds.

Abdominal stretch I
Lie on back with arms in "T" position. Raise both legs to 90°. Lower legs to touch right hand, hold 5 seconds. Raise legs to starting position, hold 5 seconds. Lower legs to touch left hand, hold 5 seconds. Raise legs, hold 5 seconds. Lower legs and relax. Repeat entire exercise.

Abdominal stretch II
Lie on back with arms in "T" position. Raise left leg to 90°, keeping knee straight. Lower left leg across the body to touch right hand; hold 5 seconds. Raise leg to 90° position, then relax. Repeat for right leg, crossing over to touch the left hand. Do exercise twice.

Gastrocnemius stretch
Lean against a wall at an angle of between 45° and 60°. Keeping heels on the floor, lean closer to the wall. Hold 15 seconds. Relax.

Groin stretch
Assume stretch position and pull ankles toward the body to increase the stretch on groin muscles.

Abductor stretch
Lift leg to the point of resistance, hold 30 seconds; relax.

Push-ups
Do at least 30.

SOURCE: Edlin, G., and E. Golanty: *Health and Wellness,* Fourth Edition © 1992. Boston: Jones and Bartlett Publishers. Reprinted by permission.

Calories Burned per Hour by Selected Activities

Activity	Body Weight		
	100 lbs	150 lbs	200 lbs
Mopping floors	144	216	288
Swimming (20 yd/min)	192	288	384
Tennis (beginner)	192	288	384
Weeding	228	342	456
Golf (carrying clubs)	270	405	540
Aerobic dancing (low impact)	276	414	552
Walking (4.5 mi)	288	432	576
Snow shoveling	312	468	624
Calisthenics	360	540	720
Jogging (5 mph)	360	540	720
Aerobic dancing (high impact)	372	558	744
Bicycling (13 mph)	426	639	852
Swimming (55 yd/min)	528	792	1,056
Cross-country skiing (8 mph)	624	936	1,248
Running (8 mph)	624	936	124

SOURCE: Latella, S., and Conkling, W. (1989). *Get in Shape, Stay in Shape.* Consumer Reports Books. Yonkers, NY. Reprinted with permission of author.

known as afterburn. The longer and more intense the exercise, the longer the basal metabolic rate (BMR) (see Chapter 1) remains elevated. Regular exercise improves overall muscle tone, contributing to a less flabby appearance.

For the woman, young or older, who is working to develop a personal fitness plan, the goal is to seek a balance among these six components of fitness. Different activities enhance these components of fitness to a greater or lesser degree.

Physical Fitness and Women— Unique Considerations

Most reference studies and books on sports medicine were derived primarily from data obtained from male subjects and thus may not actually apply to women. Women obviously have questions and concerns regarding their physiology and response to exercise that cannot be answered using data derived from studies on men. The scant information that is available on women is usually focused on elite athletes, a nonrepresentative sample of women. One of the few published reports on physical activity of women using national data showed that most women (62 percent) lead very sedentary lives (Fig. 2.2). In this report, only 22 percent of women were classified as very active. Educational level was found to be a predictor of physical activity level; women with more than 12 years of education were almost twice as likely to be very active as persons with less than 12 years of education.[5]

Psycho-social-cultural dimensions are a facet of women's exercise and physical fitness. Sociocultural prejudices have traditionally limited women's access to and full participation in sports. Historically women as "the weaker sex" have not been encouraged to attain fitness levels comparable to their male counterparts. Self-esteem and self-confidence with physical activity are developmental tasks of childhood. Young girls have traditionally not been encouraged to excel or compete in the physical arena. It was not until 1978 that Title IX mandated public schools to provide equal funding for girls' sports, and even since then, opportunities, resources, and, perhaps most importantly, encouragement for physical fitness have not been equally distributed to children, regardless of gender.

Women as Athletes

Traditionally men have excelled in physical competition against women. In general, men are able to run longer and faster, jump higher and further, lift more and longer, and so forth. The traditional assumption has been that men were inherently physically gifted while women were not. In recent years, women have become more competitive in all athletic arenas. Several questions naturally flow from these advances that seek to define gender similarities and differences in sports and exercise better. Resolution of these issues is difficult, however,

FIGURE 2.2

Percent distribution for leisure time physical activity, US women, 1985.

SOURCE: Schoenborn, C.A. (1988). Health habits of U.S. adults, 1985: the "Alameda 7" revisited. *Public Health Reports, 161*(6), 571–580.

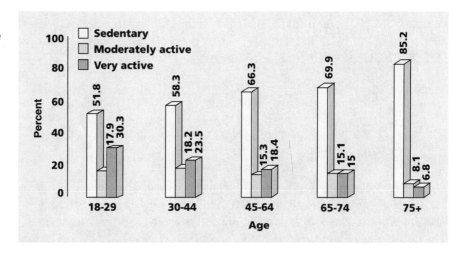

because young girls and boys have not been raised with equivalent levels of emphasis, encouragement, and training in physical fitness.

Biologically, of course, men and women are different. The influence of these differences on athletic performance is not yet well defined. There are no apparent differences between the muscles of men and women. The fact that men are stronger than women is based on the absolute quantity of their muscle mass. Individual muscle fibers, however, do not appear to be different. From a strength perspective, women appear to be about half as strong as men in the upper body areas of the shoulders, arms, and backs and two thirds as strong in the legs and lower body, primarily because men have larger muscle-fiber areas and greater **lean body weight,** total weight minus body fat. Women's naturally higher percentage of body fat, essential for reproduction and general health, may have more of an effect on their physical performance than any other factor. Typically about 25 percent of a woman's body weight is fat, compared with 15 percent for men. Women's extra body fat may be a hindrance in certain sports such as running but an advantage in others, such as swimming. In general, women also have a lower blood volume, about 5 percent less hemoglobin, smaller hearts, and less lung capacity than men.

Women have demonstrated rapid improvements in endurance sports. The gender gap difference in such sports as biking is gradually shrinking. The real issue for women and physical fitness, however, is not trying to equal or excel in male sports. Women should strive as individuals to achieve optimal personal levels of fitness. Women's bodies respond to training as quickly as do men's. It is a matter of personal responsibility to achieve the highest level of fitness commensurate with total lifestyle and personal goals. Women are increasingly being recognized as proficient athletes, whether in competition with each other or in mixed sports.

Pelvic Floor Fitness

An area usually not discussed with traditional exercise or fitness is the **pelvic floor.** The muscles that support everything inside a woman's pelvic cavity, the uterus, bladder, and rectum, form the pelvic floor. Although the muscles form a coordinated working structure, they are not really a "floor" but more like a sling, or hammock, of muscles that serve as the base, or support, for the bladder, urethra, uterus, and other pelvic organs. They are slanted at different angles and can be held with varying degrees of firmness. Many women are not even aware of these muscles. They can be "found" by interrupting a stream of urine. All of the muscles used in this effort constitute what is commonly called the "pelvic floor muscles" (Fig. 2.3). The muscles are technically known as the pubococcygeal and levator ani muscles, which encircle the urethra, vagina, and rectum in a figure-8. In addition to controlling the flow of urine, these muscles have special receptors that relay sexual sensation in the vagina.

Nearly 50 years ago, Dr. Arnold Kegel, an obstetrician/gynecologist, discovered that many of his patients, if they strengthened the muscles of the pelvic

I always thought that exercise was for jocks. I have never felt comfortable in athletic clothes. I had been very self-conscious, whenever I did anything physical. Then I started to read all this stuff about how important exercise was. I realized that it didn't matter what other people thought. At least I was going to take charge of myself. So I slowly ventured into public with my exercise program. In addition to all the benefits of exercise, an extra one happened—I am much more self-confident and I learned that I can really do what I need to do for me.

24-YEAR-OLD STUDENT

FIGURE 2.3
Pelvic floor muscles.

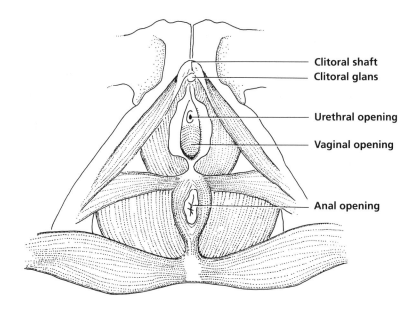

floor, could overcome **stress urinary incontinence.** Stress urinary incontinence is the involuntary leaking of small amounts of urine during sudden exertion, such as coughing, sneezing, jumping, or laughing. Dr. Kegel developed exercises, now known as Kegel exercises, to rehabilitate the muscles of women that had been damaged in birthing. Previously the only corrective modality to address the problem had been surgical repair. Now, obstetrician/gynecologists, physical therapists, and sex therapists are advocating a wider role for pelvic floor exercises, including childbirth, stress incontinence, enhanced sexual sensation, and generalized pelvic muscle conditioning.

Kegel exercises (Information Box 2.3) may help reduce the potential damaging effects of childbirth, such as tearing of the perineum, by increasing the woman's ability to relax the pubococcygeal muscle and thus increase the elasticity of the birth canal. Women who know how to exercise the pelvic floor muscles during pregnancy are also able to do the exercises after giving birth, which promotes recovery and may help prevent incontinence. The pelvic floor muscles probably cannot actually be strengthened during pregnancy because of both the relative flaccidity created by hormonal changes and the pressure exerted by the weight of the fetus. Practicing the exercises prenatally is helpful because many women experience diminished sensation in the pelvic area after birth and would find it difficult to learn the exercises at the very time that they need to be doing them most.

Kegel exercises are helpful in reducing urinary stress incontinence. Although stress incontinence usually develops after childbirth or during the final weeks of pregnancy, women can develop it at any time later in life, whether or not they have been pregnant. Individual differences in tissue strength and in the structure of the pelvis seem to be most important in predicting which women are predisposed to stress incontinence. Many physicians may approach the problem from

---

Kegel Exercises

To identify the pelvic floor muscles:

1. Try stopping a flow of urine in midstream while urinating. The muscles that are tightened in this effort are the muscles of the pelvic floor.

2. Tighten the ring of muscles around the rectum, as if trying to stop a bowel movement. The muscles that are tightened in this effort are also muscles of the pelvic floor.

3. While lying down, place a hand over the abdomen. Tighten all of the muscles of the abdomen and pelvis. Notice that the hand will move. These are *not* muscles of the pelvic floor, and they should be relaxed during Kegel exercises. During the first few practice sessions, it is helpful to check with a hand and make sure that the abdominal muscles are relaxed.

To practice Kegel exercises:

1. Deep breaths—do not forget to breathe.

2. Tighten the anal muscle, pulling inward and outward.

3. Tighten the vaginal muscle, pulling inward and outward.

4. Hold these muscles tight, counting slowly to 10, then relax.

Do Kegel exercises in sets of 5 to 10 at a time, several times a day. Build up to being able to hold the contraction for 20 seconds at a time.

---

a surgical perspective and prefer a surgical repair instead of guiding a woman through the more time-consuming natural healing and repair process.[6] This is unfortunate because some of the more common surgical problems have low success rates unless the patient has a specific anatomical abnormality.

In sex therapy, Kegel exercises may be prescribed for those women who have little or no vaginal sensation or for those women who are able to achieve orgasm with clitoral stimulation but not during intercourse. Because Kegel exercises strengthen and develop control of the pelvic floor muscles, the ability to experience sexual pleasure is enhanced.

From a prevention perspective, Kegel exercises enhance the general tone of the pelvic area, which helps counter the daily effects of gravity on the uterus, bladder, and rectum. Women who learn to do partial Kegels when lifting or with abdominal exertion may be able to avoid possible future prolapse and descending organs.

Exercise Myths

Many women avoid exercise or exercise inappropriately based on fear and misinformation about fitness, workouts, and muscles. A look at these myths shows that they are generally unfounded and potentially damaging.

Myth #1: Exercise increases the appetite.   Increased appetite is not necessarily a consequence of exercise. There is some evidence to suggest that exercise may even depress the appetite for a short while. Those who do eat more when they exercise usually add fewer calories than they burn in their workouts. Exercise raises the BMR, which remains elevated not only for the exercise period, but also for an extended time afterwards. Calories are thus consumed at a higher rate for an extended period of time as a result of the exercise.

Myth #2: Exercising special spots will reduce local fat. There is no such thing as effective "spot reduction." Although there are many gadgets and gimmicks such as girdles, corsets, weighted belts, rubberized workout suits, and specialized exercise devices, none of them will fulfill the promise of a "flat stomach" or "slender thighs" for just minutes a day (and, of course, a few dollars.) Fat tissue cannot be converted into muscle. When a woman exercises, she uses energy produced by burning fat in all parts of the body—not just around the muscles that are doing the most work. Sit-ups will not take fat off the abdomen any faster than any other body area. Sit-ups can, however, strengthen the abdominal muscles, which may help hold the abdomen in more.

Myth #3: No pain, no gain from exercise. Exercise does not have to hurt to provide benefit to the body. During the initial phase or the beginning of an exercise program or when intensifying an exercise program, some muscle discomfort is probable. Once a regular routine has been established, however, there is not a requirement to keep pushing beyond that level for benefit. It is best to avoid pain during and after exercise by intensifying workouts slowly and by beginning each session with a warm-up and ending with a cool-down.

Myth #4: Lifting weights gives women a bulky masculine physique. Because most women have relatively low levels of the hormone testosterone, it is difficult for them to build large muscles. Both men and women can build firmer rather than bulkier muscles by lifting lighter weights more times rather than heavier weights fewer times.

Myth #5: Building muscles reduces flexibility. A woman can lose flexibility by lifting weights without moving joints through their full range of motion. Properly done, weight training can actually improve flexibility. Stretching before and after using weights also helps to promote flexibility.

Myth #6: The more sweat produced, the more fat that is lost. Exercising in extreme heat or in a plastic suit will indeed promote the production of sweat and loss of weight. But sweat reflects the loss of water, not fat. The pounds lost will be soon replenished through foods and water. There is also a risk of heat exhaustion by exertion in very hot weather or in plastic clothes that do not allow sweat to evaporate. The amount of sweat produced is not a measure of energy expended. Sweating depends more on temperature, humidity, lack of conditioning, body weight, and individual variability.

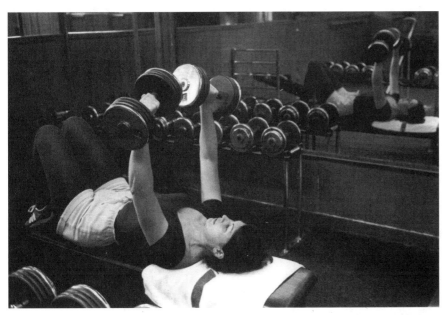

It is a common myth that a woman will develop bulging muscles if she lifts weights.

Myth #7: Exercise is not good for trimming down because weight is gained in muscle.   Aerobic exercises, such as bicycling, jogging, and swimming, burn more fat than they add muscle. With exercises like weight-lifting, muscle gain may indeed weigh more than burned off fat. The overall effect, however, is one of increased trimness because the added muscle is less dense and bulky than the lost fat. The added benefit is that the few extra pounds of muscle do not carry the health risks of excess fat.

Myth #8: Women cannot perform well while menstruating.   Most women can perform consistently throughout their menstrual cycles. Researchers have found no significant differences in physical capabilities, such as oxygen intake, throughout the menstrual cycle.

Total Fitness—Strength Training and Aerobic Exercise

Activities to improve fitness are generally referred to as conditioning programs or training regimens. A wide variety of fitness programs are possible, but they tend to fall into two major categories, **aerobic training** and **strength training.** Aerobic training increases the body's abilities to use oxygen and improves endurance. Strength training enhances the size and strength of particular muscles and body regions. Until 1990, the American College of Sports Medicine had

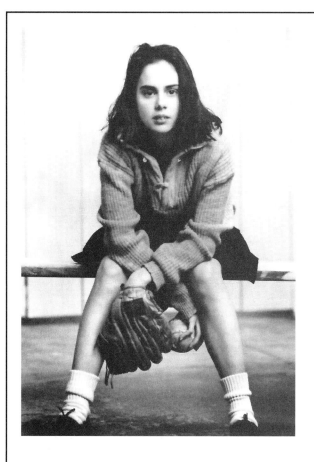

Did you ever wish you were a boy?

Did you? Did you for one moment or one breath or one heartbeat beating over all the years of your life, wish, even a little, that you could spend it as a boy? Honest. Really. Even if you got over it.

Did you ever wish that you could be a boy just so you could do *boy things* and not hear them called *boy things,* did you want to climb trees and skin knees and be third base and not hear the boys say, Sure, play, but that means you have to *be* third base.

Oh *ha ha ha.*

But did you ever wish you were a boy

just because there were *boys,* and there were *girls* and they were *them,* and we were, well,

we weren't them, and we knew there must be a difference because everybody kept telling us there was. But what was it?

You never knew. Like you *knew* that you were a girl *(you run like a girl you throw like a girl you girl you)* and that was great, that was swell, but you   *(continued)*

FIGURE 2.4

Women as athletes.

Reprinted with permission of NIKE, Inc.

primarily advocated basic aerobic activities. While maintaining its aerobic focus, however, the new program has been revised to include strength training at least twice a week. It is now realized that the best fitness program is one that combines aerobic exercise with strength training. Both types of exercise provide unique benefits. Stated simply, strength training builds muscle and bone, and aerobic exercise improves cardiovascular fitness. When both aerobic and strength training are combined, maximum benefits are derived. Coupled with a low-fat diet, the combination program may also be the most efficient way to lose weight. In addition to burning calories while working out, the resultant muscle mass from strength training serves to boost the BMR further (see Chapter 1) because muscle consumes more energy than does fat.

Circuit training is a variation of the aerobic-strength combination. Promoted by many health clubs, the idea behind circuit training, or aerobic weight training, is to raise the heart rate by lifting moderate amounts of weight quickly and

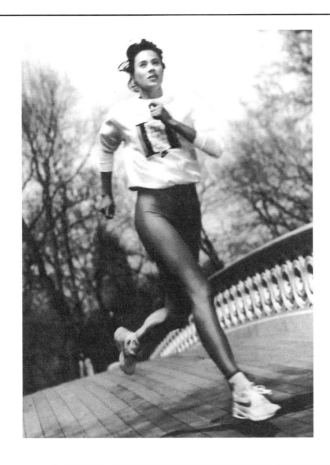

couldn't help wondering what it would be like if you... had been...a *boy.*

And if you could have been a boy, what difference would it have made? Would it have made you faster, cuter, cleaner? And if you *were* a boy, this incredibly bouncing boy, what boy would you have been? All the time knowing no two boys are alike any more than all girls are.

So you wake up. And you learn we all have differences (Yes!) You learn we all have similarities (Right!) You learn to stop lumping everybody in the world into two separate categories, or three, or four, or any at all (Finally!) And you learn to stop beating yourself over the head for things that weren't wrong in the first place.

And one day when you're out in the world running, feet flying dogs barking smiles grinning, you'll hear those immortal words calling, calling inside your head *Oh you run like a girl*

and you will say shout scream whisper call back *Yes. What exactly did you think I was?*

Just do it.

skipping the rest period between exercises. Many people, however, find that the workouts are too exhausting if they do not rest between sets.

Strength Training

For the past two decades, health experts have stressed the importance of regular aerobic exercise, such as jogging or cycling, to maintain a healthy heart and a healthy weight. Although aerobic exercises are excellent for the heart and lungs, such exercises do not provide much benefit to the upper body, where half of the muscles are located. Total fitness requires more than aerobic exercise; it also requires muscle-building. In previous years, strengthening muscles was something that concerned only bodybuilders and was done generally out of vanity. Currently fitness experts, including the American College of Sports Medicine, recommend strength training for health reasons—for women as well as men. Strength training, similar to aerobic exercise, can help prevent or delay many of the declines associated with aging or inactivity. The "use it or lose it" adage applies with all muscle groups.

Strength training does not necessarily mean lifting massive weights to build bulging muscles. Such "power lifting" has nothing to do with fitness and may actually be injurious. Weight training calls for working out against moderate resistance to tone muscles and build muscle endurance. The resistance can be provided by free weights, dumbbells or barbells, or weight machines. Body weight can also be used as resistance, as in calisthenics such as push-ups or pull-ups.

There are many benefits to strength training. Muscle strength and muscle endurance are important for women. Well-toned muscles help maintain good posture and may help prevent injuries. Both muscle strength and muscle endurance can be enhanced together through a process known as **progressive resistance training.** It calls for gradually increasing resistance, usually in the form of weights, to normal body motion. The weights are heavy enough to contract the muscles at tensions close to maximum and are progressively increased as the muscles develop. Each group of muscles is worked but not the same muscles each day. Resting between sets and working slowly and smoothly through the entire range of muscles reduces the chance of injury and subsequent soreness. At least a day of rest is required between sets for each specific muscle group.

Most people start losing muscle tissue (and gaining body fat) in their thirties, particularly if they are inactive. Maintaining muscle strength produces obvious benefits in all activities of daily living from lifting items to physical activity by increasing stamina and self-confidence. Strength training is particularly valuable for women because it also increases bone density and thus helps to delay or minimize osteoporosis and the vulnerability to fractures. Injury prevention is another important benefit of strength training for many musculoskeletal injuries, especially those that are induced by exercise, such as runner's knee or shin splints. These injuries are due in part to muscle weakness and imbalances as well as joint instability. Such conditions are often corrected with strength training. Exercise is essential for maintaining a strong back and protecting it from injury. Lower back pain often results from weakness of back and abdominal muscles, both of which help support the back. Poor posture can also contribute to back problems, and strength training may help improve posture.

Women tend to have less muscle mass than men, especially in the upper body, because of hormonal differences, because they are generally smaller than men, and because of their different normal activities. Women can work out, however, and gain strength at the same rate as men. Many women have avoided strength training out of fear of becoming "muscle bound." A moderate program will not create obvious muscle bulk in men or women but will result in a firmer, trimmer physique. Muscle fitness is described in terms of muscular endurance and muscular strength. Light resistance with many repetitions primarily builds endurance, the ability to contract a muscle repeatedly in quick succession. Heavy resistance with few repetitions primarily increases muscle strength and size. A basic strength training routine is described in Information Box 2.4.

Workout tips for women and strength training include a warm-up before each workout with a stretching routine. It is important to start with light weights that can be comfortably lifted 10 to 15 times a set. Progressive resistance training calls for gradually increasing the weight and the number of repetitions.

Aerobic Exercise

Aerobic exercise significantly raises the heart rate and provides benefits unique from strength training. Aerobic exercise seems to lower body cholesterol levels and blood pressure more than strength training. It also improves cardiovascular fitness, the ability of the heart and lungs to supply the muscles with oxygen, a benefit generally not derived from strength training.

Components of Exercise

Improvement in exercise capacity is related to three essential variables—intensity, duration, and frequency. Exercise **intensity** is the work per unit of time. Intensity can be measured by the output of sweat—if there is no sweat, the activity needs more intensity. More important than sweat per se is that the exercise must be intense enough to reach and maintain the **target heart rate,** the exercise heart rate needed to produce a training effect, for 20 to 30 minutes each workout. Exercise **duration** is affected by intensity and the purpose of the exercise. If aerobic conditioning is the goal, the 20- to 30-minute intensity is still in effect. If the purpose of the program is to lose body weight and fat, however, duration is the key, and longer, slower sessions are preferable to shorter, more intense activity. **Frequency** is measured by regularity and is the pivotal issue in any exercise program. Exercising 3 to 5 days a week rather than one hard workout improves the likelihood of meeting training objectives. Alternating light and heavy workout sessions is another component for successful fitness improvement. The body responds best to a conditioning program that alternates light and heavy demands. This approach reduces the risk of injury, provides several relaxing exercise sessions each week, and allows the body to repair fully between workouts.

Maximum and Target Range Heart Rates

It is best to exercise at a pace that forces the heart to pump beyond its usual output. One way to determine this is to check if the heart rate is beating within the target heart range, which is fast enough to insure that the activity pushes the heart muscle to the point of improving fitness but not so fast that the heart will become exhausted within too short a time or place the person in a danger zone. (See Self-Assessment 2.1 to determine maximum and target heart rates.) By checking the pulse during or immediately after exercise, it is possible to

---

SELF-ASSESSMENT 2.1

Maximum and Targeted Heart Rates

To determine *Maximum Heart Rate (MHR):*

Take age (years) and subtract it from 220.

A 25-year-old woman would have an MHR of 195.

To determine *Targeted Range:*

Multiply MHR by 0.60 to determine low end.

Multiply MHR by 0.90 to determine high end.

A 25-year-old woman would thus have a range of 117–175.

Basic Strength Training Routines

These four muscle-building exercises work all of the major muscle groups in the upper body. For a basic program:

Do one set of these exercises twice a week.
Start with a weight that can be raised only about 8 times; when it is fairly easy to do 12 repetitions, change to a heavier weight that can be raised about 8 times; repeat.

General guidelines:

Begin each session with a warm-up.
Breathe steadily and slowly during the session.
Exhale during the lift or body raise.
Inhale during the return to the standing position.
Perform the repetitions slowly.
Stop if there is any pain or injury.
Cool down after the session.

Modified Sit-ups

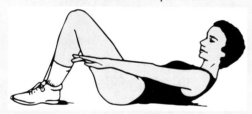

General guidelines:

Lie on back with palms face down.
Bring knees up; keep feet flat on floor.
Raise shoulders until base of shoulder blades lift off floor.
Return to starting position.

Increase resistance:

Once 12 repetitions can be easily done, lock hands behind the head and lift upper body farther off the floor.
Do sit-ups on an incline with buttocks higher than head.

Biceps-Curl

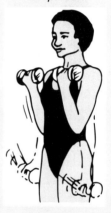

General guidelines:

Stand straight with back straight and knees slightly bent.
Hold weights at side, palms facing forward.
Slowly curl weights up and in toward chest.
Slowly lower them back to the side position.

Increase resistance:

Once 12 repetitions can be easily done, increase the weight until 8 can be done again.

calculate if the exercise is at the appropriate intensity. An exercise program that keeps the heart rate within the range provides a training effect in as safe a manner as possible. If the heart does not reach the lower limit of the target heart range during an exercise activity, increase the intensity by exercising more vigorously. If the heart rate exceeds the upper limit of the target heart range, particularly in the early phases of an exercise program, reduce the intensity to stay within range.

Modified Push-ups

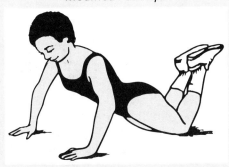

Upright Row

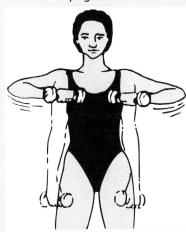

General guidelines:

Lie face down on floor, palms next to shoulders, legs bent with feet pointed upward.

Keep back straight and raise upper body from the knees until arms are almost straight—elbows should not be in a locked position.

Lower the body until it almost touches the ground. Repeat.

Increase resistance:

Once 12 repetitions can be easily done, place something under the knees to elevate them.

General guidelines:

Stand tall, back straight and knees slightly bent.

Hold weights in front of the thighs, palms facing legs.

Slowly raise weights to the armpits, without rotating wrists.

Return weights to thighs.

Increase resistance:

Once 12 repetitions can be easily done, increase the weight until 8 can be done again.

Warm-Up and Cool-Down

A **warm-up** is essential before any aerobic or strength training session. Warming up prepares the body for exercise by gradually increasing the heart rate and blood flow, raising the temperature of the muscles, and improving muscle function. It may also decrease the chance of sport injury. Stretching is not a wise way to begin a workout. Stretching cold muscles increases the risk of injury. Sudden exercise without a gradual warm-up can lead to an abnormal heart rate and blood flow and changes in blood pressure, which can be dangerous, especially for older exercisers.

There are two techniques for warming up. Activities such as jogging in place or stationary cycling are full body warm-ups. Because they use the large muscle groups, these general warm-ups are most effective for elevating deep muscle temperature. Full body warm-ups are essential before stretching or working with weights. Specific warm-ups are slightly less vigorous rehearsals of the sport or exercise that is to be performed. Specific warm-ups are particularly effective in preparing both physically and psychologically for activities involving skill and coordination. A 5- to 10-minute warm-up is usually sufficient to raise body temperature, which is generally indicated by the presence of a light sweat.

A **cool-down** is as important as the warm-up. It is best to slow down gradually by taking a slow lap around the track or pool, pedaling more slowly, or gently stretching for 5 to 10 minutes. Not only does this reduce muscle stiffness, but also it can prevent the sudden drop in blood pressure that occurs when vigorous activity is abruptly stopped.

Many Options of Aerobic Exercise

Regular exercise is important. The form it takes is of secondary importance. Many women find that they are able to maintain their interest in exercise by changing their physical activity on a regular basis to avoid boredom. Seasonal variations and access to recreational facilities also influence exercise decision making. The following examples are currently popular forms of aerobic exercise enjoyed by many women.

1. *Jogging* is generally viewed as a pace somewhere between a fast walk and a run. Technically jogging is a pace slower than a 9-minute mile. Jogging is the classic aerobic exercise because it helps strengthen the heart and lungs, boost stamina, and improve circulation. (Information Box 2.5)

2. *Cross-country skiing simulators* are another popular form of aerobic exercise. The advantage of this type of activity is that both lower and upper body workout is achieved simultaneously. This total body exercise promotes excellent cardiovascular and musculoskeletal fitness. As with stair climbing, there is minimal joint impact.

3. *Bicycling,* whether indoors on a stationary bike or outdoors, can be an excellent cardiovascular conditioner as well as an effective way to control weight.

4. *Stairs* have evolved as perhaps the hottest aerobic activity of the 1990s. The basic conditioning principles for any aerobic workout apply to stair-climbing. The session should include a warm-up and cool-down period. Stairs in buildings or stair machines offer the same fitness opportunity.

INFORMATION BOX 2.5

1.5-Mile Run Test Times for Women

Fitness Category	Age (in years)					
	13–19	20–29	30–39	40–49	50–59	60+
Very poor	>18:31	>19:01	>19:31	>20:01	>20:31	>21:01
Poor	16:55–18:30	18:31–19:00	19:01–19:30	19:31–20:00	20:01–20:30	21:00–21:31
Fair	14:31–16:54	15:55–18:30	16:31–19:00	17:31–19:30	19:01–20:00	19:31–20:30
Good	12:30–14:30	13:31–15:54	14:31–16:30	15:56–17:30	16:31–19:00	17:31–19:30
Excellent	11:50–12:29	12:30–13:30	13:00–14:30	13:45–15:55	14:30–16:30	16:30–17:30
Superior	<11:50	<12:30	<13:00	<13:45	<14:30	<16:30

SOURCE: Cooper, K.H. (1982). *The Aerobics Program of Total Well-Being.* New York: M. Evans & Co.
From *The Aerobics Program for Total Well Being* by Kenneth H. Cooper, M.D., M.P.H. Copyright © 1982 by Kenneth H. Cooper. Used by permission of Bantam Books, a division of Bantam Doubleday Dell Publishing Group, Inc.

A major advantage of stair-climbing, particularly with the machines, is that there is less impact on the joints and feet than with many other forms of aerobic exercise.

5. *Swimming* is an excellent way to strengthen and tone the muscles in various parts of the body as well as promote aerobic fitness. Swimming, however, does not appear to be as effective an exercise modality for losing weight as other forms of exercise. Studies indicate that swimmers may actually need to retain body fat as heat-preserving insulation.[7]

6. *Aerobic dance* is an exercise modality that combines music with kicking, stretching, bending, and jumping, to deliver the same benefits as running, cycling, or swimming. The activity can be done at home alone, with video tapes, or in organized classes. Aerobics can be especially good for cardiovascular fitness but presents risks to the joints and feet. Low-impact aerobics have evolved in response to the many reported injuries of traditional aerobic activities. Low-impact aerobics replace jogging and jumping with steps that minimize the risk of injury or joint trauma. The third generation of aerobics, called "nonimpact aerobics," combines techniques of modern dance and martial arts with a focus on cardiovascular fitness.

Walking—the Best Exercise?

Walking emerged from the 1980s as the survivor of several fitness fads. Walking is user-friendly, easily adaptable, and inexpensive, knowing no age or geographical boundaries. Walking's wide appeal may stem from a number of studies that indicate the regularity and duration of an activity may be far more crucial in

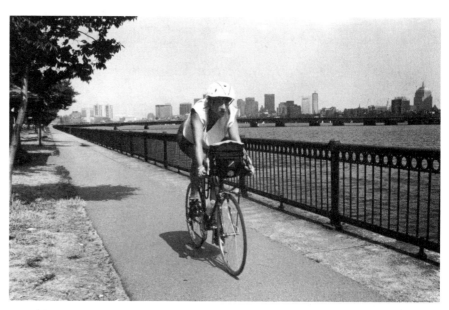

Aerobic exercise can take many forms. It is not limited to running or exercise classes.

determining good health than the intensity. The traditional standard advice has been that to improve aerobic power, a person needed to attain 70 percent of the maximum heart rate and keep it there for 20 to 30 minutes, three times a week. Studies now suggest that regular, moderate (30 to 40 percent of maximum heart rate) exercise performed over a lifetime may produce more benefits than several years of intense aerobic activity. Walking is an easy, safe, simple, and enjoyable way to stay healthy. At a moderate to brisk pace for 30 to 45 minutes a day, walking lowers the risk of heart disease, lowers blood pressure, helps control adult-onset diabetes, guards against osteoporosis, helps keep weight under control, and helps reduce stress. Walking rarely causes the kind of injuries associated with jogging. Most problems with walking can be avoided by simply wearing good walking shoes, warming up beforehand, practicing good walking technique, and working up slowly to the desired pace.

Exercise and Aging

Exercise becomes increasingly important with age. Many of the problems commonly associated with aging, such as increased body fat, decreased muscle strength and flexibility, loss of bone mass, lower metabolism, and slower reaction times, are often signs of inactivity that can be minimized or even prevented by exercise. In addition to improving the six basic elements of physical fitness previously discussed, exercise provides another benefit of special importance to women. Exercise provides a protective factor in the prevention of osteoporosis (see Chapter 12). The combination of weight-lifting and aerobic exercise seems to be the best combination for prevention of this chronic debilitating condition of women.

Exercise Abuse

The pressures to be svelte and physically fit bombard women from multiple directions. Being healthy and fit are desirable and noble goals, but occasionally individuals become so zealous in the pursuit of fitness that injury results. Exercise abuse occurs when exercise or fitness becomes the "A number 1" priority, exceeding family, friends, work, and education, or when athletic injuries are ignored. An **overuse syndrome** occurs when a body part or the entire body is exercised beyond its biological limit to the point of injury. Common overuse injuries affect the muscles, tendons, ligaments, joints, and skin. The most common causes of overuse injuries are excessive exercising, faulty technique, and poor equipment. "Going for the burn" is dangerous because the pain of overexertion is the body's message that something is wrong, and that problem should be addressed, not ignored. Some women may exercise to such a degree that they stop menstruating. This condition, known as **athletic amenorrhea**, usually is the direct result of excessive exercise and an abnormally low ratio of body fat to body weight. The long-term consequences of prolonged athletic amenorrhea include the early onset of osteoporosis and its resultant risk for injury and debilitation.

Anabolic steroid use is another form of exercise abuse. **Anabolic steroids** are synthetic derivatives of the male hormone testosterone. Steroid use has become particularly popular among teenage males, but many women use them as well. Men and women who use steroids in conjunction with heavy resistance training increase their muscle and bone mass but may also experience severe physical and psychological side effects. The documented adverse physical effects for women of steroid use include enlargement of the clitoris, beard growth, baldness, deepened voice, and breast diminution. Other side effects of steroid use include an increased risk of heart disease and stroke, increased aggression, liver tumors and jaundice, and acne. The acquired immunodeficiency syndrome (AIDS) epidemic has added another liability to steroid use: the increased risk of human immunodeficiency virus (HIV) transmission with shared needles. The psychological effects of long-term, high-dose anabolic steroid use may lead to a preoccupation (addiction) with drug use, difficulty stopping, drug craving, and withdrawal symptoms when the drugs are stopped.[8] Clearly anabolic steroids should be totally avoided.

Maintaining a Personal Exercise Program

Women, like men, do not have difficulty starting exercise programs; they have difficulty maintaining them. The benefits of exercise are so important that

I really don't like to run so I have avoided exercise. I guess I believed that if it wasn't running, then it didn't count as exercise. A friend invited me biking a year ago and it sounded like fun. The next thing I knew I was seriously biking. Now I really look forward to my weekend trips. I'm planning a long trip for next summer. I learned that exercise does not have to be boring. I am doing this because it is fun. The exercise benefits are a great secondary gain.
22-YEAR-OLD LAW STUDENT

SELF-ASSESSMENT 2.2

Determining Baseline Level of Fitness

A woman's baseline level of fitness can be determined by scoring in each of the following four major areas:

Area	Test	Procedure	Scoring Process
Aerobic Fitness	1.5 mi run	After a warm-up, complete a 1.5 mile walk/run around a measured track. For older or inactive women, this test should be delayed until regular exercise has become part of the daily routine	See Information Box 2.5
Abdominal Strength and Endurance	60 sec sit-up	Lie flat on floor with knees bent and feet close to the buttocks. Raise to a "sit" where chest touches knees. Return to start position. Do as many as possible in 60 seconds	*Adequate level* Age: 19–29, 33 or more 30–39, 29–32 40–49, 8–32
Lower Body Flexibility	Toe-touch	Keep feet together and knees straight. Bend forward at the hips and touch thumbs on the floor. Bend slowly without bouncing	Adequate level is the ability to touch the floor with any part of the hand
Body Fat	Pinch test	Using the index finger and thumb, take a deep pinch of skin and fat on the back of the upper arm, thigh, back of upper leg, and the abdomen	A pinch of more than an inch at any site indicates excess fat

exercise should be considered a permanent part of life. The form of exercise is not as important. Exercise fads come and go, and it is possible to try them all. It is better to switch to a different form of exercise when one form becomes boring or dull. Several factors should be considered when selecting an exercise program. A program should clearly fit into a woman's lifestyle and goals. Finding time is another important factor—when excuses dominate, it is time to reconsider the program or reprioritize commitments and obligations. Because about 60 percent of new exercisers drop out within the first 3 months, an exercise log may help motivate and reinforce the effort. Keeping track of time or distance can show improvement and progress toward improvement goals. Self-Assessment 2.2 provides an easy way to ascertain the base level of fitness from which goals can be established and improvement can be measured. By involving family and friends, the commitment for fitness becomes more "real," and such individuals can provide support and encouragement during low or especially busy times. Goals and rewards for specific milestones also often serve to provide additional reinforcement and incentive to maintain the momentum and progress. When boredom occurs, variety may be the answer. By rotating activities, such as biking and walking, or tennis and softball, boredom is less likely to occur. Finally, the benefits of exercise—physical and psychological—are constant reminders of the value of exercise, and they serve to maintain the effort.

Summary

Most women spend most of their waking hours in sedentary activity. By incorporating regular physical activity and exercise into their daily routine, women can improve their levels of fitness, improve their overall quality of life, and reduce their risk of chronic disease and premature death. These are dramatic benefits to activity that can also be pleasurable.

Philosophical Dimensions: Exercise and Fitness

1. It has been argued that women who are physically active are healthier and therefore at lower risk of chronic disease and early mortality. Should they have to pay the same insurance rates as those women whose lifestyles place them at greater risk for illness?

2. It has been argued that the physical fitness craze has been detrimental to the women's movement because it has added another layer of pressure to conform to an "ideal" body shape or size. Is that true?

CURRENT EVENTS

Exercise—Perspective of the 1990s

Throughout the 1970s and 1980s, exercise meant aerobic exercise—activities such as running and cycling that enhance cardiovascular fitness by building a stronger heart and lungs. There was an "elitist" perception to exercise—*only* running or aerobic exercise really counted, and one had to "go for the burn." Experts advised that workouts of 20 to 30 minutes at a near maximum exercise heart rate were necessary to produce fitness benefits. Although not disputing the value of such intense exercise periods, scientists recently have found that workouts as brief as 10 minutes, if done often enough, can result in improved levels of fitness. This news is especially encouraging for women on tight schedules. Another reason to opt for low-to-moderate intensity programs is that people tend to stick with them better over a longer period of time. Those who try to perform an activity at the highest intensity possible may be working at a pace that is too strenuous, thereby setting themselves up for injury,

exhaustion, and discouragement. A more contemporary perspective on exercise is that almost anything goes as long as the individual is active and burning calories. One does not have to be a marathon runner to be physically fit. Running and aerobic classes will continue still to attract participants, but gentler activities are more accepted as fitness modalities. These modalities include a host of activities such as low-impact aerobics, ballroom dancing, and walking. Strenuous sports such as cross training, mountain biking, and rock climbing are attracting more participants each year. The keys to a successful exercise program are simple:

- It is never too late to start.
- Maintaining a level of activity, even minimal, is better than no activity.
- Using the whole body maximizes benefits.

3. What can be done to improve the attitude of young women towards exercise and physical fitness?

References

1. Blair, S.N., Kohl, H.W., Paffenbarger, R.S., Clark, D.G., Cooper, K.H., Gibbons, L.W. (1989). Physical fitness and all-cause mortality. *Journal of the American Medical Association, 262*(17), 2395–2401.

2. Harris, S.S., Caspersen, C.J., DeFriese, G.H., and Estes, E.H. (1989). Physical activity counseling for healthy adults as a primary prevention in the clinical setting. *Journal of the American Medical Association, 261,* 3590–3598.

3. Kaplan, J.P., Caspersen, C.J., and Powell, K.E. (1989). Physical activity, physical fitness, and health: time to act. *Journal of the American Medical Association, 262,* 2437.

4. Editor. (1990). Exercise and mental health. *University of Texas Lifetime Health Letter, 2*(8), 2.

5. Schoenborn, C.A. (1988). Health habits of U.S. adults, 1985: the "Alameda 7" revisited. *Public Health Reports, 161*(6), 571–580.

6. Nowlin, J. (1990). The pelvic floor: a new research frontier. *Women's Health and Fitness News, 4*(9), 3–4.

7. Editor. (1989). To lose weight, walk, don't swim. *Tufts University Diet and Nutrition Letter, 7*(2), 2.

8. Kashkin, K.B., and Kleber, H.D. (1990). Hooked on hormones? *Journal of the American Medical Association, 262*(22), 3166–3170.

9. Kashkin, K.B., and Kleber, H.D. (Dec. 8, 1989). Hooked on hormones? An anabolic steroid addiction hypothesis. *JAMA 262*(22), 3166–70.

Resources

AEROBICS INTERNATIONAL RESEARCH SOCIETY

12330 Preston Road
Dallas, Texas 75230
800-635-7050

AGING HEALTH POLICY CENTER

University of California
  N631Y
San Francisco, CA 94143
415-666-5902

AMERICAN RUNNING AND FITNESS ASSOCIATION

2001 S Street NW Suite 540
Washington, DC 20001
202-667-4150

PRESIDENT'S COUNCIL ON PHYSICAL FITNESS AND SPORTS

450 5th St NW Suite 7103
Washington, DC 20001
202-272-3430

WOMEN'S SPORTS FOUNDATION

342 Madison Avenue
Suite 728
New York, NY 10017
800-227-3988

CHAPTER

3

Alcohol

CHAPTER OBJECTIVES

On completion of this chapter, students should be able to discuss:

1. The prevalence of alcohol consumption in the United States today.

2. How women's alcohol consumption has been viewed historically.

3. How cultural factors influence alcohol consumption.

4. How social phenomena contribute to alcohol consumption by women.

5. How social phenomena contribute to women's access to alcohol treatment services.

6. How social stigmas contribute to the problems women have with alcohol.

7. How alcohol presents incalculable costs to society.

8. The concept of co-dependency.

9. The difficulties in ascertaining the physiological effects of alcohol on women.

10. The basic physiological effects of alcohol on the body.

11. The danger of additive effects of addictive behaviors.

12. The unique physiological effects of alcohol on women.

13. How alcohol has a detrimental effect on women's reproductive health.

14. The significance of blood alcohol concentration.

15. The patterns of chronic alcohol abuse.

16. The symptoms of alcoholism.

17. The psychological approaches to understanding alcoholism.

18. The basic treatment dimensions of alcoholism.

19. Special alcohol treatment issues for women.

20. How women can exercise responsible decision making with regard to alcohol.

Introduction

Alcohol, the most widely used drug in the United States, is prevalent throughout life today. Every woman must decide for herself whether she is going to use alcohol and if she is going to use it, how she will use it, not abuse it. Overall, about 10 percent of all Americans abuse alcohol. According to the National Institute on Alcohol Abuse and Alcoholism, 1 in 20 American women has a drinking problem, and women account for a third of the alcoholics in the United States. Most women use alcohol, although it is impossible to calculate the exact extent of alcohol use and abuse by women. Alcohol is known to play a role in the lives of most women, including adolescents and young adults. For example, 57 percent of women aged 18 to 25 acknowledge using alcohol in the previous month (Fig. 3.1). Alcohol is the largest drug problem on college campuses, where between 87 and 93 percent of students drink, including females. Some encouraging news, however, is that there has been a downward trend in per capita alcohol consumption in the United States since 1981.[1] Research on substance abuse by women has been plagued by delay and methodological flaws, which make accurate assessment of the current total problem of women and alcohol difficult.

Alcohol Trends and Issues

Although alcohol consumption is generally considered a personal and private issue, the effects of alcohol consumption permeate all sectors and dimensions of society.

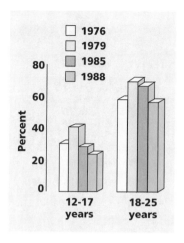

FIGURE 3.1

Percentages of female youth and young adult use of alcohol in last month before survey, selected years.

SOURCE: Adapted from *Statistical Handbook on Women in America,* compiled and edited by Cynthia Taeuber, with permission from The Oryx Press, 4041 N. Central at Indian School Rd., Phoenix, AZ 85012, (602) 265-2651.

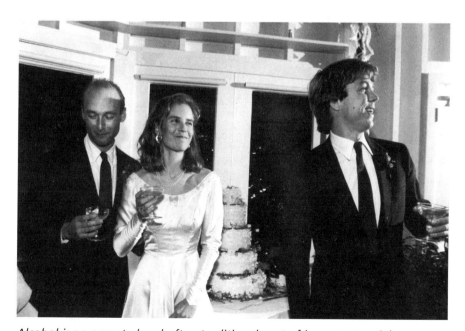

Alcohol is an accepted and often traditional part of important social events.

Myths and Misconceptions about Alcohol

Alcohol is an aid to relaxation and sleep.

Alcohol reduces discomfort.

Alcohol increases sexual arousal.

Alcohol improves sociability.

Alcohol consumption is sophisticated, glamorous, and fun.

Historical Overview

Alcohol has been a constant component of American life since colonial days. Attempts to control, restrict, or abolish alcohol in the United States have all met with failure. In 1919, the 18th Amendment to the Constitution was ratified in an attempt to stop the rapid growth of alcohol addiction. During this time, crime, corruption, and a general disregard for the law flourished, while illegal sales of bootlegged beverages and prescription "medications" prevailed. Prohibition was officially repealed in 1933 by the 21st Amendment. Attitudes toward alcohol and alcoholism have changed over time as well. During the nineteenth and early twentieth centuries, most people who opposed alcohol consumption believed that alcoholics were morally weak. Women were traditionally viewed as the moral and righteous component of society, and as such, female alcoholism or drunkenness was inconsistent with this impression. These simplistic approaches are no longer as widely accepted, and although myths about alcohol and women still abound (Information Box 3.1), there is a greater awareness of the complexities of alcoholism. The public admissions of alcoholism by prominent women such as Betty Ford, Elizabeth Taylor, and Mary Tyler Moore have served to legitimatize alcohol as a personal and pervasive health problem of women.

Epidemiological Data and Trends

Because there were few studies of women and alcohol before 1980, it is difficult to compare recent data with earlier baselines. National data indicate that overall alcohol consumption by women has dropped somewhat in recent years (Fig. 3.2). About three-fifths of American women drink alcohol. Women constitute about 25 percent of the problem drinkers in the United States. Women both initiate drinking and develop patterns of drinking behavior later in life than do

FIGURE 3.2

Female alcohol consumption status, 18 years and older, selected years.

SOURCE: Adapted from *Statistical Handbook on Women in America*, compiled and edited by Cynthia Taeuber, with permission from The Oryx Press, 4041 N. Central at Indian School Rd., Phoenix, AZ 85012, (602) 265-2651.

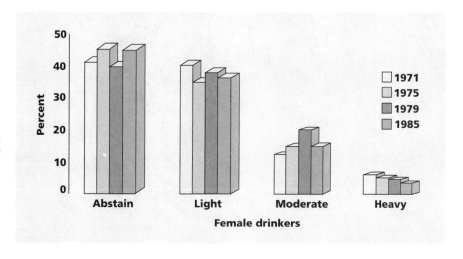

men. Also, women are older than men when they develop drinking problems.[2,3] Although women are less likely to drink and generally drink less, the proportion of women who drink, particularly those under age 35, has increased. Nearly 80 percent of working women, 21 to 34 years of age, drink alcohol. Approximately 20 percent of college women have a drinking problem. Women (and men) are most likely to drink between the ages of 21 and 34. Education and income are predictors of alcohol consumption. The higher the level of education and income, the more likely the person is to drink either moderately or heavily. The greatest percentage of abstainers have less than an eighth grade education. Geography and occupation are predictors of alcohol consumption as well. There are proportionately more drinkers in New England, in the middle Atlantic area, and on the West Coast than elsewhere, although female frequency of alcohol consumption is highest in the West and Northeast.[4] Cities and suburbs have nearly double the proportion of moderate drinkers than small towns and rural areas. Farm owners have the lowest proportion of drinkers, whereas professionals and businessmen have the highest.

It is difficult and often not practical to make generalizations about alcohol consumption among racial/ethnic classifications that represent considerable diversity. Drinking patterns have been shown to be different within varying demographic, economic, and psychosocial circumstances.[5] Nevertheless, generalizations do provide a frame of reference and some insight into alcohol consumption patterns. National data on racial/ethnic distributions of alcohol consumption show some similarities and some differences. African American women and white women have similar drinking patterns, although African American women are more likely to be abstainers and, if they drink, less likely to drink heavily (Fig. 3.3). Forty-six percent of African American women are abstainers compared with 34 percent of white women.[3,6] Racism, unemployment, poverty, and substandard housing have been identified as contributing

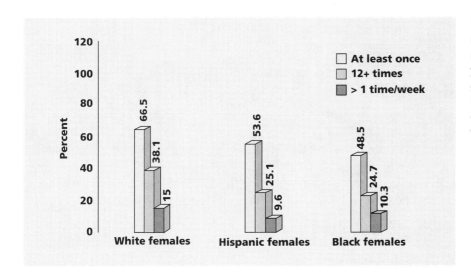

FIGURE 3.3

Use of alcohol by females by race/ethnicity within the past year (1988).

SOURCE: USDHHS (1989). National Institute on Drug Abuse. *National Household Survey on Drug Abuse: Population Estimates 1988.*

variables to alcohol problems among African American women.[7] These conditions are often compounded by a lack of access to health care services, and when services are provided, a lack of sensitivity to culture-related and gender-related issues contributes to less effective treatment.

Cultural factors influence the prevalence of alcoholism because the perception of drunken behavior as deviant depends on the culture in which it occurs. It has been suggested that when drinking is a part of family rituals or ceremonies and when there is great disapproval of public drunkenness, there is a corresponding lower prevalence of heavy drinking. Cultural/gender influences also contribute to alcohol consumption patterns. For example, there are dramatic differences in alcohol consumption between male and female Hispanic Americans. More than 70 percent of Hispanic American women are abstainers or drink less than once a month, and almost the same percentage of Hispanic American men are drinkers. About 18 percent of Hispanic American men and 6 percent of Hispanic American women experience alcohol-related problems.[8] As with Hispanic Americans, rates of alcohol consumption vary with the country of origin. Generally, however, alcohol consumption among Asian Americans is the lowest of all major racial and ethnic groups in the United States.[9] Native Americans experience considerable variability in alcohol consumption patterns. Some tribes almost totally abstain, and others have disproportionately heavy alcohol consumption patterns. Conditions, however, consistent with alcohol-related problems among both Native Americans and Alaska Natives, such as unintentional injuries, chronic liver disease and cirrhosis, homicide, and suicide, are among their 10 leading causes of death.[10]

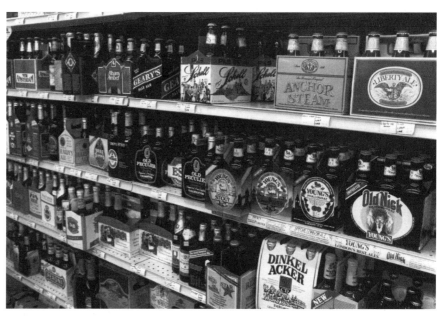

Alcohol is available in many forms.

Psychosocial Dimensions of Alcohol and Women

Social phenomena contribute to alcohol consumption by women and also influence their access to recovery services. Society's double standard for women prevails in alcoholism. A harsher stigma has always been placed on the addicted woman than on the addicted man. Society is more likely to excuse or tolerate an alcoholic man, whose drinking may be attributed to his high-pressure job, family responsibilities, demanding wife and children, and so forth. But there is little tolerance or sympathy for women who drink excessively. The popular media and folklore portray a male drunk as a comical and lovable character, but a drunken woman is considered loose, weak, and immoral. This double standard extends into the treatment arena. The greater social sanctions against alcoholism in women make them less willing to seek help and others less willing to recognize that they need help. Women who do develop alcoholism are viewed as sicker and more deviant than are male alcoholics.[11] Because alcoholic women violate the stereotype of feminine behavior, they distress their families and friends and even the health professionals who might support them. The people who would ordinarily assist a woman's efforts to recover may deny that she is an alcoholic, to protect her and themselves from social embarrassment or disgrace.

Social stigmas discourage women from seeking the help they need to overcome drinking problems. Women with alcohol problems have traditionally been judged more harshly then men with similar problems, and this may help to explain why women have a tendency both to deny their dependence and to seek help. Studies have found alcoholic women to feel more guilt and anxiety about their drinking than alcoholic men. The "housewife drinker" reportedly resorts to alcohol because of loneliness, boredom, and stress.[12] These women are usually better able to hide their addiction and maintain some semblance of a normal life. Among employed women, reasons for drinking vary with the type of job. Women who work for economic necessity identify financial stress, boredom, lack of challenge, discrimination, and powerlessness as common problems. Employed women who are alcoholics tend to leave their jobs before they are fired, either to avoid discovery or because they are physically or mentally unable to continue working.[12] The highest rates of alcohol-related problems are found among young, unemployed women, single or married, who have a heavy drinking partner. Minority women are more likely than white women to suffer from low social status and its attendant stresses. Although the literature has only a paucity of research on studies on alcohol and drug use among lesbians, lesbian women may be at greater risk of alcohol problems related to social disapproval of their sexual choice and to their social environment, which may center on bars and drinking as a meeting milieu.[13,14] Depression has been found to be associated with alcohol consumption and suggested as a factor in the alcohol drinking behavior of women. As in the age-old question of the chicken and egg, it is difficult to establish whether alcohol is a symptom of or a consequence of depression.

I knew I couldn't be an alcoholic. I had a good job and I drank only wine. I certainly don't look like an alcoholic, whatever that look is. It took a long time for me to admit that I really was dependent on that wine. I needed it every day just to dull the world.

30-YEAR-OLD WOMAN

Alcohol-Related Social Problems

Alcohol is involved with:

22,000 annual motor vehicle fatalities

50% of all murder victims and 85% of offenders

70% of fire and burn victims

65% of all suicide attempts

70% of all drowning victims

75% of assault cases (both offenders and victims)

50% of rapes

72% of robberies

33–50% domestic violence cases

SOURCE: Adapted from USDDHS (1987). Special Report to the U.S. Congress on Alcohol and Health. (ADM 87-1519.) Washington, DC: US Government Printing Office.

Societal Costs of Alcohol

Alcohol use is not benign with its effects on society. With more than 10 million adults in the United States with drinking problems, the economic, social, and personal costs of alcohol-related crimes, accidents, illnesses, and deaths are profound (Information Box 3.2). It has been estimated that the cost of alcohol abuse and dependence was $116.9 billion in 1983, with more than 60 percent attributed to lost employment and productivity reductions. Fifteen billion dollars were associated with direct alcohol-related health costs.

The costs to society from alcohol cannot all be measured in terms of dollars. Human costs are incalculable. Government estimates indicate that at least 3 percent of all deaths may be attributed to alcohol-related causes. Increased awareness and legislation have started to slow the annual 20,000 automobile fatalities attributed to drunk driving. Recent data suggest that women are experiencing greater involvement in alcohol-related driving incidents.[15] Alcohol contributes to nearly half of the lives lost each year in car accidents, burns, falls, drownings, and choking accidents. Alcoholics have a suicide rate 6 to 15 times greater than average, and alcohol is implicated in nearly half of all violent deaths, including homicide and suicide.

Alcohol contributes significantly to the personal and family violence picture. In heavy drinking situations, women are more vulnerable to rape and other forms of physical abuse. Drinking contributes 45 to 68 percent of spouse abuse cases and 38 percent of child abuse cases. Alcohol is involved in 83 percent of all arrests. About 30 percent of the nation's state prison inmates drank alcohol heavily before committing rapes, assaults, or burglaries. Alcohol has a generation cyclic effect. Children of alcoholics are more likely to suffer abuse, to have psychological or emotional problems, to become alcoholics, and to marry alcoholics.

Advertising and the glorified image of alcohol consumption impact women and society. The overall image of alcohol has changed from a generation ago, when martini lunches were almost standard fare in the executive sector. Alcohol remains a multibillion dollar American industry, which has developed aggressive and targeted advertising campaigns to the female market. Advertising implies that alcohol and romance go hand-in-hand. Studies have found women to report an increased willingness to engage in sexual activities after they had been drinking. Most women, however, indicate that they tend to enjoy sex more when they have not been drinking.[16]

Co-dependency

The concept of co-dependency is important for many women who become embroiled within the chaos of another person's life. The term co-dependent is used to describe a person obsessed, tormented, or dominated by the behavior of others. Growing out of the older notion of "co-alcoholic," a term once applied to the wives of heavy drinkers, the premise of co-dependency is that everybody in an alcoholic's family is diseased. Consciously or unconsciously, and to their lifelong detriment, co-dependents interact with the drinker and "enable" this person to drink. Co-dependents often feel helpless, miserable, hopeless, and angry as they accept the victim role. A woman may be co-dependent in a relationship with a lover, spouse, parent, child, or friend. A co-dependent typically feels responsible for the behavior and mood of the other. The co-dependent must learn how to separate her own life from that of the addictive person's. The recovery from co-dependence is similar to recovery from alcohol in that only the co-dependent can take the necessary steps toward her own recovery. A co-dependent must learn not to try to control someone else's life and to stop playing the victim role. Many co-dependents have received useful support and encouragement from various programs, such as the Twelve Step Program of Al-Anon, a support group for family and friends of alcoholics.

While offering help to people in distress, the co-dependency movement can be a valuable adjunct therapy. Little hard scientific data, however, are available on the subject. To have a hypothesis and a small amount of evidence that labels large groups of people as diseased may be helpful to a few, but it is potentially harmful and exploitative as well. Clearly additional research is indicated on this subject.

I feel responsible for John's drinking. He really has no one else who understands and helps him. I try to be patient each time he is drunk and clean up the mess. I keep thinking that if I just try harder in understanding maybe he won't have this problem.

35-YEAR-OLD WIFE

Effects of Alcohol

Physiological Effects of Alcohol*

Although the advertising would seem to suggest otherwise, alcohol is a powerful and potentially addictive drug. It functions as a central nervous system depressant that effectively impairs all major body systems. When consumed in small quantities, alcohol has a mild relaxing effect, but larger quantities result in compromised sensory motor coordination, judgment, emotional control, and reasoning capabilities. Alcohol contributes to significant morbidity and mortality among Americans (Fig. 3.4). Individuals who have three to five drinks a day have a 50 percent higher mortality rate than those who have two or fewer drinks a day. Said another way, the average life span of alcoholics is reduced by 12 years, both because of alcohol-related disorders and because of the higher incidence of accidents and suicides.[19] Alcohol contributes to several illnesses,

---

*AUTHORS' NOTE: Despite the growing concern about alcohol and drug addiction in the United States, relatively little is known about the cause and development of these problems in women. Much of the existing information has been extrapolated from research on men, and most theoretical perspectives have been developed by male researchers studying men. Until recently, most studies of women and alcohol focused on the impact of a woman's chemical dependency on children, spouse, and family life. With the few studies available on women, findings are frequently limited and inconsistent because of methodological flaws, including problems in conceptualization of variables, definitions of terms, research design, instrumentation, sampling, and data analysis techniques.[17,18]

FIGURE 3.4

Physiological effects of alcohol.

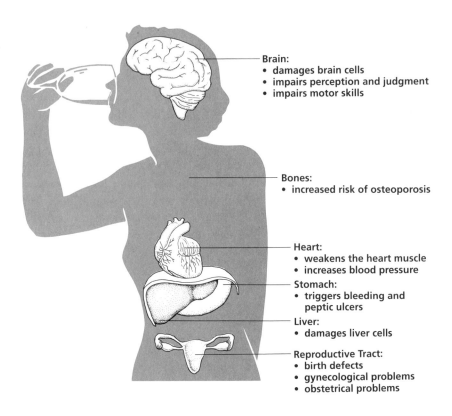

Brain:
• damages brain cells
• impairs perception and judgment
• impairs motor skills

Bones:
• increased risk of osteoporosis

Heart:
• weakens the heart muscle
• increases blood pressure

Stomach:
• triggers bleeding and peptic ulcers

Liver:
• damages liver cells

Reproductive Tract:
• birth defects
• gynecological problems
• obstetrical problems

most notably liver disease, cancer, and cardiovascular disease. As seen in Information Box 3.3, because alcohol circulates throughout the body, nearly all bodily functions can be affected by increased alcohol consumption. Alcohol is quickly and directly absorbed into the bloodstream through the walls of the stomach and upper intestine. In the stomach, alcohol triggers the secretion of acids that irritate the lining. With chronic consumption, peptic ulcers and gastric bleeding may result. It usually takes about 15 minutes for alcohol to reach the bloodstream, and peak effect occurs in 1 hour. Once in the bloodstream, alcohol is quickly carried to the liver, heart, and brain. Alcohol is a **diuretic,** a substance that expedites the elimination of fluid from the body. The liver is the most vulnerable organ to alcohol because it metabolizes alcohol. Heavy drinking may lead to alcoholic **hepatitis,** inflammation and destruction of liver cells. Alcohol is metabolized by the liver at a constant rate, regardless of what is done to speed "sobering up." Chronic alcohol consumption inhibits the production of both white blood cells, which fight off infection, and red blood cells, which carry oxygen to all organs and tissues of the body. Alcohol stimulates liver cells to attract white blood cells, which normally travel throughout the bloodstream engulfing harmful substances and wastes. White blood cells can actually cause irreversible damage to the body if they attack and invade body tissue. This mechanism is believed to occur with **cirrhosis,** severe irreversible scarring and destruction of liver cells, which presents in 10 to 15 percent of chronic drinkers. In later stages with increased scarring and destruction of liver cells, the liver loses its ability to remove bilirubin from the body, and jaundice results. Jaundice

Complications from Chronic Alcohol Consumption

Cancer:
   Cancer of the liver, larynx, esophagus, stomach, colon, breast, and skin (malignant melanoma)

Cardiovascular effects:
   Hypertension, stroke, and cardiovascular disease

Organ damage:
   Brain, stomach, colon, pancreas, and kidneys

Diabetes

Fetal alcohol syndrome

Impotency and infertility

Diminished immunity

Sleep disturbances

presents as a yellowing of the skin. As the liver continues to fail, the person experiences **edema,** the accumulation of fluid in body tissues, and uncontrolled bleeding may occur. The liver eventually fails completely, resulting in coma and death.

Chronic alcohol consumption is also associated with cardiovascular damage. Heavy drinking increases the workload of the heart and reduces coronary blood flow to the heart muscle. This decreases cardiac output, and the heartbeat develops **arrhythmias,** erratic heartbeats, which may lead to cardiomyopathy and damage of the heart valves and musculature.

Perhaps the most dramatic effects of alcohol are on the brain and behavior. Alcohol produces multiple effects. Being a central nervous system depressant, alcohol alters the activity of brain neurons, resulting in impaired sensory, motor, and cognitive function. A common initial response to alcohol is a feeling of being "up." In low doses, alcohol first affects brain regions that inhibit or control higher order behavior. Concurrent effects may also be loss of concentration, memory, discrimination, and fine motor control; mood swings; and emotional outbursts. Moderate amounts of alcohol have disturbing effects on perception and judgment. Visual acuity is impaired, and eyes become more sensitive to light and glare. The ability to differentiate sounds and judge their directional source is impaired. Impaired psychomotor skills are a major consequence of alcohol consumption. Although drinking may increase interest and reduce inhibitions in sex, alcohol has been shown to impair a man's ability to achieve or maintain an erection and a woman's ability to achieve orgasm. The anesthetic effect of alcohol may create diminished perception of pain and temperatures, and serious injuries or temperature extremes may go unnoticed in someone who has been drinking heavily. Additional drinks result in a progressive reduction in behavioral activity. This reduction can lead to sleep, general anesthesia, coma, and even death.

Alcohol is particularly dangerous when combined with other drugs, such as depressants and antianxiety medications. Alcoholics may present to physicians with a spectrum of physical and emotional concerns. The physician may prescribe medications without knowing the full extent of concurrent alcohol use.

Female alcoholics more frequently report sleeplessness and anxiety than male alcoholics. The drugs most commonly abused by alcoholics are stimulants, opiates, hypnotics, and antianxiety agents.[20] Of the 100 most frequently prescribed drugs, more than half contain at least one ingredient that interacts adversely with alcohol. Because alcohol and other psychoactive drugs affect overlapping areas of the brain, combining them can produce an effect greater than that expected of either drug (Information Box 3.4).

INFORMATION BOX 3.4

Alcohol and Drug Interactions

Type Drug	Examples	Possible Effects
Analgesics (narcotic)	codeine, Demerol, Percodan	Increased CNS depression possibly leading to respiratory arrest and death
Analgesics (nonnarcotic)	aspirin, Tylenol, ibuprofen	Gastric irritation and bleeding Increased susceptibility to liver damage
Antidepressants	Tofanil, Petofrane, Triavil	Increased CNS depression, decreased alertness
Antianxiety drugs	Valium, Librium	Increased CNS depression, decreased alertness
Antihistamines	Actifed, Dimetapp, cold medications (prescribed and over-the-counter)	Increased drowsiness
Antibiotics	penicillin, erythromycin	Nausea, vomiting, headache Some antibiotics are rendered less effective
*CNS Stimulants	caffeine, Dexedrine, Ritalin	Somewhat counters depressant effect of alcohol but do not influence level of intoxication
Diuretics	Lasix, Diuril, Hydromox	Reduction in blood pressure with possible lightheadedness
Psychotropics	Tindal, Mellaril, Thorazine	Increased CNS depression possibly leading to respiratory arrest
Sedatives	Dalmane, Nembutal, Quaalude	Increased CNS depression possibly leading to respiratory arrest and death
Tranquilizers	Valium, Miltown, Librium	Increased CNS depression, decreased alertness and judgment

*CNS, Central nervous system.

Heavy alcohol consumption generally leads to multiple nutrition problems for the chronic user. Alcohol has no nutritive value, only "empty calories" (Information Box 3.5). Because alcohol dulls the senses of taste and smell, drinkers often skip meals and develop nutritional deficiencies. Chronic consumption also disrupts normal digestive processes, resulting in **gastritis**, inflammation of the stomach lining; stomach ulcers; and intestinal lesions, which interfere with the metabolism of vitamins and minerals. These malnourished states may predispose chronic alcoholics to certain diseases of the nervous system. Alcoholism has been associated with vitamin deficiencies, most notably thiamine (B_1). This deficiency is believed to play a critical role in diseases of the neurological, digestive, muscular, and cardiovascular systems. Thiamine deficiency also plays a role in **Wernicke's syndrome,** which is characterized by a clouding of consciousness, double vision, involuntary and rapid movements of the eyes, lack of muscular coordination, and decreased mental function. **Korsakoff's psychosis** is another nervous system disease associated with malnutrition and alcoholism. This condition can be traced to degenerative changes in a specific brain region, the thalamus, as a result of B complex deficiencies, especially B_{12} and thiamine. Korsakoff's psychosis generally presents with disorientation, memory failure, failure to learn new skills, and hallucinations. Korsakoff's psychosis and Wernicke's syndrome are often manifested simultaneously in an alcoholic. Permanent brain damage resulting from chronic alcohol consumption may be a major source of mental deterioration in adults. Chronic heavy drinkers may suffer memory losses, may be unable to think abstractly or recall names of common objects, and may not be capable of following simple instructions. The deterioration caused by alcohol can be stopped or even reversed if drinking stops.

A renewed controversy has arisen over the beneficial effects of alcohol. Several studies have shown moderate drinkers to live longer and healthier lives than both alcoholics and abstainers. Moderate drinkers may actually have healthier hearts than heavy drinkers or abstainers from alcohol. Moderate drinkers have been found to suffer fewer heart attacks, have less atherosclerotic buildup, and be less likely to die of heart disease. These studies have not focused on women, so the findings may not be generalizable to women. In addition, many researchers remain skeptical of the findings. Hypertension studies have found inconsistent effects of alcohol with gender and racial differences. Women in one study who averaged fewer than two drinks a day had lower blood pressure than nondrinkers. Women in general and white men who had more than two drinks had higher blood pressures. There are interesting implications to each of these findings that are not yet well understood.

Heavy drinkers have lowered resistance to pneumonia and other infectious diseases. Malnutrition may be a factor, but lowered resistance also occurs in well-nourished heavy drinkers. Heavy drinking appears to interfere directly with bone marrow activity, in which various blood cells are formed. The suppression of the bone marrow contributes to alcoholic anemia, in which red and white blood cell production cannot keep pace with the need. Heavy drinkers are also likely to develop alcoholic bleeding disorders.

INFORMATION BOX 3.5

Calories in Alcoholic Beverages (per serving)

Wine cooler	220
Beer	150
Mixed drinks	150
Sherry	125
Wine	110
Gin, vodka, rum, rye, or whiskey (80 proof)	100
Light beer	100
Cordials or liqueurs	75
Light wine	65

An additive effect of addictive behaviors can occur. Addictive behaviors may be combined, as in the case of a person who smokes cigarettes and drinks heavily. Alcohol may be a cocarcinogen, enhancing tobacco's cancer-causing effects. The risk of cancer generally increases with the amount of alcohol consumed and the number of cigarettes smoked. In these cases, alcohol may act as a promoter for cancers in the lungs, pancreas, prostate, and intestines. Chronic heavy drinking is also linked with an increased risk of cancer of the mouth, esophagus, stomach, liver, and bladder.

As with tobacco usage, research indicates that women who regularly use drugs also tend to drink more heavily than women who report no regular drug use. Similarly, significantly more regular drug users have been found to be heavy drinkers.[21] The long-term physiological effects of combining alcohol and drugs have not yet been well studied. It is unlikely, however, that such effects are beneficial.

Special Physiological Effects of Alcohol on Women

In addition to experiencing the general effects of alcohol previously discussed, women also experience unique direct and indirect physiological effects of alcohol consumption. The penalties for chronic excessive drinking are particularly severe for women. Alcoholic women experience a higher mortality rate, i.e., premature death, than alcoholic men.[22] In one study, 12 years after treatment, the mortality rate of female alcoholics was found to be 4.5 times that of the general population (6.7 for African American women and 3.9 for white women). Deaths from accidents and violence were significantly higher than in the general population, as were deaths from digestive disorders such as cirrhosis and pancreatitis.[23] Higher morbidity rates are also experienced by alcoholic women because the physiological effects of alcohol on women are more detrimental than on men. Women who drink less and for shorter periods of time than men have been found to experience greater physiological consequences.[24,25] Hypothetical explanations for the greater morbidity include higher concentrations of alcohol in the blood because of women's smaller blood volume, higher ratio of fat to lean tissue, more rapid rate of absorption into the bloodstream, and effects of the menstrual cycle.[26] Some evidence indicates that liver disease is more common among female alcoholics and occurs at younger ages than in male alcoholics and that this damage occurs with lesser amounts of alcohol ingestion over a shorter period of time.[24,27,28] Physiologically women appear to produce lower levels of **alcohol dehydrogenase,** the enzyme responsible for ethanol metabolism. As a result, women absorb about 30 percent more alcohol than men do into their bloodstream before it can be metabolized in the liver.[29] The alcohol reaches their brains and other organs more quickly, resulting in both more rapid intoxication than in men as well as more organ-specific ethanol toxicity. In alcoholic women, the stomach seems to stop digesting alcohol at all, which may explain why women alcoholics are more likely to suffer liver damage than men. For a woman of average size, one drink has the same effect as two for the average-sized man.

Hormone levels play a role in alcohol metabolism. Studies have indicated that the menstrual cycle and oral contraceptive use influence blood alcohol levels. The rate of alcohol metabolism and peak blood level attained with a standard dose of alcohol may vary depending on estrogen levels. The rate of alcohol elimination is slower in women taking oral contraceptives, and peak blood levels appear to be reached just before onset of menstruation.[30,31] These variances may help explain why some women have difficulty predicting their response to alcohol and their feelings of loss of control over their responses.

Alcohol consumption has also been associated with breast cancer. Studies have found that women who regularly consume as few as three drinks a week had a 30 percent greater chance of developing breast cancer than those who seldom or never drank. Another study found a 50 percent higher risk of breast cancer among women drinking even small amounts of alcohol and a 100 percent increase in breast cancer risk among those having three or more drinks a week. Based on these findings, may clinicians are advising women with other risks of breast cancer to stop or reduce significantly their consumption of alcohol.

Alcohol consumption has also been associated with osteoporosis. Alcohol can block the absorption of many nutrients, including calcium. As women become older, their risk of osteoporosis increases. Heavy drinking appears to worsen the condition.

Alcohol can have a detrimental influence on reproductive health and pregnancy. Alcohol use during pregnancy has been identified as the leading preventable cause of birth defects.[32] Although alcohol crosses the placental barrier, its effects on the developing fetus are variable because of variance in the degree and timing of exposure, genetic differences in maternal metabolism of alcohol, maternal nutritional status, and possible interaction with other drug compounds. Women who drink have a higher than average number of gynecological and obstetrical problems, including amenorrhea, hysterectomies, miscarriages, and infertility, and women who are alcoholics or who drink heavily during pregnancy have a higher rate of spontaneous abortion, suggesting that alcohol is toxic to developing embryos.[12,33] A special direct effect of alcohol and women is **fetal alcohol syndrome** (FAS). FAS is a term coined to describe a condition distinguished by specific physical and mental abnormalities in infants born to mothers who drank heavily during pregnancy. Approximately 50 percent of women who are heavy drinkers (defined as those who have three or more drinks a day three or more times a week) may deliver a baby with at least some of the characteristics associated with the condition. These include low birth weight and distinctive facial characteristics that vary with the severity of the disease, such as small head size, low nasal bridge, small nose, small midface, droopy eyelids, very thin upper lip, and a wide space between the nose and upper lip. Long-term developmental deficiencies are also associated with FAS and include mental retardation and poor sensorimotor development. In 1990, the term **fetal alcohol effect** (FAE) was proposed for use when some but not all of the FAS criteria are present in a child. The prevalence of FAS is estimated to be between 1 and

3 cases per 1,000 births.[34] African American and Native American women have the highest incidence of FAS. Some plains tribe Native Americans have FAS rates as high as 10 per 1,000 live births.

Alcohol appears to act in concert with other factors in the development of FAS in infants. These factors include differences in the degree of prenatal exposure to alcohol, maternal drinking patterns, possible genetic susceptibility to FAS, differences in maternal metabolism of alcohol, time of gestation during heavy alcohol consumption, interactions of alcohol use with other drugs and medications, and the nutritional status of the mother. One study of 204 abusive prenatal drinkers found five babies with symptoms of FAS.[35] Factors other than alcohol consumption might account for this discrepancy. It has been suggested that the fetus may be especially vulnerable during the first trimester of pregnancy, when central nervous system development occurs, and during this vulnerable period, effects on the infant may be more related to peak blood ethanol level in the mother rather than overall consumption throughout the pregnancy. Without further information, no safe level of alcohol consumption can be established for women during pregnancy.

Alcohol plays an indirect role in many unwanted pregnancies and sexually transmitted diseases (STDs). With impaired judgment and reasoning from intoxication, contraception may be forgotten or ignored, judgment may be distorted, and danger may not be perceived. In addition to unwanted pregnancies and STDs, alcohol plays a significant role in acquaintance rape cases and incidents of pressured sex.

Properties of Alcohol

Pure alcohol is a colorless liquid obtained by fermentation of a liquid containing sugar. **Ethyl alcohol (ethanol)** is the type of alcohol found in alcoholic beverages. Different drinks contain varying amounts of alcohol (Information Box 3.6). Nearly the same amount of alcohol is present in a 12-oz bottle or can of beer (5 percent alcohol), 4 oz of table wine (12 percent alcohol), 2.5 oz fortified wine (20 percent alcohol), and 1 oz (50 percent alcohol) of distilled spirits (Information Box 3.7; Fig. 3.5). The American Heart Association has recom-

---

INFORMATION BOX 3.6

Alcohol Content in Beverages

Serving Size	Beverage	Alcohol by Volume, %
12 oz	Light beer	2.4
12 oz	Beer	3.2
4 oz	Wine	12.0
3 oz	Martini (gin and vermouth)	40.0

INFORMATION BOX 3.7

Blood Alcohol Concentrations

BAC	Effects
0.02–0.4	No overt effects. Feelings of muscle relaxation and slight mood elevation
0.05–0.06	Relaxation and warmth; slight increase in reaction time and slight decrease in fine muscle coordination
0.08–0.10	Balance, speech, vision, and hearing slightly impaired; euphoria feelings; increased loss of motor coordination
0.11–0.12	Difficulty with coordination and balance; distinct impairment of mental facilities and judgment
0.14–0.15	Major impairment of mental and physical control; slurred speech, blurred vision, and lack of motor skill
0.20	Loss of motor control; substantial mental disorientation
0.30	Severe intoxication with minimum conscious control of mind and body

Greater levels lead to unconsciousness, coma, and death from respiratory failure

SOURCE: Drug Abuse and Mental Health Administration.

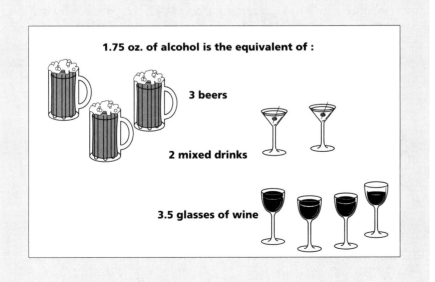

FIGURE 3.5

Equivalents of 1.75 oz of alcohol.

mended that alcohol should not account for more than 15 percent of the total daily calories consumed by an individual, up to a maximum of 1.75 oz daily.

Blood Alcohol Concentration

An essential question in terms of both immediate and long-term consumption is not yet answered: "What is a safe level of alcohol?" The best immediate physiological indicator of safe drinking is the amount of alcohol present in the blood. This amount is known as **blood alcohol concentration** (BAC). BAC is used by clinicians and law enforcement officials to determine if a person is legally "drunk." BAC is expressed in terms of the percentage of alcohol in the blood. A BAC of 0.10 indicates that there are approximately 10 parts of alcohol to 10,000 other blood components. As seen in Information Box 3.8, a BAC of 0.10 results in significant compromise of mental and psychomotor capabilities. Many factors affect BAC and an individual's response to alcohol. The amount of alcohol and the rate at which it is consumed is an important factor. The more alcohol that is consumed, the higher the BAC. Alcohol that is consumed quickly places increased demand on the liver, and BAC levels rise higher than if alcohol is consumed more slowly. Food slows absorption by covering some of the membranes through which alcohol would be absorbed and prolonging the time the stomach takes to empty. The type of drink is another factor. Obviously the stronger the drink, the faster and higher BAC levels will rise. Mixed drinks are absorbed more slowly than straight drinks. Body size is another important factor. A larger person becomes drunk more slowly than a smaller person who is drinking the same amount at the same rate. Age also influences BAC, with higher levels presenting in elderly persons who have consumed the same quantities as a younger adult. BAC is also influenced by race, with Asian Americans and Native Americans unable to break down alcohol as quickly as whites. In addition to higher BACs, many experience effects such as nausea and flushing when they drink. Physical tolerance is an important dimension of drinking. With regular alcohol consumption, more and more alcohol is required to achieve the same desired psychological effect, although motor coordination and judgment are impaired at the same level. After several years of drinking, some individuals develop "reverse tolerance" and actually become intoxicated after drinking only a small amount of alcohol.

Alcoholism

Alcoholism has officially been recognized as a disease for more than 20 years. The traditional definition of an **alcoholic** is a person whose consumption of alcohol interferes with a major aspect of her life. Alcoholism has recently been redefined as a primary, chronic disease with genetic, psychological, and environmental factors influencing its development and manifestations. Common warning signs of alcoholism are summarized in Information Box 3.9. Alcoholism generally appears between ages 20 and 40 but can present in

---

INFORMATION BOX 3.8

What Is a "Standard" Drink?

12 ounces of beer

3–5 ounces of wine

1 ounce hard liquor

Each contains the same amount of alcohol, 0.5 oz or 12 g.

SOURCE: National Institute on Alcohol Abuse and Alcoholism, *Alcohol Alert, 16*(PH315) April 1992.

Warning Signs of Alcoholism

Having 5 or more drinks a day

Needing a drink to start the day

Denial of alcohol problem

Sleep problems

Changing brands or going on the wagon to control drinking

Depression and paranoia

Failure to recall what happened during a drinking episode

Dramatic mood swings

Doing things while drinking that are regretted afterward

Experiencing the following symptoms after drinking: headaches, nausea, stomach pain, heartburn, gas, fatigue, weakness, muscle cramps, irregular or rapid heart rate

---

childhood or early adolescence. When alcohol is not available to an alcoholic, withdrawal occurs. Withdrawal symptoms may include physical trembling, sweating, high blood pressure, delusions, and hallucinations.

Women exercise considerable variability in their drinking patterns. Some women may drink once a month or only on special occasions. Others drink three or four times a month and have two to four drinks at a time. "Moderate" drinkers usually drink a small amount (one drink or less) at least once a week or have a total of two to four drinks three or four times a month. Women with heavier patterns of alcohol consumption usually have a "drinking problem." Chronic alcohol abuse is usually manifested as one of the following patterns:

■ Daily intake of large amounts of alcohol.

■ Regular heavy drinking on weekends.

■ Periods of sobriety between binges of daily heavy drinking that may last for weeks or months.

There is no technical distinction between problem drinkers and alcoholics: Both are impaired by their drinking behavior. Alcohol is a problem when the individual is no longer able to control when and how much drinking takes place. Clinical diagnosis of alcoholism is based on the presence of at least three of the following symptoms, persisting for a month or more or occurring repeatedly over a longer period of time:

■ Alcohol taken in large amounts over a longer period than desired.

■ Persistent desire to quit drinking or one or more unsuccessful attempts to cut down or quit alcohol.

■ Spending considerable time obtaining, using, or recovering from alcohol.

- Continued drinking despite social, psychological, or physical symptoms such as ulcers caused or worsened by alcohol.

- Development of tolerance—needing at least 50 percent more alcohol than in the past to achieve intoxication.

- Withdrawal symptoms when alcohol intake is curbed.

- Drinking to avoid or relieve withdrawal symptoms.

The cause of alcoholism is not known. Metabolic, biochemical, cultural acceptability, stress, or dietary factors may be involved. Heredity plays a role that is not yet well defined. Alcoholism has been found to be four to five times more common among the children of alcoholics. Women alcoholics are less likely than men alcoholics to have had alcoholic parents or siblings. Support for a genetic factor of alcoholism has been found in studies that show a child, male or female, of an alcoholic, adopted at birth by nonalcoholic parents is at greater risk of developing alcoholism than is a child of a nonalcoholic placed in a similar home.[36,37] The role of environment is considered to be a factor in alcoholism as well. Children may perpetuate alcohol consumption patterns by role modeling the drinking patterns of their parents. Stress and traumatic experiences may influence drinking patterns. Some individuals start heavy drinking as a self-treatment for psychological problems such as dependence. Once addicted, they may not be able to stop their drinking behavioral patterns.

There are several psychological approaches to understanding alcoholism. Many psychiatrists believe that alcohol abuse is a symptom of a personality disorder and that the drinking of alcohol is the person's way of seeking relief from stress. Because alcohol distorts reality and helps one avoid discomfort or pain, the act of drinking reinforces drinking behavior, and the cycle of abuse begins. Some researchers have identified traits associated with alcoholism. These traits include a history of antisocial behavior, high levels of depression, and low self-esteem.[38] It is not clear whether these personality characteristics predispose one to alcoholism or whether they are the result of years of abuse. Other studies have found alcoholics to have certain expectations regarding alcohol, often seeing it as a "magic elixir" that can enhance sexual pleasure or performance, provide power and aggressiveness, and loosen up inhibitions to function more effectively at parties and social functions.

Alcoholism is seen as a progressive and fatal condition characterized by continuous or periodic impaired control over drinking, preoccupation with the drug alcohol, use of alcohol despite adverse consequences, and distortions in thinking, most notably denial. Most cases of alcoholism can be described in four stages, which usually evolve over a period of several years. In the prealcoholic phase, alcohol consumption is characterized by social drinking with an eventual evolvement into occasional drinking to escape tension and frustration. The early alcoholic phase follows, during which drinking itself becomes increasingly significant to the drinker. The very act of drinking becomes a pattern of behavior to the point where the drinker is uncomfortable in nondrinking situations and seeks out a drinking situation as a substitute. **Blackouts,** of either short or long duration, may occur during this phase, when the drinker will experience a loss of memory of what occurred while drinking. The loss of memory may be associated with intoxication or about the drinking events. The true alcoholic phase is characterized by alcohol dominance. Family relationships and friendships may deteriorate. A cycle of self-pity and increased drinking may occur. Unable to stop after one drink, the alcoholic believes that drinking is the most important activity. In complete alcoholic dependence, the drinker experiences complete physiological addiction to alcohol. Severe withdrawal symptoms occur if maintenance levels of alcohol are not consumed. The alcoholic in this stage is in danger of the severe alcohol medical complications.

Treatment Dimensions

The most difficult and significant step for an alcoholic is for that person to admit to an alcohol problem. Often the alcoholic is shielded from the truth by well-intended friends or family out of fear, embarrassment, loyalty, or hope. Unconsciously they may conspire to keep the alcoholic that way. Confrontation, either personal or via an accident or drunk driving conviction, that makes the individual acknowledge the alcohol problem is often a turning point in seeking assistance. Recovery from alcoholism is enhanced when the person has a strong emotional support system, including concerned family, friends, and employer.

Alcoholism is a complex problem, and each case must be treated with sensitivity to its unique situation and contributing factors. Standard treatment programs focus on the relief of physiological dependence but do not eliminate the underlying disease. Individual personality, psychological, and sociocultural factors must be addressed to help the alcoholic regain control of her life. There are more than 7,000 alcohol treatment programs in the United States. Three steps in the treatment of alcoholism are generally recognized:

- Management of acute intoxication episodes.
- Correcting chronic health problems associated with alcoholism.
- Changing long-term behavior.

The most successful treatment modalities combine different approaches and provide ongoing support for people learning to live without alcohol. Many alcohol treatment facilities assist clients in overcoming their physical addiction to alcohol and helping them through their withdrawal symptoms (Information Box 3.10) through detoxification programs. Most withdrawal symptoms generally disappear within 5 to 7 days. If heavy drinking has occurred for more than 10 years, withdrawal symptoms increase in severity, with delusions, hallucinations, and severely agitated behavior. These symptoms are known as **delirium tremens** (DTs). DTs are more likely to occur in drinkers suffering from malnutri-

INFORMATION BOX 3.10

Alcohol Withdrawal Symptoms

Irritability
Agitation
Depression
Lack of concentration
Body tremors
Nausea and vomiting
Generalized weakness, achiness
Sweating
Fever
Dry mouth
Elevated blood pressure
Headache
Anxiety
Puffy, blotchy skin
Fitful sleep with nightmares
Brief hallucinations

tion, fatigue, depression, or other physical illness. Detoxification programs are generally available in medical or psychiatric hospitals. Psychological addiction is usually addressed immediately after the detoxification process is completed.

The correction of chronic health problems associated with alcoholism requires the medical management of those conditions, such as cirrhosis and polyneuritis, that are complications of alcoholism. Changing the long-term behavior of alcoholics is actually more complex than treatment for the physiological or withdrawal phase or the management of associated chronic conditions. Behavior changes promoted include the encouragement of skill development in assertiveness training, stress management, problem solving, and relaxation. Several specific treatment modalities have evolved, and many programs provide combinations of specific treatment modalities.

1. *Intermediate care units* are generally located in hospitals or at separate treatment facilities. They usually provide 2 to 6 weeks of intensive treatment, which may include individual and group psychotherapy, family therapy, fitness, relaxation training, biofeedback, and spiritual counseling. Some units include Alcoholics Anonymous (AA) meetings in addition to formal instruction about alcoholism.

2. *Small group therapy* is another form of alcoholism treatment. Groups are generally conducted by a professional therapist with a focus on understanding members' alcohol behavior patterns.

3. *Alcoholics Anonymous* is a fellowship of recovering alcoholics and is the best known of alcohol treatment programs. Members help each other maintain sobriety. The underlying premise of AA is that members are powerless when it comes to alcohol. AA meetings are held daily throughout major cities and communities. A 12-step process provides the foundation for the philosophy and activities of the group. Al-Anon and Alateen are parallel organizations that provide support to persons who live with alcoholics. Al-Anon is primarily for spouses and other relatives, and Alateen has a focus for children of alcoholics. Chapter organizations are usually listed in telephone directories or in newspaper classified sections.

4. *Women for Sobriety* is a national self-help program based on the premise that female alcoholics have different and often more severe problems than male alcoholics. Most groups have about 10 members and meet regularly in one of the member's homes.

5. *Family therapy* provides a mechanism for dealing with an individual's alcohol problem as well as underlying family problems that may be contributing to the drinking behavior. Al-Anon is an example of a national self-help family therapy program. It helps an alcoholic's adult family members cope with the problem of alcoholism. Alateen is a similar self-help group, providing support for the teenage children of alcoholics.

6. *Aversion therapy* has been used in various forms for alcohol treatment since the turn of the century. Electric shock therapy is an example of aversion

therapy, but it has demonstrated little long-term effectiveness as an alcohol treatment modality. Emetic drugs, which result in nausea and vomiting when taken in combination with alcohol, have demonstrated limited success. Antabuse (disulfiram) specifically causes nausea when alcohol is consumed. If the person taking Antabuse does not drink, there are no problems. If alcohol is consumed at all while taking it, however, extreme nausea results. If a large amount of alcohol is consumed while taking Antabuse, it is possible to become dangerously ill.

7. *Antidepressive and antianxiety drugs* are sometimes prescribed early in alcohol recovery programs. Other drugs often prescribed include nutritional supplements to counter some of the nutritional deficiencies associated with alcoholism.

8. *Behavioral therapy* programs attempt to reverse the reinforcement pattern of drinking so abstinence or moderate drinking brings rewards or avoids punishment. Techniques used in behavioral therapy include aversion therapies, assertiveness training, development of coping skills, relaxation techniques, biofeedback, blood alcohol discrimination training, and controlled drinking. Analysis of drinking behavior focuses on cues and stimuli, attitudes and thoughts, specific drinking behavior, and consequences of drinking. Because these variables are complex and highly individualized, they require careful assessment and specifically tailored interventions.

9. *Controlled drinking* has been proposed as a treatment modality in lieu of total abstinence. Some researchers have proposed that it is a more reasonable approach because relapse rates are so high with traditional treatment programs that focus on total alcohol abstinence. Studies on controlled drinking programs have produced inconsistent findings. One major study found that women with less severe alcohol problems were able to keep their drinking at a moderate level.

Long-term success rates with alcohol treatment programs are not impressive. Most programs report a 80 percent success rate after 1 year, but studies indicate about a 25 percent long-term (permanent) success rate.

Special Alcohol Treatment Issues for Women

As discussed earlier, social stigma discourages women from seeking the help they need to overcome alcohol problems. Women alcoholics who enter treatment programs have special needs. Treatment programs for women must be culturally sensitive and incorporate issues such as age, socioeconomic status, drug use, and sexual orientation into their format. Strategies that have been proposed for assisting women in addressing their alcohol problems include use of culturally appropriate, nonstigmatized language; development of supportive case management; implementation of a mentoring or buddy system; expansion of child-care services; and creation of a multimedia campaign that educates women.

Treatment programs for female alcoholics must also take into account the age of onset of alcoholism, generational experience, early life history, and current age of patients to be fully effective.[39]

Informed Decision Making for Women

Alcohol consumption is a personal responsibility issue. Personal responsibilities include being able to ascertain and acknowledge that an alcohol problem may be present (Self-Assessment 3.1). Many women are unwilling to acknowledge that they have a problem with alcohol (Information Box 3.11). Recognizing the warning signs of alcoholism and seeking early treatment intervention are important (see Information Box 3.9). Women who do acknowledge a problem with drinking often find it difficult to learn how to drink alcohol moderately. Several suggestions provide a framework for decision making and skills development for moderate drinking behavior. First and foremost, it is important to set a limit and stick to it. A limit of one or two drinks a day may be a reasonable amount. The development of alternatives to drinking is a critical task to avoid turning to alcohol when upset or depressed. Alcohol neither "fixes" the problem nor provides an "escape." During or after drinking, it is best to avoid performing tasks, particularly driving, that require skilled reactions. Drinking should not be the focus of any activity. When drinking becomes the primary focus, there is a significant risk for serious long-term alcohol problems. Communication skills are an important component of moderate drinking. Learning to say, "no, thank you, I have had enough to drink" is an important step in exercising personal power and control over drinking behavior. Alcohol should facilitate

---

INFORMATION BOX 3.11

Reasons Women Drink

Relaxation
Alcohol slows body activities and women do feel less tense after a drink.

Celebration
Alcohol is a traditional component of family celebrations and important events.

Romance
Alcohol lowers inhibitions and produces a relaxing effect. Yet, ironically, alcohol can interfere with sexual response.

Social activity
Alcohol is often a reason for social events, "getting together for a drink" or an "enhancer" of social events. Women often feel sexier, wittier, and more confident with drinking.

Advertising
The advertising media portray alcohol as the essential ingredient for sex or a good time.

National Council on Alcoholism Self Test: Do You Have a Drinking Problem?

1. Do you occasionally drink heavily after a disappointment or a quarrel, or when your parents give you a hard time? yes _____ no _____

2. When you have trouble or feel pressured at school, do you always drink more heavily than usual? yes _____ no _____

3. Have you noticed that you are able to handle more liquor than you did when you were first drinking? yes _____ no _____

4. Did you ever wake up on "the morning after" and discover that you could not remember the evening before, even though your friends tell you that you did not pass out? yes _____ no _____

5. When drinking with other people, do you try to have a few extra drinks that others don't notice? yes _____ no _____

6. Are there certain occasions when you feel uncomfortable if alcohol is not available? yes _____ no _____

7. Have you recently noticed that when you begin drinking you are in more of a hurry to get the first drink than you used to be? yes _____ no _____

8. Do you sometimes feel a little guilty about your drinking? yes _____ no _____

9. Are you secretly irritated when your family or friends discuss your drinking? yes _____ no _____

10. Have you recently noticed an increase in the frequency of your memory blackouts? yes _____ no _____

11. Do you often find that you wish to continue drinking after your friends say that they have had enough? yes _____ no _____

12. Do you usually have a reason for the occasions that you drink heavily? yes _____ no _____

13. When you are sober, do you often regret things you did or said while drinking? yes _____ no _____

14. Have you tried switching brands or following different plans for controlling your drinking? yes _____ no _____

15. Have you often failed to keep the promises you've made to yourself about controlling or cutting down on your drinking? yes _____ no _____

16. Have you ever tried to control your drinking by changing jobs or moving to a new location? yes _____ no _____

17. Do you try to avoid family or close friends while you are drinking? yes _____ no _____

18. Are you having an increasing number of financial and academic problems? yes _____ no _____

19. Do more people seem to be treating you unfairly without good reason? yes _____ no _____

20. Do you eat very little or irregularly when you are drinking? yes _____ no _____

21. Do you sometimes have the shakes in the morning and find that it helps to have a little drink? yes _____ no _____

22. Have you recently noticed that you cannot drink as much as you once did? yes _____ no _____

23. Do you sometimes stay drunk for several days at a time? yes _____ no _____

24. Do you sometimes feel very depressed and wonder whether life is worth living? yes _____ no _____

25. Sometimes after periods of drinking, do you see or hear things that aren't there? yes _____ no _____

26. Do you get terribly frightened after you have been drinking heavily? yes _____ no _____

Those who answer yes to two or three of these questions may wish to evaluate their drinking in these areas. "Yes" answers to several of these questions indicate the following stages of alcoholism:

Question 1–8: *Early Stage:* Drinking is a regular part of your life.

Questions 9–21: *Middle Stage:* You are having trouble controlling when, where, and how much you drink.

Questions 22–26: *Beginning of the Final Stage:* You no longer can control your desire to drink.

the social event, not be the social event. When drinking, a woman should savor the company, the experience, the food, and so forth, not just the drink. Pacing alcohol is important as well. Bingeing Friday night on a week's worth of alcohol is not the same as moderate paced drinking throughout the week. Alcoholic beverages are not good or wise thirst quenchers. A glass of water, tea, or soft drink can effectively quench a thirst before having an alcoholic beverage. Food should be consumed before drinking, so it is a good idea to eat something before going to a party or meeting someone for a drink. Solo drinking is not a good idea. Although it may seem relaxing, other means, such as exercise, meditation, music, or TV, provide generalized relaxation without the risk of dependency.

Helping others to drink in moderation is also a personal responsibility issue. When entertaining and serving alcoholic beverages, it is perhaps wiser to avoid having an open bar and to offer nonalcoholic beverages as well. Serving diluted drinks may help limit alcohol consumption. It is not wise to push drinks or to refill empty glasses quickly. Measuring drinks and knowing how much alcohol is being served can be a reminder the limit is near or has been reached. Food helps to slow the absorption of alcohol and should be encouraged first, particularly if guests have not eaten for a while. Perhaps the single most important responsibility is never to serve alcohol to a guest who seems intoxicated and never permit an intoxicated person to operate a vehicle. Assuming responsibility includes making contingency plans for intoxication. If it occurs despite efforts to prevent it; assume responsibility for the health and safety of guests by providing transportation home or overnight accommodations. The early identification of designated drivers helps ensure safe transportation for partygoers.

Knowing what to do when someone else is drunk is another dimension of personal responsibility. It is important to keep the person still and comfortable. Do not attempt to walk, run, or exercise the drunk person, and do not try to keep the person awake. Any abrupt or unnecessary movement may cause the person to fall or faint with resulting injury. Do not permit the person to drive or operate any machinery. Stay with the person if he or she is vomiting. If the person is lying down, turn the head to the side and protect the person from swallowing the vomit. Monitor the breathing status. If there are any signs of unconsciousness or respiratory problems, seek immediate medical attention. Keep calm; speak in a clear, firm, and reassuring manner; and do not transfer any anxiety to the person who is drunk. Explain any movement or approach to the person. A person who is drunk may be unpredictable and violent. Do not attempt to administer any food, drinks, or drugs or give the person a cold shower. The only thing that sobers a drunk person is time.

Summary

Alcohol use is prevalent throughout life today as the most widely used drug in the United States. Every woman must decide for herself whether she is going

INFORMATION BOX 3.12

Alcohol Wisdom

Alcohol does not fix problems. Using alcohol to escape problems creates bigger problems.

Alcohol's effects may be compounded when taken with any other drug, including prescribed or over-the-counter medications. It is particularly dangerous to combine alcohol with other depressant drugs.

Monthly cycle variances may compound the effects of

alcohol. Many women are especially vulnerable just before menstruation.

Alcohol impairs psychomotor control. Drinking and driving (or operating any vehicle) should be avoided.

Food consumed before and during alcohol consumption may help to slow the effects of alcohol.

to use alcohol and if she is going to use it, how she will use it, not abuse it. Understanding oneself, being "alcohol-wise" (Information Box 3.12), and knowing the consequences of drinking alcohol are the first steps in controlling the situation. Alcohol wisdom and assuming personal responsibility for oneself are the foundation skills to manage alcohol consumption effectively.

CURRENT EVENTS

Moderate Drinking—Benefits and Risks

Enoch Gordis, M.D.
Director, National Institute on Alcohol Abuse and Alcoholism
Alcohol Alert 16(PH315) April 1992

Moderate drinking levels are defined as up to two drinks a day for men and one drink a day for women. Recent studies suggest that there are both benefits and risks associated with moderate consumption of alcohol. Additional research is needed to clarify the many questions posed by this confusing situation. In light of the confusion, current guidance from the National Institute on Alcohol Abuse and Alcoholism is:

"Current advice to individuals should acknowledge that there are tradeoffs involved in each decision about drinking: reducing risk of developing coronary artery disease, for example, may be offset by risk of developing another alcohol-related health condition. In general, if an individual is drinking "moderately" and does not fit into one of the special risk categories (women who are pregnant or trying to conceive; people who plan to drive or engage in other activities that require attention or skill; people taking medications, including over-the-counter medications; recovering alcoholics; and persons under the age of 21), there is no reason to do anything different. Similarly, individuals who are not yet drinking (young adults who have recently turned 21, for example), and are not at special risk, can be told that "moderately drinking" will probably not be harmful. (Abstinent individuals, however, should not be advised to begin to drink two drinks a day solely to protect against coronary heart disease.) Finally those who are at higher risk (because of a family history of alcoholism, for example) must be made aware of the tradeoffs involved in decisions to drink."

Philosophical Dimensions: Women and Alcohol

1. Who is responsible when a drunk driver has a motor vehicle accident and someone is killed?

2. Should pregnant women be permitted to drink alcohol?

3. Is it a sign of personal weakness or strength for a person to admit that she has a problem with alcohol?

4. What measures indicate that a person is drinking reasonably?

5. What specific actions can a host(ess) do to serve alcohol responsibly?

6. How do societal expectations about alcohol differ for women and men?

7. What should a friend do/say when a friend consumes at least two or three beers every day but insists that daily drinking in moderation is not a problem?

References

1. Brooks, S., Williams, G., Stinson, F., and Noble, J. (1989). *Surveillance Report #13: Apparent per capita alcohol consumption, national, state, and regional trends, 1977–1987.* Washington, DC: US Department of Health and Human Services.

2. Hesselbrock, M.N. (1981). Women alcoholics: a comparison of the natural history of alcoholism between men and women. In National Institute on Alcohol Abuse and Alcoholism, *Evaluation of the alcoholic: Implications for research, theory, and practice.* (Research Monograph #5; DHHS Pub. No. ADM 81-1033.) Washington, DC: US Government Printing Office.

3. Schoenborn, C.A., and Cohen, B.H. (1986). Trends in smoking, alcohol consumption, and other health practices among U.S. adults, 1977 and 1983. *Advance Data, 118,* 1–13.

4. National Institute on Drug Abuse (1989). *National Household Survey on Drug Abuse: Population Estimates, 1988.* (DHHS Pub. No. ADM 89-1636.) Washington, DC: US Government Printing Office.

5. Bradstock, K., Forman, M., Binkin, N., Gentry, E., Hogelin, G., Williamson, D., and Trowbridge, F. (1988). Alcohol use and health behavior lifestyles among U.S. women: the behavioral risk factor surveys. *Addictive Behaviors, 13*(1), 61–71.

6. Herd, D. (1989). Drinking by black and white women: results from a national survey. *Social Problems, 35* (5), 493–505.

7. Thorton, C.I., and Carter, J.H. (1988). Treating the black female alcoholic: clinical observations of black therapists. *Journal of the National Medical Association, 80*(6), 644–647.

8. Caetano, R. (1989). Drinking patterns and alcoholic problems in a national sample of U.S. Hispanics. In *The Epidemiology of Alcohol Use and Abuse Among U.S. Minorities* (pp. 147–162). (NIAAA Monograph No. 18. DHHS Pub. No. ADM 89-1435.) Washington, DC: US Government Printing Office.

9. Sue, D. (1987). Use and abuse of alcohol by Asian Americans. *Journal of Psychoactive Drugs, 19*(1), 57–66.

10. Rhoades, E.R., Hammond, J., Welty, T.K., Handler, A.O., and Amler, R.W. (1987). The Indian burden of illness and future health interventions. *Public Health Reports, 102* (4), 361–368.

11. Reed, B.G. (1987). Developing women-sensitive drug dependence treatment services. Why so difficult? *Journal of Psychoactive Drugs, 19*(2), 151–164.

12. Sandmaier, M. (1980). *The Invisible Alcoholics.* New York: McGraw-Hill.

13. O'Halleran, G.K. (1989). Alcoholism, chemical dependency and the lesbian client. *Women and Therapy, 8*(1/2), 131–144.

14. Nicoloff, L.K., and Stiglitz, B.A. (1987). Lesbian alcoholism: etiology, treatment and recovery. In Boston Lesbian Psychologies Collective (Eds.), *Lesbian psychologies. Explorations and challenges* (pp. 283–293). Chicago: University of Illinois Press.

15. Shore, E.R., McCoy, M.L., Toonen, L.A., and Kuntz, E.J. (1988). Arrests of women for driving under the influence. *Journal of Studies on Alcohol, 49*(1), 7–10.

16. Johnson, N.P., Robbins, K.H., Hornung, C.A., et al. (1990). Characteristics of women alcoholics. *Substance Abuse, 11*(1), 23–29.

17. Vanicelli, M. (1985). Treatment outcome of alcoholic women: the state of the art in relation to sex bias and expectancy effects. In S.C. Wilsnack and L.J. Beckman (Eds.), *Alcohol problems in women: antecedents, consequences, and interventions* (pp. 369–412). New York: Guilford Press.

18. Vanicelli, M., and Nash, L. (1984). Effects of sex bias on women's studies on alcoholism. *Alcoholism: Clinical and Experimental Research, 8,* 334–336.

19. USDHHS (1984). *Fifth special report to the U.S. Congress on Alcohol and Health.* (DHEW Pub. No. ADM 84-1291.) Washington, DC: US Government Printing Office.

20. Schuckit, M.A., and Morrissey, E.T. (1979). Drug abuse among alcoholic women. *American Journal of Psychiatry, 136*(4B), 607–610.

21. Russell, M., and Coviello, D. (1988). Heavy drinking and regular psychoactive drug use among gynecological outpatients. *Alcoholism: Clinical and Experimental Research, 12*(3), 400–406.

22. Lindberg, S., and Agren, G. (1988). Mortality among male and female hospitalized alcoholics in Stockholm 1962–1983. *British Journal of the Addictions, 83,* 1193–1200.

23. Smith, E.M., Cloninger, R., and Bradford, S. (1983). Predictors of mortality in alcoholic women: a prospective follow-up study. *Alcoholism: Clinical and Experimental Research, 7*(2), 237–243.

24. VanThiel, D., and Gavaler, J. (1988). Ethanol metabolism and hepatotoxicity.

Does sex make a difference? In M. Galanter (Ed.), *Recent developments in alcoholism* (pp. 291–304). New York: Plenum Press.

25. Hasin, D., Grant, B., and Weinflash, J. (1988). Male/female differences in alcohol-related problems: alcohol rehabilitation patients. *The International Journal of the Addictions, 23*(5), 437–448.

26. Dunne, F. (1988). Are women more easily damaged by alcohol than men? [letter to the editor]. *British Journal of the Addictions, 83*(10), 1135–1136.

27. Hill, S.Y. (1980). Biological consequences of alcohol use in women. In *Alcoholism and Alcohol Abuse among Women: Research Issues.* (Research Monograph No. 1 of the National Institute on Alcohol Abuse and Alcoholism, USDHHS.) Washington, DC: US Government Printing Office.

28. Tuyns, A.J., and Pequignot, G. (1984). Greater risk of ascitic cirrhosis in females in relation to alcohol consumption. *International Journal of Epidemiology, 13*(1), 53–57.

29. Frezza, M., DiPadova, C., Pozzato, G., et al. (1990). High blood alcohol levels in women. *New England Journal of Medicine, 322*(2), 95–99.

30. Jones, B.M., and Jones, M.K. (1984). Ethanol metabolism in women taking oral contraceptives. *Alcoholism: Clinical and Experimental Research, 8*(1), 24–28.

31. Zeiner, A.R., and Kegg, P.S. (1981). Menstrual cycle and oral contraceptive effects on alcohol pharmakinetics in Caucasian females. *Currents in Alcoholism, 8,* 47–56.

32. USDHHS (1991). *Healthy people 2000: National health promotion and disease prevention objectives.* (DHHS Pub. No. (PHS) 91-50212.) Washington, DC: US Department of Health and Human Services.

33. Van Thiel, D. (1983). Effects of ethanol upon organ systems other than the central nervous system. In B. Tabakoff, P.B. Sutker, and C.L. Randall (Eds.), *Medical and social aspects of alcohol abuse.* New York: Plenum Press.

34. USDHHS. (1990). *Seventh Special Report to the U.S. Congress on Alcohol and Health.* Washington, DC: National Institute on Alcohol Abuse and Alcoholism.

35. Sokol, R.J., Miller, S.I., and Reed, G. (1980). Alcohol abuse during pregnancy: an epidemiologic study. *Alcoholism: Clinical and Experimental Research, 447,* 87–102.

36. Ward, D.A. (1990). *Alcoholism, Introduction to Theory and Development.* Dubuque, IA: Kendall Hunt Publishing Co.

37. Bohman, M., Sigvardsson, S., and Cloninger, C.R. (1981). Maternal inheritance of alcohol abuse. *Archives of General Psychiatry, 38,* 965–969.

38. Marlatt, G.A., Baer, J.S., Donovan, D.M., and Kivlahan, D.R. (1988). Addictive behaviors: etiology and treatment. *Annual Review of Psychology, 39,* 223–252.

39. Gomberg, E.S.L. (1989). Alcoholic women in treatment. Early histories and early problem behaviors. *Advances in Alcohol and Substance Abuse, 8*(2), 133–147.

Resources

SUBSTANCE ABUSE AND MENTAL HEALTH SERVICES ADMINISTRATION (SAMHSA)

5600 Fishers Lane
Rockville, MD 20857
301-443-2403
  Substance Abuse
  Prevention
301-443-0365

ALCOHOLICS ANONYMOUS

This is perhaps the best-known self-help alcohol treatment program, with more than 50,000 groups across the United States. Local meetings are held in communities throughout the United States. Participants may remain anonymous— only first names are used. *Al-Anon* and *Alateen* are support groups that help families and friends of problem drinkers. Meeting times and groups are announced in newspapers, church bulletins, and community flyers. See white pages of telephone directory or write/call:

ALCOHOLICS ANONYMOUS

PO Box 459
Grand Central Station
New York, NY
212-686-1100

AL-ANON AND ALATEEN

PO Box 862
Midtown Station
New York, NY, 10018
212-302-7240
800-356-9996

ALCOHOL HOTLINE

1-800-ALCOHOL

BACCHUS (BOOST ALCOHOL CONSCIOUSNESS CONCERNING THE HEALTH OF UNIVERSITY STUDENTS)

This college-based organization promotes responsible drinking among university students who choose to drink. They support responsible party hosting and employ creative educational approaches to promote alcohol awareness.

CHILDREN OF ALCOHOLICS FOUNDATION

200 Park Avenue
31st Floor
New York, NY 10166
212-351-2680

COMMUNITY ALCOHOL AND DRUG TREATMENT PROGRAMS

Most community hospitals and drug treatment programs sponsor outpatient alcohol treatment programs and support groups. Information is available in the yellow pages of telephone directories under "Alcoholism" and "Drug abuse/treatment."

MOTHERS AGAINST DRUNK DRIVERS (MADD)

An organization founded by a mother of a traffic victim killed by a drunk driver, MADD has a national network of more than 200 local chapters. MADD attempts to provide education about alcohol's effects on driving and to influence legislation and enforcement of laws related to drunk drivers.

MADD

669 Airport Freeway
Suite 300
Hurst, TX 76053
817-268-6233
800-438-6733

NATIONAL ASSOCIATION FOR CHILDREN OF ALCOHOLICS (NACoA)

31706 Coast Highway
Suite 201
South Laguna, CA 92677
714-499-3889

NATIONAL CLEARINGHOUSE FOR ALCOHOL INFORMATION

PO Box 2345
Rockville, MD 20852
301-468-2600
800-729-6686

NATIONAL COUNCIL ON ALCOHOLISM

Provides leadership in public education, advocacy of enlarged government involvement in alcohol prevention and treatment, and consultation services, particularly to industry.

12 West 21st St
New York, NY 10010
212-206-6770
800-622-2255 (hotline)

NATIONAL INSTITUTE ON ALCOHOL ABUSE AND ALCOHOLISM (NIAAA)

Provides policy guidance for federal action on alcohol-related problems and channels funds for research, training, prevention, and development of community-based services for the

treatment of alcoholics, a national information and education program, and other special projects.

5600 Fishers Lane
Rockville, MD 20857
301-443-3860

REMOVE INTOXICATED DRIVERS (RID)

PO Box 520
Schenectady, NY 12301
518-372-0034

STUDENTS AGAINST DRIVING DRUNK

An organization composed mostly of high school students whose goal is to reduce drinking deaths among teens. Students help to educate other students about the consequences of combining drinking and driving. They promote the SADD Lifetime Contract between students and their parents to provide trans-portation for each other if either is unable to drive safely after consuming alcohol.

SADD

PO Box 800
Marlboro, MA 01752

WOMEN FOR SOBRIETY, INC.

Support group for women with drinking problems. About 450 self-help groups located across the United States.

PO Box 618
Quakertown, PA 18951
215-536-8026

CHAPTER

4

Drug Use

CHAPTER OBJECTIVES

On completion of this chapter, students should be able to discuss:

1. Drug use in the United States from a historical perspective.

2. Drug use in women from an epidemiological perspective.

3. How women are especially vulnerable to problems with medically prescribed psychotherapeutic drugs.

4. How society's double standard for women prevails in drug use.

5. How the concept of co-dependency may have a negative spin for women.

6. Societal costs of drug use in the United States.

7. The differences between physiological and psychological drug dependence.

8. The mechanisms for drug entry into the body.

9. How legal drugs can be misused or abused.

10. The risks and effects of stimulant drug use.

11. The risks and effects of depressant drug use.

12. The risks and effects of antianxiety drug use.

13. The risks and effects of marijuana use.

14. The risks and effects of psychedelic and hallucinogenic drug use.

15. The risks and effects of narcotic drug use.

16. The risks and effects of inhalant drug use.

17. The risks and effects of designer drug use.

18. What is known and not known about drug use by women.

19. How sex has evolved as a currency in the drug epidemic.

20. How prescription drugs present special problems to women.

21. How drug overuse and misuse are particular problems among older women.

Introduction

Drug use has become pervasive throughout American life. Drugs are consumed for legitimate health reasons, such as fighting off infections and pain relief. Drugs taken for "fun" or pleasure are known as recreational drugs. Most people associate recreational drugs with illegal substances, but legal substances such as alcohol, tobacco, and caffeine as well as many legal prescription drugs (amphetamines and tranquilizers) are also considered to be recreational drugs. All drugs, whether legal or illegal, prescribed or purchased over-the-counter (OTC), are complex compounds that alter body activities. Drug users are affected physically, psychologically, mentally, financially, and socially. Society is affected with an

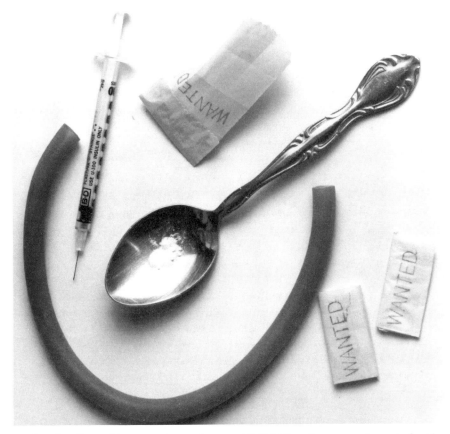

Society is affected by an estimated annual $44 billion in economic costs for the drug problem today.

estimated $44 billion in economic costs annually attributed to drug problems. Women are uniquely affected throughout the spectrum of drug issues. An understanding of drugs, medications, dependency, and treatment issues within a biological-social-cultural context provides a foundation for understanding how drugs impact the quality of women's health.

Drug Trends and Issues

Drug use is pervasive throughout contemporary American society. The use includes compounds taken for legitimate medical reasons and those taken for a desired psychological effect. Women are especially vulnerable to the consequences of drug use. A review of drug trends and issues reveals a complex multidimensional issue with devastating implications for women's health.

Historical Overview

Drugs are generally defined in terms of their legal or illegal status. It is interesting to note that the legal status of drugs changes with time, customs, and beliefs. In the 1920s and 1930s, alcohol was illegal and marijuana was legal. The reverse is true today. In the early 1900s, opium, morphine, and cocaine were openly advertised and sold as "remedies" in the form of tonics, syrups, and elixirs. Coca-Cola was originally sold as both a remedy and refreshing beverage, containing cocaine until 1906, when the cocaine was replaced by caffeine. The use of drugs by women has correspondingly changed over time. It has been proposed that changes in the patterns and intensity of drug use among women have been related to major transitions in their lives and how they are perceived by society.[1]

Epidemiological Data and Trends*

Women use all types of illicit drugs, but across age groups, the prevalence of illicit drug use by women is less than illicit drug use by men (Fig. 4.1). The 1985 National Household Survey on Drug Abuse conducted by the National Institute on Drug Abuse (NIDA) found that approximately 15 percent of

*AUTHORS' NOTE: Despite the growing concern about drug addiction in the United States, relatively little is known about the cause and development of these problems in women. Much of the existing information has been extrapolated from research on men, and most theoretical perspectives have been developed by male researchers studying men. Many estimates of drug dependency are based, at least in part, on numbers of persons in treatment, but because many women never receive treatment, estimates may be low. Until recently, most studies of women and drug dependence have focused on the impact of a woman's chemical dependency on children, spouse, and family life. With the few studies available on women, findings are frequently limited and inconsistent because of methodological flaws, including problems in conceptualization of variables, definitions of terms, research design, instrumentation, sampling, and data analysis techniques.

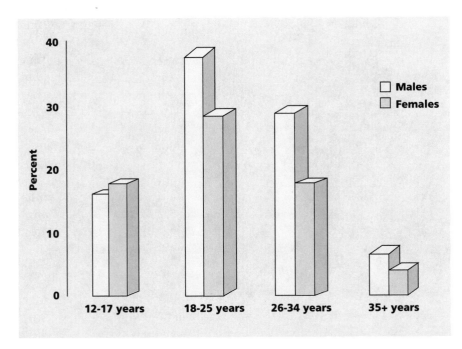

FIGURE 4.1

Comparison of male/female lifetime illicit drug use.

SOURCE: NIDA (1989). *National Household Survey on Drug Abuse: 1988 Population Estimates.* (DHHS Publication No. (ADM) 89-1636.) Washington, DC: US Government Printing Office.

American women between the ages of 15 and 44 years were substance abusers.[2] More recent data (1991) are similar, indicating that 13.4 percent of 18 to 25-year-old women have used any illicit drug in the past year (Information Box 4.1). Cocaine use by women appears to be underestimated, however, according to the increase in calls by women to the national cocaine hotline, where women represented one-third of all calls in 1983 and one-half of all calls in 1985.[3]

INFORMATION BOX 4.1

Illicit Drug Use by Women, 1991

Age (years)	Use (%)		
	Ever Used	**Past Year**	**Past Month**
12–17	18.9	13.7	6.6
18–25	52.8	27.0	13.4
26–34	57.0	14.7	6.6
35 +	23.8	5.7	2.3
Total	33.5	11.1	5.0

SOURCE: Adapted from National Institute on Drug Abuse (1992). *National household survey on drug abuse; population estimates.* (DHHS Pub No (ADM) 92-1887.) Washington, DC: Alcohol, Drug Abuse and Mental Health Administration. p. 19.

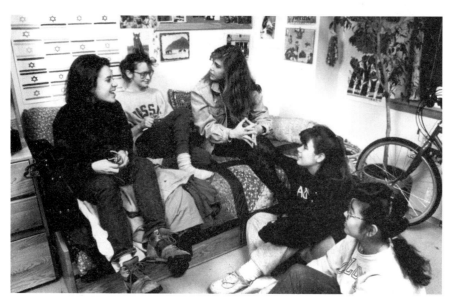

There is no particular stereotype of a drug-dependent woman.

It is difficult and often not practical to make generalizations about drug use among racial/ethnic classifications, which represent considerable diversity along lines of subgroups, socioeconomic strata, and age levels. Drug use patterns have been shown to be different within varying demographic, economic, and psychosocial circumstances.[4] Nevertheless, generalizations do provide a frame of reference and some insight into drug use patterns. National data on racial/ethnic distributions of drug use show some similarities and some differences. A data analysis on the National Longitudinal Survey of Youth (NLSY) examined the relationship between early adolescent (14 to 15 years) conduct disorder and late adolescent (18 to 19 years) alcohol and drug use. The study found that delinquency in early adolescence is a predictor of substance use in late adolescence. The study also found that white female adolescents were more involved in delinquent activity and alcohol and illicit drug use than African American female adolescents.[5] Lifetime rates of cocaine and marijuana use by women show higher use by white females than either African American or Hispanic American females[2] (Figs. 4.2 and 4.3).

The major exception to the generalization that drug use by males exceeds that of females is in regard to the use of medically prescribed psychotherapeutic drugs, such as sedatives, tranquilizers, stimulants, and analgesics. The fact that they are prescribed does not necessarily mean that these medications are used in a therapeutic sense, that is, in a manner consistent with prescribed instructions. Information Box 4.2 shows the percent of male and female lifetime users of psychotherapeutic drugs by type of use and age. Among youths aged 12 to 17 years, females have higher rates of nonmedical use of sedatives, stimulants, and analgesics. These findings generate many questions about why women disproportionately and inappropriately use these medications from such a young

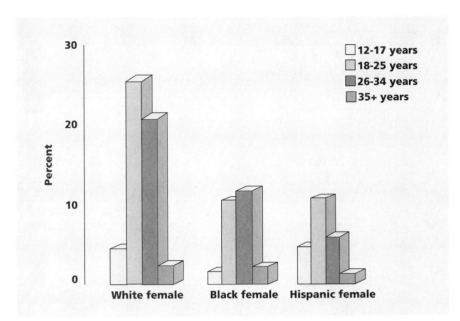

FIGURE 4.2

Lifetime use of cocaine by females and race/ethnicity, 1985.

SOURCE: NIDA (1988). *National Household Survey on Drug Abuse, 1985.* (DHHS Publication No. (ADM) 88-1586.) Washington, DC: US Government Printing Office.

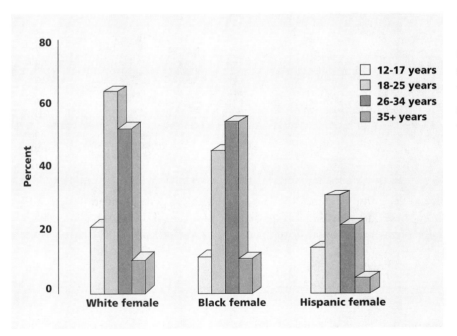

FIGURE 4.3

Lifetime use of marijuana by females and race/ethnicity, 1985.

SOURCE: NIDA (1988). *National Household Survey on Drug Abuse, 1985.* (DHHS Publication No. (ADM) 88-1586. Washington, DC: US Government Printing Office.

age. Unfortunately, the data currently available do not provide the answers to these complex, multifaceted questions.

Determining the extent to which drug use contributes to illness (morbidity) and death (mortality) among women is another difficult task. Drug use information is not always requested or volunteered when women are ill. The Drug Abuse Warning Network (DAWN) is a surveillance system designed to monitor drug-related visits to hospital emergency rooms in several major metropolitan

---

INFORMATION BOX 4.2

Percent of Lifetime Users of Psychotherapeutic Drugs by Type of Use, Age, and Sex

| Drug Class and Type of Use | Percent Use by Age | | | | | | | |
| | 12–17 Years | | 18–25 Years | | 26–34 Years | | 35+ Years | |
	Male	Female	Male	Female	Male	Female	Male	Female
Sedatives								
Nonmedical	48	54	72	55	52	28	17	0.3
Prescribed	41	42	8	31	28	57	75	99
Both	10	4	20	14	20	15	8	1
Tranquilizers								
Nonmedical	39	24	46	29	23	6	5	0.4
Prescribed	52	71	36	58	57	86	91	99
Both	9	5	18	13	20	7	4	0.5
Stimulants								
Nonmedical	55	79	92	67	81	23	39	4
Prescribed	29	17	7	21	9	57	53	92
Both	16	4	1	12	10	20	8	4
Analgesics								
Nonmedical	8	13	10	3	4	1	2	0
Prescribed	81	83	69	85	81	93	94	99
Both	12	4	20	12	15	6	4	1

SOURCE: National Institute on Drug Abuse (1986). *Research Monograph No. 65.* Washington, DC: US Government Printing Office. p. 87.

---

areas of the United States. It is not possible to calculate population percentages from these data, but the data do demonstrate a steady rise annually in absolute numbers of women with drug-related emergencies from 1985 (Fig. 4.4).

Sociocultural Dimensions of Women and Drug Use

Despite the growing concern about drugs and drug addiction in the United States, relatively little is known about the cause and development of these problems in women. Of the studies that do exist, most have focused on the impact of women's addiction on children, spouse, and family life. Particular emphasis has been given to the health problems of the fetus and infant born to a mother who uses drugs. There is a need for specific research attention to the diversity of women. An area that is receiving recent AIDS research interest but that has not generated much data to date is intravenous drug use among women. Female intravenous drug users (IVDUs) are a poorly understood, little studied group. Sexual preference data with drug use are also nonexistent.

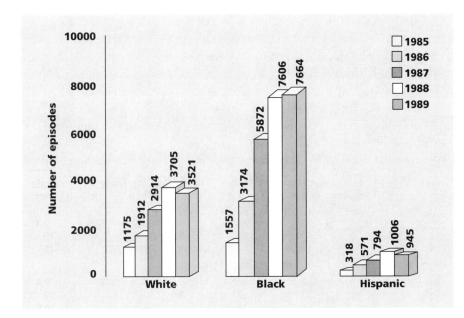

FIGURE 4.4

Cocaine-related emergency room episodes, females in selected metropolitan areas, 1985–89.

SOURCE: USDHHS (1991). *Health United States, 1990.* (DHHS Pub. No. (PHS), 91-1232.) Washington, DC: US Government Printing Office, p. 127.

Although the number of HIV-infected lesbian IVDUs may be relatively small, lesbians are a significant subpopulation of IVDUs in some cities and may represent a group that is not likely to be reached with prevention efforts that target either gay men or the heterosexual community.[6] Older women also present unique drug issues. Research indicates that the rate of heavy drinking among women generally declines after age 50, but polypharmacy, the dual use of alcohol and prescription drugs, continues to be a significant problem.

Society's double standard for women prevails in drug use. Harsher stigma has always been placed on the addicted woman than on the addicted man. In a comparison of attitudes of the 1920s and attitudes of the present, society's view of female cocaine users was and is that of a social deviant.[3] The greater social sanctions against addiction in women make them less willing to seek help and others less willing to recognize and intervene to provide help. Studies indicate that significant life stresses, such as divorce, loneliness, and dissatisfaction with a career, may exacerbate tendencies to abuse alcohol and other substances.[7] High prevalences of sexual abuse and physical abuse have been found in drug-dependent women.[8] Additional issues, such as low self-esteem, self-depreciation, anxiety, and conflict, have also been identified as precursors that often lead to and sustain drug abuse among women.

The relationship between alcohol use, drug use, and age may be different for women than it is for men. Although studies have shown that women who regularly use drugs also tend to drink more heavily than women who report no regular drug use, it also has been noted that older women are more likely to use psychoactive drugs, whereas younger women are more likely to drink heavily. This finding held true despite the relatively consistent use of alcohol and drugs in various age groups.[9]

Co-dependency (Information Box 4.3), the sense of being "other-focused," often occurs with women who feel responsible or who facilitate the drug use of someone else. A potential gender bias may be present with the concept of co-dependency. Co-dependency is often assumed to exist in the significant other, spouse, and immediate family members of an addicted person. Although this process may have some therapeutic value in that it may help individuals deal with another's drug dependency, it creates problems from a research and gender-bias perspective. Little research has been conducted on the process of developing behaviors or mechanisms to cope with a loved one who is alcoholic or addicted. There is little understanding of the behaviors, attitudes, or psychological states of co-dependents. This process may have a negative spin for women because most of those identified as addicted are men, and because men are represented disproportionately in treatment programs, the enabling and co-dependency concepts are most frequently associated with female significant others of alcoholic and drug-dependent men.

Cultural dimensions influence drug use and treatment issues for women. For example, studies indicate that Puerto Rican women experience a significant use of alcohol and noninjected drugs. This is compounded by a risk for HIV infection because of multiple sexual partners, frequent change of sexual partners, low rates of condom use, and relationships with IVDUs. Cultural norms, however, dictate that these women must bear the burden of raising children and keeping the family together, even at the cost of their own well-being.[10] Given these conditions and responsibilities, the likelihood that these women

---

INFORMATION BOX 4.3

Co-Dependency

A person (friend, spouse, partner, parent) may, without meaning to, allow or enable the addict to remain dependent on drugs through enabling behaviors, which may include:

Rescuing:	Overprotective behavior that permits the addict to use drugs at home to avoid being discovered or at risk elsewhere.
Rationalizing:	Acceptance and explanation of the addict's behavior; making excuses for the behavior.
Shielding:	Covering up for addicts, running interference for them at work, school, and for obligations
Controlling:	Personally attempt to control addict's use of drugs with bribes or rewards (money, favors, sex)
Covering:	Taking over chores, job responsibilities, paying bills or giving/loaning addict money to buy drugs
Cooperating:	Becoming involved in buying, selling, testing, preparing, or using the drug

would seek traditional drug rehabilitation treatment or be able to remain in a traditional program is quite remote.

Societal Costs of Drug Use

In addition to the high costs paid at the personal level by drug users, there are also greater costs to society at large. Drug use is not benign in its effects on society. Drug abuse takes a toll on those who do not use or abuse drugs. Addicts may turn to crime and violence to finance their habits. They risk their lives and the lives of others when they operate vehicles or machinery while under the influence of drugs. The costs to society from drug use cannot all be measured in terms of dollars. Human costs are incalculable. "Crack babies" are an example of societal costs associated with drug use. Not only do babies born to crack-dependent mothers suffer from physical deformities, behavioral dysfunction, and developmental difficulties, but also they require medical care and special education, both of which further strain already faltering systems. Some major cities are reporting that 20 percent of newborns show the effects of drugs. Often in crack-plagued ghettos, where the effects of perinatal addiction are most visible, many mothers continue to use crack after birth, and the family unit continues to face a life of neglect, poverty, and violence.[11]

Overview of Drugs

A drug is any chemical other than food that is purposely taken to affect body processes. Drugs may be therapeutic, taken to improve or extend life by treating illness or by providing relief from physical or mental distress. Using a drug for a purpose other than that for which it was originally intended is **drug misuse.** Drug misuse includes taking more or less of a prescribed drug or using a friend's or outdated prescribed medication. Excessive drug use that is inconsistent with accepted medical practice is **drug abuse.** The dangers of using a particular drug are often associated with the drug's ability to cause addiction, or **physical dependence.** Many legal drugs, including barbiturates, tranquilizers, analgesics, opiates, alcohol, and tobacco, are addicting and cause physical dependence. Besides physical dependence, drugs can create a **psychological dependence,** called habituation. Habituation is the repeated use of a drug because the user finds that each use increases pleasurable feelings or reduces feelings of anxiety, fear, or stress. The habituation becomes detrimental when the person becomes so consumed by the need for the drugged state of consciousness that all energies are directed to compulsive drug-seeking behavior.

Psychoactive drugs are drugs that alter thoughts, feelings, perceptions, and moods. Legal and illegal psychoactive drugs are used to cope with mental and emotional problems as well as to alter moods and behaviors. Misuse of a psychoactive drug can grow into abuse and physical or psychological addiction. Addiction occurs when an individual relies on drugs to cope with life or if the drugs are interfering with normal living. The effects of psychoactive drugs depend on several factors, including how the drug enters the body, drug action, and the presence of other drugs in the body.

There are several modalities by which drugs can enter the body. The most common way of taking a drug is oral administration, taking the drug in capsule, tablet, or liquid form in the mouth and swallowing it. Drugs taken orally do not reach the bloodstream as quickly as the other means. Drugs may also enter the body through the lungs, either by sniffing a powder, such as cocaine, or by inhaling gases, aerosol sprays, or fumes from solvents or other compounds that evaporate quickly. Inhaling drugs can produce serious, even fatal consequences. With the use of a syringe, drugs may also be injected **subcutaneously,** under the skin; **intramuscularly,** into the muscle tissue; or **intravenously,** directly into a vein. An intravenous injection results in the drug getting into the bloodstream immediately. Intramuscular and subcutaneous injections are slower in action.

There is variability in the types of action from drugs and the ways in which drugs can interact with other drugs (Fig. 4.5). A drug may act locally, as does Novocain used by a dentist. It may also act in a general way, throughout the body system, for example, alcohol and its effect on the central nervous system. The drug may have a selective form of action, such as an antacid, by having a greater effect on one specific organ or system than on others. Drugs may also have a **cumulative** effect, meaning that when it is taken in faster than the body can metabolize and excrete it, the impact of the drug is heightened. Alcohol is also an example of a cumulative drug.

Several factors also influence the effects of a drug. Individual differences are an important consideration because each person responds differently to different drugs at different times and in different settings. The underlying emotional state at the time the drug is taken may be intensified by the drug; for example, a woman who is feeling depressed may feel more depressed. Generalized physical conditions such as a cold or pregnancy may make the body more vulnerable to the effects of a drug. Genetic differences among individuals may also account for varying drug responses. Mindset has been shown to play a role in drug effects. Someone who snorts cocaine to enhance sexual pleasure may feel more stimulated simply because that is what she expects to happen. Social setting may also influence drug effects. Drug effect at a noisy crowded party is different from the effect produced at an intimate subdued event.

Tolerance is the body's ability to withstand the effects of a drug. Continued use results in increased tolerance and decreased responsiveness, so larger and larger doses become necessary to achieve a constant effect. Larger doses increase the risk of **toxicity,** the level of a drug at which it becomes poisonous to the body. Toxicity may result in either temporary or permanent minor or major body damage or death. Individuals initiate drug use for a variety of reasons (Information Box 4.4). Most users prefer a specific drug but use several others. This is called **polyabuse.** The average user who enters treatment is on five different drugs. The more drugs used, the greater the chance of side effects, complications, and possible life-threatening situations.

INFORMATION BOX 4.4

Why People Abuse Drugs

Curiosity

Boredom

Psychological needs

Peer influence

Imitating role models (parents, older adults)

Availability of drugs

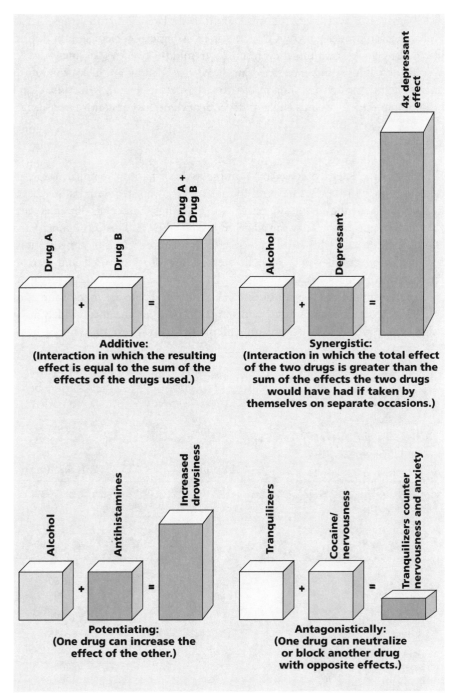

FIGURE 4.5

Interactive effects of drugs.
(1) **Additive** (interaction in which the resulting effect is equal to the sum of the effects of the drugs used). (2) **Synergistic** (interaction in which the total effect of the two drugs is greater than the sum of the effects the two drugs would have had if taken by themselves on separate occasions). Example: Mixing barbiturates and alcohol has up to four times the depressant effect that either drug has alone. (3) **Potentiating** (one drug can increase the effect of the other). Example: Alcohol can increase the drowsiness caused by antihistamines. (4) **Antagonistically** (one drug can neutralize or block another drug with opposite effects. Example: Tranquilizers may counter some of the nervousness and anxiety produced by cocaine.

Illegal Drugs

Drugs are often categorized by their legal or illegal status. Illegal drugs are those that an individual is not authorized to have. Examples of illegal or "illicit" drugs include marijuana, cocaine, and heroin. Illegal drug production and

I don't really know how I got into drugs. It started with friends and was fun. I was curious and thought it was something I could easily handle. It ran away with me. I didn't realize how desperate I had become until I was arrested for stealing. I couldn't believe that I was in jail.

22-YEAR-OLD WOMAN

distribution is a worldwide effort. Despite a declared "war on drugs," drug availability continues to grow. No sector of American society is immune to illegal drugs. By the time they reach their middle twenties, as many as 80 percent of young adults have tried an illegal drug. Some are lucky enough to satisfy their curiosity and not return to drugs; others are less fortunate and become caught in a vicious circle of dependency and loss of control over drugs.

Legal Drugs

Whether a drug is legal or illegal has nothing to do with its proven pharmacological action or with the personal and social dangers associated with its use. Legal drugs include alcohol, nicotine, caffeine, OTC drugs, and drugs obtained with a medical prescription. They can all be misused or abused. The OTCs most often abused include pain relievers, sedatives, and stimulants. Prescription medications such as amphetamines and anabolic steroids are often misused and lead to serious consequences.

Caffeine should also be considered a legal drug. There are many sources of caffeine (Information Box 4.5), and it may be one of the most widely used drugs in the world. As a stimulant, caffeine helps to relieve drowsiness, helps

---

INFORMATION BOX 4.5

Sources of Caffeine

Substance	Amount	Caffeine (mg)
Coffee		
Brewed, drip	1 cup	115
Brewed, percolator	1 cup	80
Instant	1 cup	65
Decaffeinated	1 cup	3
Tea		
Brewed	1 cup	40–60
Instant	1 cup	30
Cocoa	1 cup	50
Soft drink	1 can	36–55
Weight-control products		
Dex-A-Diet II	1	200
Dexatrim	1	200
Diuretics		
Aqua-Ban	1	100
Chocolate bar	1	20
Excedrin	32 mg	65
Nodoz	1 tablet	100

in the performance of repetitive tasks, and improves mental capacity for work. Caffeine also raises the basal metabolic rate. In addition, caffeine has been shown to trigger anxiety, insomnia, irregular heartbeat, faster breathing, upset stomach and bowels, dizziness, and headaches. Heavy caffeine users who suddenly stop using caffeine may experience headaches, irritability, and fatigue.

More than $10 billion are spent each year by Americans on OTC drugs and remedies. By taking higher than recommended doses or by taking them for different purposes for which they were intended, individuals misuse OTC drugs. Side effects may result from this misuse, particularly if the OTCs are used in combination with other drugs, including alcohol. For example, alcohol enhances the effects of OTCs (see Chapter 3), such as increasing the drowsiness associated with antihistamines and the stomach irritation associated with aspirin. The most frequently misused OTCs are painkillers, sedatives, and stimulants. Painkillers are also known as **analgesics** and include such compounds as aspirin, acetaminophen, and ibuprofen. Drugs that relax the central nervous system to relieve anxiety or induce sleep are known as **sedatives**. Most OTC sedatives are actually antihistamines—allergy medications, which cause drowsiness as a side effect. OTC **stimulants** usually contain about as much caffeine as one or two cups of coffee. Side effects from stimulants are similar to the side effects of coffee, which include increased alertness, irritability, and nervousness.

Prescribed medications are also legal drugs. They can be obtained only through the authorization of a licensed physician or dentist. Prescribed medications that are most abused include sleeping pills, antianxiety medications, opiates, amphetamines, and steroids. In small doses, sedatives such as Seconal and Nembutal produce a calming effect. In larger doses, they induce sleep. Valium, Librium, and similar compounds function as muscle relaxants and antianxiety medications. The sedative or relaxant effect of one tablet of each is roughly the equivalent to the effect of one alcoholic drink. Prescription **opiates** are analgesics composed of morphine or codeine.

Amphetamines are another category of prescribed medications. They were once widely prescribed for weight control because they result in appetite suppression and stimulate the central nervous system. Hyperactive children may be prescribed Ritalin, a drug that helps increase attention span. In narcoleptics, people who experience irresistible attacks of sleepiness, amphetamines can prevent sudden episodes of sleep in dangerous situations, such as operating machinery or driving a car. A serious side effect of amphetamines is the additional strain placed on the cardiovascular system, which can lead to severe cardiovascular damage.

Anabolic steroids, which are synthetic derivatives of the male hormone testosterone, are powerful compounds prescribed for treatment of burns and injuries. They have been increasingly illegally misused by athletes and others who want to appear athletic. For males, the potential side effects of anabolic steroids include an increased risk of heart disease or stroke, liver tumors and jaundice, acne, breast enlargement, testicular atrophy, and impotency. Women who take anabolic steroids risk a deepened voice, breast reduction, and beard growth. Both men and women run a risk of HIV transmission when needles are shared

I started using tranquilizers to help me get through school. All the pressure of final exams was really too much for me. Then I needed them to help me survive a new and stressful job. I had to be creative with the lies I told various doctors to get the prescriptions. I couldn't admit that I had a problem. I just knew that I couldn't get through the day without my pills.

28-YEAR-OLD WOMAN

for steroid injection. Anabolic steroid users can become increasingly aggressive and paranoid. Studies have shown steroids to be addictive substances that create the same problems with dependence and withdrawal as cocaine.

Physiological Effects and Risks of Drug Use

No drug use is benign. At a minimum, all psychoactive drugs affect the central nervous system. In addition to the direct physiological effects and risks of drug use, there may be additional risks associated with the administration of drugs to the body. The process of using needles to inject drugs presents serious risks beyond those of using drugs. Many diseases, including hepatitis and HIV, can be transmitted from one person to another via contaminated injection equipment. The effects and risks of drugs are summarized in Information Box 4.6.

Stimulants

Stimulants affect the central nervous system and increase the heart rate, blood pressure, strength of heart contractions, blood glucose level, and overall muscle tension. All of these effects result in additional stress on the body. *Cocaine* has become a popular stimulant drug. Approximately 5 million Americans use cocaine, with 3 million users estimated to be addicted. Cocaine is also known as "coke," "lady," or "snow." It is sold as a crystalline powder. Cocaine is ingested by snorting, smoking ("free-basing"), and injection. Each method can produce serious effects, but smoking and injection are the most dangerous. The immediate effects of cocaine last 5 to 15 minutes because it is rapidly metabolized by the liver. With repeated use, the brain becomes tolerant to cocaine, and users need more of the drug to get high. Physical effects of cocaine include headaches, exhaustion, shaking, blurred vision, nausea, loss of sexual desire, and impotence. Loss of appetite from regular cocaine use can be quite severe, leading to dramatic weight loss and malnutrition.

Crack is a smokable mixture of cocaine and baking soda. It is also known as "rock." Crack is generally smoked in a glass water pipe. Because it sets off rapid ups and downs, crack causes a powerful chemical and psychological dependence. Crack users often need another "hit" within minutes of the previous one. Crack users often become active, paranoid, and dangerous. Smoking crack doused with liquid phencyclidine (PCP) is known as "space-basing" and has had very detrimental effects on behavior.

Amphetamines are manufactured chemicals that act as stimulants of the central nervous system. They are generally in pill form and sold under a variety of names. Chronic users may grind and sniff the pills or capsules or make a solution for injection. A smokable form of methamphetamine, more addictive and which produces an intense physical and psychological high, is known as "ice." Amphetamines speed up body processes, increasing blood pressure and heart rate, dilating pupils, and decreasing appetite. High doses may result in an irregular heart rate, tremors, loss of coordination, loss of consciousness, heart failure, and death. Prolonged use may result in psychosis, paranoia, and violence.

Depressants

Drugs that relax the central nervous system are called **depressants, sedatives, or hypnotics.** The most widely used form of depressants is alcohol (see Chapter 3). *Barbiturates* are also depressants. They are used medically for inducing relaxation and sleep, relieving tension, and treating seizures. They may also be administered intravenously as a general anesthetic. Low doses of barbiturates produce mild intoxication and euphoria and decrease alertness and muscle coordination. With a higher dose, slurred speech, decreased respirations, cold skin, weak and rapid heartbeat, and unconsciousness may result. Barbiturate side effects include drowsiness, impaired judgment and performance, and a hangover that may last for hours or days. Regular barbiturate use leads to physical dependence. Barbiturate addicts tend to be sleepy, confused, or irritable. Depressants have a synergistic effect when they are mixed together. Barbiturates are a factor in nearly one-third of all reported drug-related deaths. As the user builds up tolerance, the likelihood of a potentially fatal overdose increases. Barbiturate withdrawal is a time-consuming process and medically difficult to manage. Withdrawal symptoms include anxiety, insomnia, delirium, and convulsions. Systemic dependence is so critical that occasionally an abrupt ending of barbiturate use leads to death.

Antianxiety Drugs

Antianxiety drugs, *benzodiazepines,* are primarily prescribed to treat tension or muscular strain. The *dicarbamates* produce sedation for up to 10 hours or longer. Similar to the barbiturates, high doses of these drugs result in slurred speech, drowsiness, and stupor. Physiological and physical dependence on antianxiety drugs may occur within 2 to 4 weeks. Withdrawal symptoms from antianxiety drugs may include coma, psychosis, and death.

Cannabis (Marijuana)

Cannabis, known as *marijuana,* "pot," or "grass," is mixture of crushed leaves and flowers of the *Cannabis sativa* plant. Hashish is also an extract of cannabis but is 2 to 10 times as concentrated as marijuana. Tetrahydrocannabinol (THC) is the primary psychoactive ingredient. Marijuana is considered to be an illegal drug in most places. Marijuana use has been falling ever since the late 1970s. In 1990, 42 percent of college students reported using it, compared with 51 percent in 1980. Cannabis is being used experimentally as a legal medical therapy for severe nausea in cancer patients receiving chemotherapy. Studies are also being conducted to evaluate the effectiveness of marijuana in reducing pressure within the eye in glaucoma and in treating muscle spasticity. Marijuana

I am clean now, but I had a heavy street habit for several years. I really didn't care what happened to me. I just lived for my daily hits. I was pretty careless about other things too. I got pregnant and had a baby. He is in a home now and he will never be normal. He is that way because of the drugs that I did. I would change the past if I could but I can't. I did learn though that I had to take care of myself and that meant giving up the drugs. It wasn't easy. I am still afraid but I can't go back and risk repeating that whole scene again.

30-YEAR-OLD WOMAN

Summary of Effects and Risks of Drugs

Cocaine and Crack

Names	"Coke," "snow," "lady," "rock"
Physiological effect	Speed up physical and mental processes; create sense of heightened energy and confidence
Health effects	Headaches, exhaustion, shaking, blurred vision, nausea, seizures, loss of appetite, loss of sexual desire, impotence, impaired judgment, hyperactivity, babbling, paranoia, violence
Long-term risks	Nasal damage (if snorted); lung damage (if smoked); hepatitis and HIV (if injected); damage to heart and blood vessels; chest pain; heart attack; disruptions in cardiac rhythm; stroke; damage to liver
Special risks to women	Increased danger of miscarriage and physical and mental impairment of the fetus; increased risk of congenital malformations, fetal deaths, and SIDS

Amphetamines

Names	Benzedrine ("bennies"), dextroamphetamine (Dexedrine, "dex"), methamphetamine (Methedrine, "meth," "speed"), Desoxyn ("copilots"), methylphenidate (Ritalin), pemoline (Cylert), phenmetrazine (Preludin)
Physiological effect	Speed up physical and mental processes; lessen fatigue; boost energy; sense of excitement
Health effects	Loss of appetite; blurred vision; headache and dizziness; sweating; sleeplessness; trembling; anxiety and suspiciousness; delusions and hallucinations
Long-term risks	Cardiovascular damage—hypertension, stroke, heart failure; malnutrition, vitamin deficiencies; skin disorders; ulcers; sleeplessness; fever; brain damage; depression; violent behavior; fatal overdose
Special risks to women	Not yet determined

Barbiturates

Names	Pentobarbital (Nembutal, "yellow jackets"), secobarbital (Seconal, "reds"), thiopental (Pentothal), amobarbital (Amytal, "blues" "downers"), phenobarbital (Luminal, "phennies"), methaqualone ("love drug," Quaalude, "ludes," "Q,"), sopor ("Sopors")
Physiological effect	Mild intoxication, drowsiness, lethargy, decreased alertness
Health effects	Drowsiness, poor coordination, slurred speech, impaired judgment, hangover, confusion, irritability; cold skin; depressed respirations; rapid heart rate
Long-term risks	Disrupted sleep, impaired vision; increased risk of fatal overdose with increased use
Special risks to women	Risk of birth defects and subsequent behavioral problems if used during pregnancy

Antianxiety Drugs

Names	Benzodiazepines: chlordiazepoxide (Librium), diazepam (Valium), oxazepam (Serax), flurazepam (Dalmane); dicarbamates: meprobamate (Equanil, Miltown)
Physiological effect	Slows down central nervous system
Health effects	Slurred speech, drowsiness, stupor
Long-term risks	Physical and psychological dependence; possible fatal overdose; withdrawal can lead to coma, psychosis and death
Special risks to women	Menstrual irregularities and failure to ovulate have been reported

Marijuana and Hashish

Names	Marijuana ("pot," "grass," "maryjane"), hashish
Physiological effect	Relaxes the mind and body; heightens perceptions
Health effects	Increased heart rate; dry mouth and throat; impaired perceptions and reactions; lethargy; nausea; disorientation, possible hallucinations, heightened anxiety
Long-term risks	Psychological dependence; impaired thinking, perception, memory, and coordination; increased heart rate and hypertension; compromised immunity
Special risks to women	Prenatal use may lead to fetal effects, including small head, poor growth, lower birth weight

Psychedelics

Names	LSD ("acid"), mescaline, PCP ("angel dust," "peace pill"), designer drugs
Physiological effect	Alters perceptions and produces hallucinations
Health effect	Increased heart rate, hypertension, fever, headache, nausea, sweating, and trembling; delusions and unpredictable violence
Long-term risks	Possible flashbacks, psychological dependence; stupor, coma, convulsions, heart and lung failure; brain damage
Special risks to women	Effects on fetus unknown

Inhalants

Names	Depends on specific product
Physiological effect	Temporary feelings of well-being; giddiness; hallucinations
Health effect	Nausea, sneezing, coughing, nosebleeds, loss of appetite, decreased heart and breathing rates; impaired judgment; loss of consciousness
Long-term risks	Hepatitis, liver and kidney failure; respiratory impairment; blood abnormalities; possible suffocation
Special risks to women	Not yet determined

Opiates/Synthetic Narcotics

Names	Opium, morphine, codeine; heroin ("horse," "junk," "smack," "downtown"); methadone (Dolophine, "meth," "dollies"); hydromorphone (Dilaudid, "little D"); oxycodone (Percodan, "perkies"); meperidine (Demerol, "demies"); propoxyphene (Darvon)
Physiological effect	Relaxation of the central nervous system; pain relief; temporary sense of well-being
Health effect	Nausea and vomiting; restlessness; reduced respirations; lethargy; weight loss; slurred speech; mood swings; sweating
Long-term risks	Physical dependence; malnutrition; compromised immunity; hepatitis, HIV; skin lesions; fatal overdose
Special risks to women	Higher risk for preterm labor, intrauterine growth retardation, and preeclampsia

is generally smoked in a cigarette ("joint"). The high from marijuana depends on how long the smoke is held in the lungs and the concentration of THC in the marijuana. In low to moderate doses, the effects from marijuana are similar to the effects of alcohol and some tranquilizers. In contrast to alcohol, however, marijuana at low doses does not dull sensation, but it may cause slight alterations in perception. The immediate physical effects of marijuana include an increased heart rate, bloodshot eyes, and dry mouth and throat. High doses diminish the ability to perceive and react and cause sensory distortion. Hashish users may experience vivid hallucinations and LSD-like psychedelic reactions, and some people experience acute panic attacks.

Psychedelics and Hallucinogens

Hallucinogenic drugs create changes in perceptions and thoughts. A common feature of a hallucinogenic experience is that the drug suspends normal psychic mechanisms that integrate the self with the environment. Some of the more common effects induced by hallucinogenic drugs include changes in mood, sensation, perception, and relations. Hallucinogenic drugs produce tolerance to the psychedelic effects but do not create physical dependence or produce symptoms of withdrawal, even after long-term use. As with most psychoactive drugs, however, there is a danger of psychological dependence.

Peyote and lysergic acid diethylamide *(LSD)* are hallucinogens. Mescaline is the active ingredient in peyote, a spineless cactus with a small crown, or button, that is dried and then swallowed. Mescaline affects the brain within 30 to 90 minutes, and effects may persist for 12 hours. The average dose may produce vivid hallucinations. LSD ("acid") is also ingested orally and produces hallucinations, including bright colors and altered perceptions of reality. The effects generally begin within 30 minutes and may last up to 12 hours. The hallucinogenic experience, or "trip," is characterized by slight increases in body temperature, heart rate, and blood rate; sweating; chills; and sometimes headaches and nausea. A "bad trip" may result in an acute anxiety reaction that may trigger panic, depression, confusion, fear of insanity, and distorted thoughts and perceptions. LSD users have injured or killed themselves by jumping out of windows or throwing themselves in front of automobiles. Although there is no evidence that LSD creates physical dependence, there is evidence of psychological dependence. The most common delayed reaction of LSD is flashback, in which individuals re-experience the perceptual and emotional changes originally produced by the drug.

PCP (phencyclidine, "angel dust," "peace pill," "lovely," "green") is manufactured as a tablet, capsule, liquid, flake, spray, or crystalline white powder that can be swallowed, smoked, sniffed, or injected. Sometimes it is sprinkled on other drugs and smoked. A fine powder form of PCP can be snorted or injected. According to NIDA, although use of other drugs has generally declined, PCP use has increased among teenagers. The greatest danger from PCP is the behavioral toxicity, what it causes users to do to themselves and to others. It can trigger psychotic attacks that turn normal people temporarily insane and sometimes violent. Because of its delusional effects, users think that they have superhuman strength and abilities; because of its anesthetic effects, they feel no pain. The effects of PCP are unpredictable. PCP may trigger violent behavior or irreversible psychosis. Physiological effects with low doses include double vision, nausea, and muscular incoordination. Higher doses may produce a stupor that lasts for several days, increased heart rate and blood pressure, flushing, sweating, dizziness, and numbness. Taking large amounts can lead to convulsions, coma, heart and lung failure, ruptured blood vessels in the brain, and death.

Narcotics

Narcotics include the opiates—*opium and its derivatives, morphine, codeine, and heroin*—and some other nonopiate synthetic drugs. All narcotics have sleep-inducing and pain-relieving properties. They may be used medically for pain relief, but they have a high potential for abuse. All narcotics relax the user and when injected may produce an immediate rush. They may also result in restlessness, nausea, and vomiting. With large doses, the skin becomes moist, cold, and bluish, and the pupils become smaller. Respirations slow, and the user may not be awakened. Death is possible. Over time, opiate users may develop heart infections, skin abscesses, and congested lungs. Infections from unsterile equipment increase the risk of hepatitis, tetanus, and HIV. Dependence is likely to develop with long-term use. Withdrawal can begin within 4 to 6 hours from last dose for an addict, with symptoms of uneasiness, abdominal cramps, diarrhea, chills, sweating, and nausea. The intensity of withdrawal symptoms depends on the severity of the addiction.

Synthetic narcotics include methadone, which has been used to help heroin addicts kick their habit. Findings on the effectiveness of methadone have been mixed. Two semisynthetic derivatives of morphine include hydromorphone (Dilaudid) and oxycodone (Percodan), which have 5 to 10 times the painkilling effect of morphine. Propoxyphene (Darvon), a synthetic narcotic, is a somewhat less potent painkiller than codeine. In low doses, it is no more effective than aspirin, but in high doses, it produces a euphoric high, which increases its abuse. NIDA estimates that Darvon kills more people each year than does heroin.

Inhalants

Inhalants are chemicals that produce vapors with psychoactive effects. Many products that are used as inhalants were not meant for inhalation. These include solvents, aerosols, cleaning fluids, and petroleum products. Most inhalants produce the same effects as anesthetics in slowing down bodily functions. At low doses, users may feel slightly stimulated, and at higher doses, they may feel less inhibited. Regular use of inhalants leads to tolerance, so the user needs increasingly higher doses to attain the desired effects. Side effects of inhalant use include local irritation to the nose, nausea, sneezing, coughing, nosebleeds, bad breath, lack of coordination, loss of appetite, decreased heart and breathing rates, and impaired judgment. Inhalants may also cause serious medical complications, such as hepatitis with liver failure, kidney failure, respiratory impairment, destruction of bone marrow and skeletal muscles, blood abnormalities, and irregular heartbeats.

Designer Drugs

Designer drugs are produced in chemical laboratories and are sold illegally. Synthetic narcotics are particularly dangerous because they are more powerful than those derived from natural substances. The risk of brain damage or fatal overdose from ingestion is correspondingly higher. MDMA (methylene dioxmethylamphetamine, or "ecstasy") is an example of a designer drug. It is somewhat related to mescaline and amphetamines. Immediate effects include a feeling of warmth and openness. Delayed responses, usually within a day, include insomnia, muscle aches, fatigue, and difficulty concentrating. MDMA has been shown to cause brain damage in laboratory animals and is suspected to cause brain damage in humans.

Special Effects and Risks for Women

Most research on illicit drug use with women has focused not on women but on the effects of women's drug use on others, particularly the fetus and infant. Understanding the physiological effects of drug use by women is a difficult problem. The elusive and multifaceted nature of addiction has inherent limitations, which are compounded by differences in female/male physiology and the psychological pressures associated with the diversity of women's roles and society's double standards. It can be stated, however, that general physiological drug effects are the same in women as men.

The general physiological effects of drug use are compounded in women by their reproductive capabilities. For example, women who are addicted to opiates are often in poor general health and have a higher incidence of chronic infections, gynecological problems, anemia, and sexually transmitted diseases, including HIV infection.[12] Because drug-dependent women often use a combination of drugs, have poor nutrition, and lack appropriate prenatal care, serious complications to mother and baby can occur. Prenatal drug exposure has detrimental effects on neonatal and infant growth and development. **Teratogens** are drugs and other substances that cause defects in developing embryos. The magnitude of drug use among pregnant women is not known.

Cocaine is dangerous for both pregnant women and their unborn babies, causing miscarriages, developmental disorders, and life-threatening complications during birth.[13] Women who use cocaine while pregnant are more likely to miscarry in the first 3 months of pregnancy than other groups of women, including those who do not use drugs and those who use heroin or narcotics. Infants born to cocaine users suffer major complications, including cocaine withdrawal and permanent disabilities. Because cocaine affects blood pressure, it can deprive a fetal brain of oxygen or cause brain vessels to burst, so the

I used to model. I was told I had to keep my weight down—really down. I tried diets and exercise, but the only thing that really helped were the pills. It wasn't that hard to get them off the street. I knew that I shouldn't take them, but I kept saying that it would only be for the next job, or the next month. I couldn't sleep and I was constantly wired. Finally I became really strange—I couldn't separate the real world and the delusions in my head. I became paranoid and violent. Maybe it was good that I lost my job. I was able to get help and realize that the pills were destroying me.

26-YEAR-OLD WOMAN

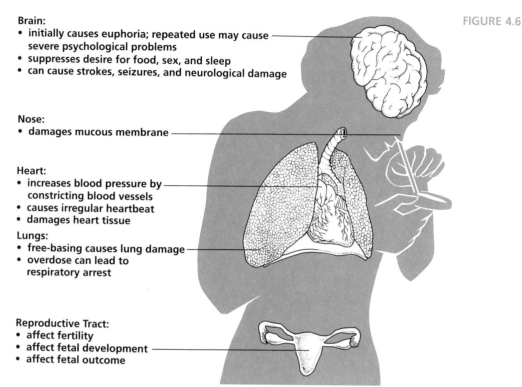

FIGURE 4.6

Brain:
- initially causes euphoria; repeated use may cause severe psychological problems
- suppresses desire for food, sex, and sleep
- can cause strokes, seizures, and neurological damage

Nose:
- damages mucous membrane

Heart:
- increases blood pressure by constricting blood vessels
- causes irregular heartbeat
- damages heart tissue

Lungs:
- free-basing causes lung damage
- overdose can lead to respiratory arrest

Reproductive Tract:
- affect fertility
- affect fetal development
- affect fetal outcome

fetus experiences the prenatal equivalent of a stroke, resulting in permanent physical and mental damage. Cocaine babies have higher-than-normal rates of respiratory and kidney problems and may be at a greater risk for sudden infant death syndrome (SIDS.) Visual problems, low birth weight, seizures, depression, lack of coordination, and developmental retardation are also common among cocaine babies. Higher rates of congenital malformations have been reported in babies born to mothers who used cocaine.[14]

Barbiturates also present problems in pregnancy. Barbiturates easily cross the placenta and cause birth defects and behavioral problems. Babies born to mothers who abused sedatives during pregnancy may be physically dependent on the drugs themselves and are more prone to respiratory problems, feeding difficulties, disturbed sleep, sweating, irritability, and fever.

Chronic use of marijuana has been shown to suppress ovulation and alter hormone levels in women. The frequent use of marijuana during pregnancy results in lower-birth-weight infants and congenital abnormalities similar to fetal alcohol syndrome (see Chapter 3), such as small head size, irritability, and poor growth.

The drug epidemic, in effect, has created a unique drug currency that further compromises women's health. In an examination of crack use among women, an association was found with the exchange of sex for drugs. Most women in the study indicated that crack had a negative effect on their interest in sex. In addition to the heightened risks of sexually transmitted diseases, including HIV, additional physical effects experienced by the women included a lack of attention to hygiene, paranoia, and loss of sleep. Caught in a vicious cycle of dependency, these women are unable to give up crack because of their constant exposure to the drug, their vulnerability, and the need to escape.[15]

Prescription drugs also present special problems for women. Women are more likely to become addicted to prescription drugs and to use them, often with alcohol, to medicate themselves to cope with anxiety, depression, and painful reactions to life stresses.[16] Women are not likely to report adverse consequences to medications when they are taken as prescribed, but problems, such as depression and becoming argumentative, do present when the medications are taken in a nonmedical manner (Information Box 4.7).

Drug overuse and misuse are particular problems among older women. Although they are generally not users of illicit drugs, older women are likely to be consumers of high levels of medications. Elderly women represent 11 percent of the general population, but they are prescribed more than 25 percent of all written prescriptions.[17] These prescriptions include estrogen replacement therapy, sedatives, hypnotics, antianxiety drugs, antihypertensive drugs, vitamins, analgesics, diuretics, laxatives, and tranquilizers. These medications are prescribed for women at a rate 2.5 times that of elderly men. The reasons for this disparity are not clear and probably involve a combination of biological, psychological, and social reasons. The potential for harmful drug interactions as a result of this myriad pattern of medication consumption is obvious. Research has found that women experience more adverse drug reactions than men, possibly owing to the combinations of these large amounts of medications.[16] Other adverse health consequences associated with drug use among older women include suicide, insomnia, affective disturbance, and impairment of cognitive

Consequences Attributed by Women to Use of Psychotherapeutic Drugs by Type of Use

Types of Problem	Percent with Problems and Types of Use		
	Nonmedical Use Only	Taken as Prescribed (medical)	Both Nonmedical and Medical
Depression	16.4	5.4	18.4
Argumentative	13.6	2.2	15.0
Auto accident	0.0	0.1	0.9
Trouble at school	6.1	0.6	9.6
Trouble at work	1.0	1.0	6.6
Medical emergency	0.0	0.1	3.2

SOURCE: National Institute on Drug Abuse (1986). *Research Monograph No. 65.* Washington, DC: US Government Printing Office, p. 89.

and motor function.[17] These consequences compromise the quality of life of older women and increase the likelihood of long-term institutionalization.

Drug Dependency

Drug dependency, alcoholism, and other self-destructive behaviors may not be separate problems but rather all symptoms of an addictive disorder. They all share common characteristics. **Dependency** refers to the attachment, physiological or psychological (or both) that a person may develop to a drug. Physical dependence occurs when physiological changes in the body's cells cause an overpowering, constant need for the drug. If the drug is not taken, the user develops withdrawal symptoms, such as intense anxiety, extreme nausea, and deep craving for the drug. Tranquilizers, painkillers, barbiturates, and narcotics may produce physical dependence. Psychological dependence is also called habituation and results in a strong craving for a drug because it produces pleasurable feelings or relieves stress or anxiety. Physical and psychological dependence do not always coexist. For example, marijuana and LSD may not create physical dependence, but continued use has demonstrated psychological dependence. **Cross-tolerance,** or **cross-addiction,** often presents with drug dependency. In this condition, a state of physical dependence exists in which psychological need for one psychoactive substance leads to dependence on similar substances.

Five primary stages in the development of drug dependency have been described. The first stage is the temptation or experimental stage, in which young adults may try drugs out of curiosity, peer pressure, the lure of excitement, or the need to rebel. The second stage occurs when the new user experiences a chemically induced "high," which is reinforced with repeated use. In the third stage, the user becomes preoccupied with the desired effect and develops frequent solo use. Behavior change becomes apparent to others at this point, and drug dependence is well established. In the fourth stage, users become preoccupied with achieving the drugs' effects. They often feel depressed, guilty, and even suicidal. Because the habit is expensive, they may have to resort to stealing or dealing to maintain the habit. In the final stage, users will do almost anything to get the drugs, and the drug consumption becomes the primary focus of their lives. The risk of overdosing and death increase steadily.

Treatment Dimensions of Drug Dependency

There are three basic approaches to drug-abuse treatment. These include detoxification, therapeutic communities, and outpatient drug-free programs. Different forms of intervention help different people and different dependencies. Detoxification is the supervised withdrawal from drug dependence, either with or without medication, in a hospital or outpatient setting. Therapeutic communities are highly structured, drug-free environments in which abusers live under strict rules while participating in group and individual therapy. Outpatient drug-free programs are available through community and treatment facilities. Self-help programs include Narcotics Anonymous (NA) and Pills Anonymous (PA), which follow the philosophy of Alcoholics Anonymous. In these programs, users admit to their helplessness and put their faith in a "higher power."

Drug dependency treatment programs must address the spectrum of physical and psychosocial issues that confront the addict. These challenges are especially difficult for women addicts, who experience an array of problems such as contraception, pregnancy, motherhood, child rearing, and health problems in addition to the underlying drug dependency. Although large-scale data are lacking, it appears that women are less likely to seek and participate in drug rehabilitation programs. Specifically opiate-dependent women have been found to be less likely to seek treatment than opiate-dependent men, and those who do seek treatment find that services to meet their needs are almost nonexistent.[18] Female clients in drug treatment centers have been shown to experience more extensive health needs than men while they are in drug treatment, particularly respiratory, genitourinary, and circulatory problems.[19,20] Female IVDUs present special challenges for recruitment and retention in treatment. Drug risk-taking behavior often has corresponding HIV risk-taking behavior. In a study of IVDUs, the women were found to have an average of 19 sexual partners in the preceding 6 months, and two-thirds of the women never used condoms.[21]

Chemical dependence treatment facilities have experienced great difficulty in recruiting and retaining women, particularly when they have children. Motherhood may be an important dimension to be incorporated in drug treatment programs for women. Despite the various levels of abuse, stigmatization, and guilt, many women value the role of motherhood, which is often linked to a woman's self-esteem.[22] Approximately 90 percent of female substance abusers are in their childbearing years. A great number of female drug users have relationships with male drug users, thereby increasing their risks for HIV infection. Chemically dependent women are also more likely to experience other traumas, such as rape and sexual and physical assault.[8] These dimensions compound the need for comprehensive treatment modalities as well as reduce the likelihood that women abusers will seek or remain in treatment. Financial concerns complicate drug treatment for women. Drug-dependent women are more likely to depend on financial assistance from public sources than drug-dependent men and are more likely to be unemployed. The employment factor may be especially significant because recovering drug-dependent men often attribute their recovery to employment-related reasons.[20] Cultural values, beliefs, societal roles, and empowerment are additional dimensions to be incorporated into drug treatment programs for women. These differences accentuate the greater need of women for supplemental financial, medical, and counseling services while they are in drug treatment.

Informed Decision Making for Women

Drug use is a personal responsibility issue. Developing personal strengths and self-confidence are the foundation for a woman to resist drugs effectively. These strengths include communication skills development and assertiveness. Knowing how to express a personal opinion, regardless of the subject, is a strength and skill in resisting the temptation to use drugs. Knowing how to cope with stress is another personal strength. Coping techniques need to be individually tailored but may include a variety of modalities, such as exercise, relaxation exercises, and visual imagery. Established coping skills help prevent turning to drugs when a difficult situation arises. Developing a range of interests is also a personal strength that may prevent a psychological need for drug use. Having personal hobbies and outside interests and being a participant and fan of specific sporting activities all foster a mental climate that reduces vulnerability to drug use. The enhancement of self-esteem is another significant personal strength that provides a foundation of drug avoidance. Self-esteem inherently evolves through the successful development of personal assertiveness, new interests, and coping techniques. Self-esteem evolves also from taking pride in personal achievements and accomplishments and further strengthens the skills to resist drug use.

Early identification and treatment offer some hope to the person who is using drugs. Unfortunately many people either fail to see or refuse to see the signals that a person is using drugs (Information Box 4.8). Knowing what to do when someone has a drug problem is another dimension of personal responsibility. The first step is to try to obtain as much information as possible about the problem. Many treatment and counseling centers offer free telephone advice on assessing the situation and learning about resources. Confronting the abuser is sometimes best handled in a group of loved ones and in the presence of a trained counselor. Outlining how the abuse has impacted each person and how much each person cares about the abuser helps to balance the information. It is unrealistic to expect

---

INFORMATION BOX 4.8

Indications of Drug Use

Abrupt change in attitude, including a lack of interest in previously enjoyed activities

Frequent vague and withdrawn moods

Sudden decline in work or school performance

Sudden resistance to discipline or criticism

Secret telephone calls and meetings with a demand for greater personal privacy

Increased frustration levels

Decreased tolerance for others

Changes in eating and sleeping habits

Sudden weight loss

Evidence of drug use

Frequent borrowing of money

Stealing

Disregard for personal appearance

Impaired relationships with family and friends

Disregard for deadlines, curfews, or other regulations

Unusual temper flareups

New friends, especially known drug dealers, and strong allegiance to these friends

SOURCE: National Institute on Drug Abuse (NIDA), National Institutes of Health. Bethesda, MD.

the abuser to quit without help. Drug dependency is a both a medical and psychological problem requiring multidisciplinary professional intervention. It is wise to offer support, but the abuser needs to know that treatment and therapy are necessary. The treatment program selected should provide a comprehensive medical evaluation as well as psychological evaluation before proceeding with an intervention. Another important consideration in selecting a drug treatment program is that it should be culturally sensitive to the client and ideally would have staff who are similar in ethnicity to the client. Abusers should not be believed when they say that they have learned to "control" their drug use. Absolute abstinence is the standard rule. Support groups are a good mechanism to maintain support and encouragement for abstinence.

Informed decision making is also an essential responsibility with prescribed and OTC medication use. Many women have little or no idea why they take certain prescribed medications, or they have multiple and vague reasons for the use of complex OTC medications. Drugs, whether prescribed or self-medicated, can have powerful adverse reactions with each other, certain foods, and lifestyle behaviors such as alcohol, tobacco and caffeine consumption. Prevention of adverse reactions with medications requires that women be well informed and sensitive to the array of possible problems and interactions. An underlying personal philosophy of medication use is a first step in problem prevention. Any drug, new or old, prescribed or purchased OTC, should be used for as short a time as necessary, unless there is evidence or medical advice that continued use is beneficial. The guiding principle of using as few drugs as possible to reduce the likelihood of adverse reactions also increases the likelihood that ones that are really necessary will be properly taken and will be able to address the underlying condition effectively. Informed women ask if a prescribed drug is really needed in the first place, whether a safer drug can be substituted, or whether a lower dose could be used to reduce or eliminate any side effects. The person taking the medications must also assume personal responsibility for understanding why the medications are needed, when and how they should be taken, and any possible adverse reactions.

Often women, particularly older women, are prescribed drugs to treat situational problems, such as loneliness, isolation, and confusion. Whenever possible, it is preferable to use nondrug approaches, such as hobbies and socializing with others, to treat these problems. Depression after the loss of a loved one is often better treated with social support from family and friends or a counselor rather than antidepressant drugs. Nondrug therapy is also preferable with conditions such as weight loss, where sound nutritional practices (see Chapter 1) have demonstrated better long-term effectiveness without the risks of drug side effects and dependencies. Increasing fiber and dietary liquids is preferable to laxative medications. Exercise is a demonstrated, nondrug, therapeutic agent for all these conditions: mild depression, weight loss, and constipation. It must be emphasized that a "no-drug" approach is not being advocated; rather informed women should carefully evaluate their expectations of the medication and determine with their physicians if a nondrug approach would be applicable. Many medications are prescribed by physicians because patients expect "a pill" to cure or resolve their problems, and the receipt of a prescription is seen by many as legitimizing the clinical visit. Honesty about drug use is another important consideration. Often women stop their medications, take them at nonregular intervals, or develop their own criteria for taking the medication. Failure to convey this information to the physician may lead to mistaken conclusions about health status, dosages, and medication effectiveness.

Medication information may be intimidating to some individuals. The names are often complex long words that make little or no sense to the user, and prescriptions, written in abbreviated Latin medical jargon, further intimidate some women. Actually medication information can be "translated" into easily understood information. A little time and patience are required. A medication worksheet or log often facilitates the process (Information Box 4.9). The work-

---

INFORMATION BOX 4.9

Medication Record

A. Prescribed Medications

A separate sheet should be completed for each prescribed medication. When dosages are changed, they should be noted.

Name of drug:
  Generic
  Brand name
  Trade name

Date prescribed:
  Date dosage changed
  Date medication restarted

Prescribed by (name and telephone):

Pharmacy and Prescription number:

Reason(s) for prescription (or change):

Dosage (how much to take each time):
  How much of drug is actually taken:

Frequency (how often is the drug to be taken):
  How often the drug is actually taken:

Time of day to be taken:

How long drug is to be taken:

Does this drug interact with certain foods?

Does this drug interact with other drugs?

New problems or concerns since taking this drug:

Symptom relief since taking the drug:

B. Over-the-Counter Medications

A separate sheet should be completed for each over-the-counter medication. When dosages are changed, they should be noted.

Name of drug:
  Generic
  Brand name
  Trade name

Date medication started:

Reason(s) for taking the medication:

Dosage (how much to take each time):
  How much of drug is actually taken:

Frequency (how often is the drug to be taken):
  How often the drug is actually taken:

Time of day to be taken:

How long drug is to be taken:

Does this drug interact with certain foods?

Does this drug interact with other drugs?

New problems or concerns since taking this drug:

Symptom relief since taking the drug:

sheet can easily be taken to the physician's office and completed during the course of a visit whenever medications are prescribed. It is a good idea to complete a worksheet on all new prescribed medications, any new OTC medications, and "old" medications. "Old" medications should be discussed with a physician as to whether they should be discarded or kept. If they are to be kept for possible future use, a medication worksheet should be completed so there is no misunderstanding about when and how to use the drug.

A medication log or worksheet should clearly specify the name of the drug in both brand and generic names because both are commonly used. Alcohol, tobacco, and caffeine use should be indicated because these drugs clearly can interact and complicate the effectiveness of prescribed and OTC medications. Because may of the most serious effects of drugs are often wrongly attributed to "being depressed" or "growing old," it is important for women to know about possible adverse drug reactions and side effects so they can be recognized and reported. Women should also know which foods and other drugs interact with the medications being taken and whether specific dietary recommendations have been identified for the medications.

SELF-ASSESSMENT 4.1

Do I Have a Drug Problem?

Carefully read and honestly answer the following questions:

1. Sometimes I am preoccupied with getting and taking a drug.   ____ yes ____ no

2. Sometimes I don't go to an important event at school or work, or a social or recreational event in order to get or take a drug.   ____ yes ____ no

3. I continue to use a drug despite the fact that I know it makes things with my family or friends worse, or it interferes with school or work activities.   ____ yes ____ no

4. I have developed a specific physical or mental condition from my drug use (example, irritated nose from cocaine).   ____ yes ____ no

5. I have repeatedly tried to cut down or eliminate my use of a drug.   ____ yes ____ no

6. I am sometimes unable to fulfill my obligations because of my drug use (family, friends, work, or school).   ____ yes ____ no

7. I feel specific symptoms when I cut back or eliminate the drug.   ____ yes ____ no

8. I sometimes take another drug to relieve withdrawal symptoms.   ____ yes ____ no

9. I sometimes use the drug in larger doses or over a longer period than recommended.   ____ yes ____ no

10. I need to take more of the drug now than I did before to get the same effect.   ____ yes ____ no

If you answered "yes" to any of these questions, it is important to seek help now with your drug problem.

Summary

Drugs are chemical substances that can provide considerable benefit in maintaining health and in treating disease. Additional research is necessary to provide a better understanding of the physiological, psychosocial, and behavioral dimensions of drug use among women. The development of comprehensive and sensitive drug treatment facilities that are available to all women is another necessity in this arena. At the individual level, women must exercise caution and wisdom with drug use. Self-Assessment 4.1 is a questionnaire women can use to determine if they have a drug problem. Every woman should weigh the risks and benefits before taking any drug. Reducing the kinds and amounts of drugs—recreational drugs; prescribed medications; OTC medications; and substances such as caffeine, nicotine, and alcohol—should be an important personal health goal.

Philosophical Dimensions: Drug Use and Women's Health

1. Should the state intervene in cases of maternal drug use? Is it fair to charge the mother who uses drugs while she is pregnant with child abuse or with the felony of delivering illegal drugs to a minor?

CURRENT EVENTS

Special Population: Older Women and Medications

National Institute of Aging Factsheet

Older women use more medications than any other segment of the population. They also have the highest rate of chronic or long-term illness such as arthritis, diabetes, high blood pressure, and heart disease. It is common for them to take many different drugs at the same time and for long periods of time. Drugs taken by older people act differently from the way they do in younger people, probably because of normal changes in body makeup that occur with age. Such changes can affect the length of time a drug remains in the body and the amount of drug absorbed by body tissues.

Precautions to be taken to reduce the risks associated with drug use include:

- Take the exact dosage prescribed.
- Ask the doctor and/or pharmacists about special concerns or properties of the medication.
- **Never** take medication prescribed for someone else.
- Tell the doctor about all other medications (prescribed and over-the-counter).
- Keep a daily record of all medications.
- Call the doctor if unusual reactions occur.

A chemical agent strong enough to cure an ailment is also strong enough to cause harm if not used wisely. If a prescribed drug seems to be doing more harm than good, do not hesitate to call the doctor. Another medicine can often be substituted.

2. List all chemicals and substances that you use to change your state of consciousness. Include caffeine, tobacco, alcohol, prescription drugs, over-the-counter drugs, and illegal drugs. Try to give up one or more of these substances for a period of time. Keep a record of how you feel and any changes that you notice in your health or behavior.

References

1. Worth, D. (1991). American women and polydrug abuse. In Roth, R. (Ed.), *Alcohol and drugs are women's issues: Volume one: A review of the issues* (pp. 1–9). Meutchen, NJ: Women's Action Alliance and The Scarecrow Press, Inc.

2. USDHHS, National Institute on Drug Abuse. (1988). *National Household Survey on Drug Abuse: Main Findings 1985.* (NIDA (ADM) 88-1586.) Washington, DC: US Government Printing Office.

3. Erickson, P.G., and Murray, G.F. (1989). Sex differences in cocaine use and experiences: a double standard revived? *American Journal of Drug and Alcohol Abuse, 15*(2), 135–152.

4. Anglin, M.D., Booth, M.W., Ryan, T.M., and Yih-Ing, H. (1988). Ethnic differences in narcotic addiction. II. Chicano and Anglo addiction career patterns. *The International Journal of the Addictions, 23*(10), 1011–1027.

5. Windle, M. (1990). A longitudinal study of antisocial behaviors in early adolescence as predictors of late adolescent substance abuse. Gender and ethnic group differences. *Journal of Abnormal Psychology, 99*(1), 86–91.

6. Cohen, J.B., Hauer, I.B., and Wofsy, C.B. (1989). Women and IV drugs: parenteral and heterosexual transmission of human immunodeficiency virus. *The Journal of Drug Issues, 19*(1), 39–56.

7. Korolenko, C.P., and Donskih, T.A. (1990). Addictive behavior in women: a theoretical perspective. *Drugs and Society, 4*(3/4), 39–65.

8. Ladwig, G.B., and Anderson, M.D. (1989). Substance abuse in women: relationship between chemical dependency of women and past reports of physical and/or sexual abuse. *The International Journal of the Addictions, 24*(8), 739–754.

9. Russell, M., and Coviello, D. (1988). Heavy drinking and regular psychoactive drug use among gynecological outpatients. *Alcoholism: Clinical and Experimental Research, 12*(3), 400–406.

10. Robles, R.R., Colon, H.M., and Gonzalez, A. (1990). Social relations and empowerment of sexual partners of IV drug users. *Puerto Rico Health Sciences Journal, 9*(1), 99–104.

11. Toufexis, A. (1991). Innocent victims. *Time, 137*(19), 56–60.

12. American College of Obstetricians and Gynecologists. (1986). *Drug Abuse and Pregnancy.* Washington, DC: ACOG Technical Bulletin #96.

13. Burkett, G., Yasin, S., and Palow, D. (1990). Perinatal implications of cocaine exposure. *The Journal of Reproductive Medicine, 35*(1), 35–42.

14. Bingol, N., Fuchs, M., Diaz, V., Stone, R.K., and Gromisch, D.S. (1987). Teratogenicity of cocaine in humans. *Journal of Pediatrics, 110,* 93–96.

15. Worth, D. (1990). *Women, sex, and crack.* Paper presented at the American Anthropological Association meeting. New Orleans, LA.

16. Hamilton, J., and Perry, B., (1983). Sex-related differences in clinical drug response: implications for women's health. *Journal of the American Medical Association, 38,* 126–132.

17. NIDA (1986). *Drugs and drug interactions in elderly women. National Institute of Drug Abuse Research Monograph #65.* Washington, DC: US Government Printing Office.

18. Handler, A., Kistin, N., Davis, F., and Ferre, C. (1991). Cocaine use during pregnancy: perinatal outcomes. *American Journal of Epidemiology, 133,* 818–825.

19. Andersen, M.D. (1980). Health needs of drug dependent clients. *Women and Health, 5*(1), 23–33.

20. Marsh, K.L., and Simpson, D.D. (1986). Sex differences in opioid addiction careers. *American Journal of Drug and Alcohol Abuse, 12*(4), 309–329.

21. Booth, R., Koester, S., Brewster, J.T., Weibel, W.W., and Fritz, R.B. (1991). Intravenous drug users and AIDS: risk behaviors. *American Journal of Drug and Alcohol Abuse, 17*(3), 337–353.

22. Karan, L.D. (1989). AIDS prevention and chemical dependence treatment needs of women and their children. *Journal of Psychoactive Drugs, 21*(4), 395–399.

Resources

SUBSTANCE ABUSE AND MENTAL HEALTH SERVICES ADMINISTRATION (SAMHSA)

5600 Fishers Lane
Rockville, MD 20857
301-443-3783

SUBSTANCE ABUSE PREVENTION ADAMHA
301-443-0365

COCAINE ANONYMOUS WORLD SERVICES

3740 Overland Avenue
Suite G
Los Angeles, CA 90034
213-559-5833

COKENDERS

1240 Powell
Emeryville, CA 94608
415-652-1772

COMMUNITY ALCOHOL AND DRUG TREATMENT PROGRAMS

Most community hospitals and drug treatment programs sponsor outpatient alcohol treatment programs and support groups. Information is available in the yellow pages of telephone directories under "Alcoholism" and "Drug abuse/treatment."

NARCOTICS ANONYMOUS

PO Box 9999
Van Nuys, CA 91409
818-780-3951

NATIONAL CLEARINGHOUSE FOR ALCOHOL AND DRUG INFORMATION

PO Box 2345
Rockville, MD 20852
301-468-2600
800-729-6686

NATIONAL INSTITUTE ON DRUG ABUSE HOTLINE

800-662-4357

NATIONAL COCAINE HOTLINE

800-COCAINE

CHAPTER 5

Smoking

CHAPTER OBJECTIVES

On completion of this chapter, the student should be able to discuss:

1. Tobacco use by women in the United States from a historical perspective.

2. Recent epidemiological trends of female smokers compared with male smokers.

3. Recent epidemiological trends with females from a daily consumption perspective.

4. Epidemiological data on smoking prevalence among women from a racial and ethnic perspective.

5. Epidemiological data on smoking prevalence from an educational and occupational perspective.

6. Epidemiological data on smoking behavior of pregnant women.

7. Epidemiological data on the prevalence of smoking among adolescent girls.

8. Why there are concerns about early initiation of smoking behavior.

9. Marketing strategies of tobacco companies toward women.

10. How tobacco companies have targeted and promoted their products in minority communities.

11. Direct and indirect costs to society from smoking.

12. Why tobacco is sheltered from additional legislative intervention or regulation.

13. How the tobacco industry has influenced the women's movement.

14. The significance of the Supreme Court decision allowing smokers to sue tobacco companies for damage.

15. How smoking contributes to cardiovascular disease in women.

16. How smoking contributes to cancer in women.

17. How smoking presents special risks during pregnancy.

18. How smoking is related to other chronic conditions in women.

19. The significance of involuntary smoking from a health perspective.

20. The three most significant compounds in tobacco smoke.

21. The variables that influence the health risks of smoking.

22. How nicotine is an addictive drug.

23. The common reasons given for women's smoking behavior.

24. The two basic strategies for quitting smoking alone.

25. The types of group smoking cessation interventions.

26. The concerns with the transdermal nicotine patch.

27. The issue of weight gain and smoking cessation.

Introduction

Cigarette smoking is simply the single most preventable cause of premature morbidity and mortality in the United States today. Tobacco causes more deaths and suffering among adults than any other toxic material in the environment. The health consequences of smoking are devastating to women's health, and the outlook is even more bleak as older women smokers progress out of their "healthy years." Although older women are beginning to quit cigarettes, younger women are initiating the habit at high rates, higher than their male peers. Smoking is a complex addictive behavior, but smokers are not the only individuals affected by tobacco use. Involuntary smokers, the nonsmoking spouses, partners, co-workers, children, and even pets of smokers who inhale either the exhaled smoke from smokers or the wafts from their cigarettes, also experience significant smoking-related morbidity and mortality. Several political, economic, marketing, legal, and cultural dimensions influence the current smoking problem among women. This chapter explores these and other dimensions of smoking to provide a comprehensive perspective of smoking as a women's health-related behavior.

Smoking Trends and Issues

Cigarette smoking does not exist in a vacuum. The prevalence of smoking is influenced by myriad historical, economic, political, legal, and sociocultural dimensions that contribute to the fabric of smoking today in the United States.

Historical Overview

Tobacco has a long history, and women have a long history of using tobacco. Tobacco was one of the New World "discoveries" of Spanish explorers 450 years ago, although archaeological and historical evidence suggests that the use of tobacco by women antedated the European consumption of the product. Tobacco became an accepted component of early colonial life, and New England colonial women reputedly smoked while performing routine domestic duties. Through the next century, tobacco was also snuffed, dipped, and chewed.

Chewing was the main form of tobacco use between 1800 and 1850 in the United States but was primarily practiced by men. Snuff dipping or "digging" was practiced among women of both upper and lower classes. Between the Civil War and World War I, tobacco use was confined mainly to adult men, but there were still a few groups of women using it. Cigarette smoking gradually increased in popularity and surpassed the practice of tobacco chewing, which peaked around 1890. Technological "improvements" to cigarettes enhanced the ease of inhalation and modified their flavor and aroma. The 1920s were a critical change period for women with radically altered social and cultural patterns. Liberal behavior of the period included automobile-based cigarette smoking, drinking, and petting. From this period, the tobacco industry began its portrayal of cigarettes as a form of rebellion, romance, and emancipation for women. Women began to smoke openly in public settings, and female cigarette smoking prevalence rates rose from 2 percent in 1930 to 34 percent in 1965.

Epidemiological Data and Trends

Today more than one in four women under the age of 25 in the United States smokes cigarettes (Fig. 5.1). Although the total percentage of cigarette smokers among women in the United States has declined since 1955, the percentage of women who are **heavy smokers,** defined as those who smoke 25 or more cigarettes a day, has actually increased to 23 percent of the adult female population.[1] Cigarette smoking rates among adult women have never reached those of men, but the prevalence rate of current women smokers peaked at 34 percent in 1965. Since 1965, the decline in current female smokers has been less dramatic than that of the male population, with approximately 27 percent of all adult women being current smokers in 1987 (Fig. 5.2). The percentage of **ever smokers** (the combination of current and former smokers), however, has remained between 45 and 46 percent since 1970 (Fig. 5.2). These data indicate that although the percentage of **former smokers** has increased among adult women between 1956 and 1985, the percentage of ever smokers has remained approximately the same, suggesting that the proportion of women who initiate smoking has not declined.

Another way of looking at the prevalence of smoking behavior among women is by cohort. A **cohort** is a group of individuals who share a common condition or characteristic. A birth cohort represents a group sharing a common specified birth year(s). Fig. 5.3 shows the lifetime prevalence of cigarette smoking by birth cohort groups for adult white women. The lifetime prevalence rates of cigarette smoking among women peaked in the cohorts born between 1930 and 1939 and 1940 and 1949. Male birth cohort data for the same years show the prevalence of cigarette smoking among men exceeds that of women for all birth cohorts except for the youngest (those born 1960 to 1963).[1] These generalizations about trends must consider the differences in the rates of cigarette smoking initiation among men and women. Historically women took up the smoking habit later than men. The prevalence of cigarette smoking is highest

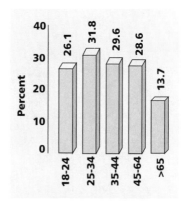

FIGURE 5.1

Current female smokers by age, 1987.

SOURCE: USDDS (1991). *Health United States, 1990.* (DHHS Pub No. (PHS) 91-1232.) Washington, DC: US Government Printing Office.

among men born between 1920 and 1929 and among women born between 1930 and 1949.

Because of differences in data collection and racial/ethnic labeling over the years, data are sometimes difficult to interpret from a racial or ethnic perspective. Cigarette smoking among African American males has always exceeded that of white males. The prevalence of cigarette smoking among African American females appears to be the same or to exceed slightly the prevalence rate among white females.[1] Reliable national data on smoking trends among Hispanic Americans are not available, but current smoking prevalence estimates for Hispanic Americans exceed those for the US population overall.[2] The smoking rates for Hispanic American women are considerably lower than the rates for Hispanic American men, but data do indicate that smoking rates have been steadily increasing among successive cohorts of Hispanic American women while decreasing among corresponding cohorts of Hispanic American men.[3] In a regional study of Chinese, Vietnamese, and Hispanic populations, dramatic differences were present, with Vietnamese women having the lowest overall smoking prevalence rates (Fig. 5.4).

Cigarette smoking prevalence rates also vary by educational level and occupational specialty, with disproportionately higher smoking rates among blue-collar workers and people with fewer years of education. In a national survey, for example, 27 percent of white-collar females were smokers, compared with 37 percent blue-collar females.[2] Although the general prevalence of smoking for all sociodemographic groups is declining, the trend is slowest among the least educated.

Because cigarette smoking is a major contributor to low-birth-weight infants and presents additional risks to mother and baby, it is important to examine the smoking prevalence rates among pregnant women. National data on cigarette smoking during pregnancy are scarce, and estimates vary. Although the overall prevalence of adult female smokers in the United States was recently calculated at 27 percent, data indicate that 29 to 43 percent of reproductive-age women

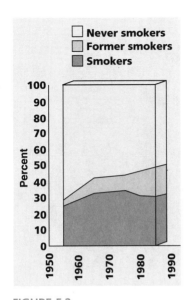

FIGURE 5.2

Adult females by smoking status, selected years.

SOURCE: *Smoking and health: A national status report. A report to Congress.* USDHHS. (HHS/PHS/CDC 87-8396.) Washington, DC: US Government Printing Office.

FIGURE 5.3

Lifetime prevalence of cigarette smoking by birth cohort.

SOURCE: National Health Interview Survey (1983). *Smoking and health: A national status report. A report to Congress.* USDHHS. (HHS/PHS/CDC 87-8396.) Washington, DC: US Government Printing Office.

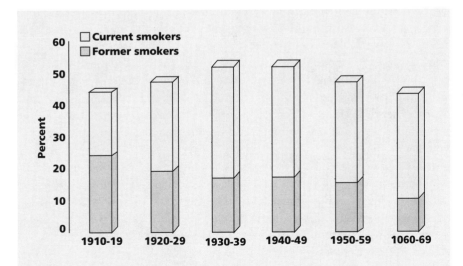

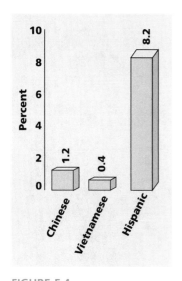

FIGURE 5.4

Percent of current smokers, Chinese, Vietnamese, and Hispanic women, California, 1991.

SOURCE: Centers for Disease Control (1992). Cigarette smoking among Chinese, Vietnamese, and Hispanics—California, 1989–1991. *Morbidity and Mortality Weekly Report.* 41(20), 362–367.

smoke.[1,4,5] These data take on added significance because of the extra risks associated with smoking and pregnancy. In general, unmarried women in the lowest age and socioeconomic categories have the highest likelihood of smoking during pregnancy.[6]

Among people age 20 and older, overall smoking prevalence has been steadily declining, but the most significant trend of women's smoking is the increasing initiation of cigarette smoking among adolescent girls. Adolescent girls are more likely to smoke than their male counterparts. In 1980, the rates of female adolescent smokers surpassed those of adolescent males for the first time. Young female smokers are smoking more cigarettes and even starting the habit younger than male counterparts. National data indicate that almost 5 percent of 12- to 14-year-olds are now smoking, representing an eightfold increase since 1968.[1] Although the trend of smoking initiation among males (with less than or equal to 12 years of education) has declined in prevalence from 46 percent in 1974 to 43 percent in 1985, the prevalence of cigarette smoking initiation of women with similar education has increased from 39 percent to 45 percent.[7] This is of significance to women's health because the younger an individual begins to smoke, the greater the likelihood of difficulty in quitting and early mortality. Earlier initiation of smoking has also been shown to be a predictor in the use of other substances, such as alcohol and illicit drugs, particularly marijuana.[8]

Marketing Dimensions

Advertising is clearly effective in perpetuating and promoting specific products to selected groups. Cigarette advertising is especially effective in increasing cigarette consumption by recruiting new smokers, enticing former smokers to relapse, making it more difficult for current smokers to quit cigarettes, and acting as an external cue or reminder to smoke.[9] Tobacco companies have been targeting specific audiences and promoting specific brands with calculated strategic effort. Cigarettes are one of the most heavily advertised and promoted products in the United States, with an annual expenditure of more than $3.3 billion.[10] Some advertising restraints against the tobacco companies have been levied, however. Direct cigarette advertisement is not permitted on radio or television, but it abounds in printed materials, particularly in publications targeting young women. These advertising and promotional campaigns include the introduction of "feminine" cigarettes, such as Capri, Eve, Satin, and Virginia Slims. The cigarettes are slim or "ultra slim" with decorative borders and sophisticated designer packaging. In addition to promoting "feminine themes," younger models are being used in cigarette advertisements. Tobacco companies also use age subtly to deny the health consequences of smoking by showing women holding happy and healthy babies or depicting several generations of adult women together in smoking situations.

Minority communities, including women, have also been aggressively singled out and targeted by the tobacco industry. Several brands are specifically targeted to the African-American community and are heavily advertised in African American–oriented media. In addition to the typical tobacco printed media advertising, tobacco industries have also sponsored civic, athletic, and cultural events directed at African-American communities. Examples of these events include the Kool Achiever Awards, honoring those committed to improving inner-city life, the anniversary of the United Negro College Fund, and the publication of "A Guide to Black Organizations," sponsored by Philip Morris.[9] Hispanic-American communities have also been targeted by the tobacco industry, although not as heavily as African-American communities. Rio and Dorado are cigarette brands specifically promoted in Hispanic-American communities.

Tobacco companies are not single-product entities, having diversified into megaconglomerate titans that have broad bases of economic and political power in the media industry. With seemingly unlimited annual advertising budgets, tobacco companies are able to exert their influence and promote journalistic complacency on tobacco-related health publications. Studies have shown strong statistical evidence that cigarette advertising in magazines, particularly women's magazines, is associated with diminished coverage of the hazards of smoking.[11]

Although the tobacco industry denies that its advertising is targeted to children and adolescents, cigarette advertising is heavy in many magazines with large adolescent readership. Furthermore, tobacco advertisers typically use image-based ads, such as Joe Camel, which are most effective with young people and have the greatest impact on children whose poor performance in school increases the distance between their ideal and current self-image. *Mirabella,* a stylish young woman's magazine, recently blasted the tobacco industry's manipulation of women, stating, "The prosperous tobacco industry makes a generous friend and a formidable foe . . . [Cigarette ads] are received at a time when a young woman's self-image is at its shakiest, and when she may be most open to a cigarette ad's nonverbal messages." Data indicate that four out of five smokers begin smoking before the age of 21.[1] Individuals who start smoking early have more difficulty in quitting, are more likely to become heavy smokers, and are more likely to develop a smoking-related disease. Many adolescents who smoke do not understand the nature of tobacco addiction and are unaware of, or underestimate, the health consequences of smoking. Current national health objectives are focused on prohibiting the sale and distribution of tobacco products to youth younger than age 19 and on restricting the forms of tobacco advertising and promotion targeting youth.[2]

Indirect advertisement of cigarettes occurs when tobacco companies sponsor events because although federal law prohibits the broadcast advertisement of tobacco products, sponsorship does allow the product name to be mentioned. For example, the Virginia Slims Tennis Tournament has the prominent Virginia Slims logo throughout the view of the camera lens, and the tournament name is frequently mentioned throughout the broadcast period.

Many communities and states have launched smoking restrictions that seek to restrict smoking to designated areas. The public campaigns to reduce smoking, heighten public awareness of the dangers of smoking, and "unsell cigarettes" pale in financial comparison to the mega media campaigns of the tobacco titans. A public campaign has been especially aggressive in California, where the rate

It's so amazing to look through the family photo album and try to image what life was like during various times. The 1950s are particularly interesting to me. But the photos always surprise me—most of the photographs have someone smoking cigarettes in them! Did everyone smoke in the 1950s?

25-YEAR-OLD WOMAN

of smokers quitting cigarettes has doubled. An aggressive advertising campaign there has stigmatized smoking as declasse and dangerous and depicts tobacco companies as loathsome. In one radio ad, a man tells his girlfriend that her yellow teeth are disgusting.

Societal Costs

Human costs are the greatest cost associated with cigarette smoking. No other avoidable condition claims more adult lives than tobacco addiction. Between 2 million and 2.5 million smokers die worldwide each year from smoking-related diseases. Additional thousands die as a result of fires caused by cigarettes and from cancers caused by tobacco consumed as snuff or chews. Almost one-fifth of all deaths in the United States can be traced to tobacco.[2] **Passive smoking,** or involuntary smoking, causes thousands of deaths each year as well. Annual tobacco-related deaths exceed the combined drug and alcohol abuse deaths; automobile fatalities; AIDS deaths; and the number of Americans killed in World Wars I and II, Korea, and Vietnam combined.[12] Smokers pay a human cost before dying as well. The smoking-related diseases of cancer, emphysema, and cardiovascular disease extract a toll of suffering and disability. In working populations, absenteeism is nearly 45 percent higher in the smoking populations than among nonsmokers.[13]

Other societal economic costs are attributable to cigarette smoking. Economic costs of smoking can be measured in two ways. Direct costs are the value of resources that could be allocated to other uses in the absence of disease; indirect costs are the value of idle resources and lost output and may be calculated in terms of morbidity and mortality. Direct costs include health care costs associated with prevention, diagnosis, and treatment of smoking-related illness; expenditures of hospital and nursing home care; professional fees and services; pharmacological preparations; research; and other public health expenditures. In 1982, an estimated total of $322 billion was spent in the United States, or 10.5 percent of the US Gross National Product.[14] Smoking has been attributed to account for specific proportions of each major cause of morbidity and mortality. Calculations indicate that annually smoking is responsible for 38 percent of direct health costs, 17 percent of morbidity costs, and 45 percent of mortality costs for the United States. For 1 year, that represents $42.2 billion dollars. These estimates do not include the costs of cigarettes (estimated at $22 billion in 1980), the costs of fires, or pain and suffering. Clearly the magnitude of costs associated with cigarette smoking exceeds reasonable or affordable boundaries.

Political and Legal Dimensions

Because tobacco is obviously a major threat to public health, the question arises as to why it continues to be so readily available and promoted. Direct smoking and involuntary smoking are responsible for considerable illness, disability, and death, yet they seemingly remain regulation free, while lesser issues like Alar on apples are regulated and banned for the public well-being. Many Americans assume that federal agencies provide comprehensive surveillance and monitoring of all drugs, products, and foodstuffs. The Department of Agriculture, the Food and Drug Administration, and other federal and state agencies do provide comprehensive quality control and assurance of products, foods, and pharmaceuticals. Every consumer knows a story about a baby crib recall, a car part recall, the removal of red dye no. 10, or some other example of government supervision to protect the public health and safety. What many consumers do not know is that tobacco has been excluded from the jurisdiction of the Food and Drug Administration. This exemption permits tobacco to be manufactured and sold to consumers without the quality control and assurance provided to other products, foods, and pharmaceuticals.

Several other political factors affect the availability of tobacco and cigarettes in American society. Cigarette taxes provide considerable revenue to state and national coffers and the loss of revenue can have an impact on legislator's willingness to lose such revenue. The federal government while supporting national objectives to reduce cigarette consumption and research on the treatment of cigarette related diseases, consistently spends federal dollars on tobacco subsidies.

Tobacco industry dollars have also funded innumerable political activities and groups, including women's advocacy groups.[15] Through this courting and fundig of some women's groups and organizations, the tobacco industry has tried to project an image of sensitivity to contemporary women's issues. Unfortunately, there has been a consistent concurrent aggressive marketing of their products to women that result in significant disability and death.

The undeniable bottom line is that cigarette smoking kills Americans and others who smoke American tobacco. It is a national and international issue of ethics versus dollars. The tobacco industry with its multibillion dollar capacity for advertising and lobbying is not about to relinquish its hold on the political system voluntarily. The legal system may present the greatest challenge to the tobacco industry. Litigation efforts have been increasing in an attempt to make the industry responsible for tobacco-related damage. An appeals court ruling preventing smokers from suing for damages from cigarettes smoked after 1966, when mandated health warnings first appeared, has been protecting the tobacco industry. The Supreme Court recently ruled, however, that smokers are allowed to sue tobacco companies. The Court ruled that a federal cigarette labeling law does not protect tobacco companies against all personal-injury suits under state law. The ruling has cleared the way for smokers to sue the tobacco industry for allegedly misleading the public about the hazards of cigarette smoking. This particular case had been watched closely because of its implications not only for health and tobacco interests, but also for the question of how explicit Congress must be for federal statutes to preempt state law.

Health Consequences for Women Who Smoke

The health consequences of smoking for women are a delayed phenomenon. Symptoms of smoking-related illness usually take years to develop, although irritation symptoms such as watery eyes, nasal irritation, squinting, and coughing develop fairly soon after smoking initiation. Smoking affects not only the person smoking, but also others in the smoker's environment, including unborn babies. Although women were once thought to be fairly immune to the ravages of cigarettes, it is realized now that women are exceptionally vulnerable to all the health consequences of smoking (Information Box 5.1; Fig. 5.5).

Morbidity and Mortality

Smoking is responsible for considerable morbidity (illness) and mortality (death) among Americans. Tobacco use has actually been officially identified as the most important single preventable cause of death and disease in our society.[3] The mortality and morbidity associated with cigarette smoking has a dose-response relationship; that is, the higher the number of cigarettes, the greater the number of health-related consequences. Information Box 5.2 presents a comparison on the percent of current smokers by the average number of cigarettes smoked per day for select years 1965 through 1985. Among both male and female smokers, there is a greater percentage of heavier smokers today than in the 1960s or 1970s. The percent of female smokers who smoked 25 or more cigarettes per day increased from 13 percent in 1965 to 23 percent in 1985.

As a result of the trends with cigarette smoking, women are now facing significant smoking-related morbidity and mortality. Because women's cigarette use did not become widespread until the onset of World War II, those women with the greatest intensity of smoking are now still in their "relatively healthy"

INFORMATION BOX 5.1

Women's Health Consequences of Smoking

Increased risk for *cancer*—lungs, larynx, oral cavity, esophagus, kidneys, and cervix

Increased risk for *COLD*—chronic bronchitis, emphysema

Increased risk for *cardiovascular disease*—myocardial infarction, chronic ischemic heart disease, arteriosclerotic vascular disease, subarachnoid hemorrhage, malignant hypertension

Complications of pregnancy and infant health—increased risk for low-birth-weight babies, fetal growth retardation, preterm babies, ectopic pregnancy, spontaneous abortion, fetal death, SIDS, and neonatal death

Other—increased risk for osteoporosis, urinary incontinence, decreased fertility, earlier menopause, peptic ulcer disease, migraine headaches, and facial wrinkles

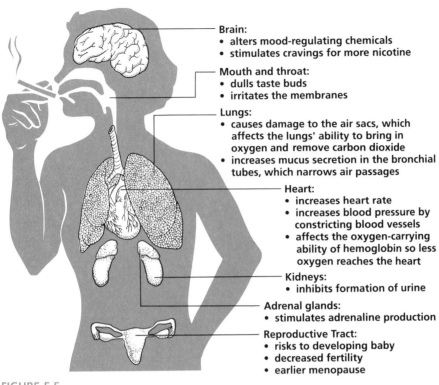

Brain:
• alters mood-regulating chemicals
• stimulates cravings for more nicotine

Mouth and throat:
• dulls taste buds
• irritates the membranes

Lungs:
• causes damage to the air sacs, which affects the lungs' ability to bring in oxygen and remove carbon dioxide
• increases mucus secretion in the bronchial tubes, which narrows air passages

Heart:
• increases heart rate
• increases blood pressure by constricting blood vessels
• affects the oxygen-carrying ability of hemoglobin so less oxygen reaches the heart

Kidneys:
• inhibits formation of urine

Adrenal glands:
• stimulates adrenaline production

Reproductive Tract:
• risks to developing baby
• decreased fertility
• earlier menopause

FIGURE 5.5

Physiological effects of cigarette smoking.

years. As these women age, however, their burden of smoking-related disease/death will continue to grow. Mortality rates vary directly with the amount smoked, the depth of cigarette inhalation, "tar" and nicotine content of cigarettes smoked, and the duration of smoking. Mortality rates also vary inversely with the age of initiation of smoking, meaning that the earlier a women begins to smoke, the shorter her life.

Cardiovascular Disease

Cigarette smoking is clearly associated with cardiovascular morbidity, accounting for 21 percent of all coronary heart disease deaths.[2] Coronary heart disease is the major cause of death among both men and women in the US. Cigarette smoking increases the risk of coronary heart disease for women by a factor of two, and in younger women, cigarette smoking may increase the risk severalfold. The use of oral contraceptives by women smokers increases the risk of myocardial infarction by a factor of approximately 35.[16] Women over the age of 35 who smoke are advised to stop smoking or change their method of contraception. Young and middle-aged women who smoke have substantially higher rates of both fatal and nonfatal stroke.[17] Other cardiovascular conditions associated with women's smoking include lower levels of high-density lipoproteins (HDL):

Percent of Cigarette Smokers by Number of Cigarettes per Day, According to Sex and Survey Year

Number of cigarettes

Males	1965	1976	1980	1983	1985
<15	30.1	24.9	24.2	23.5	28.0
15–24	45.7	44.4	41.7	42.9	42.0
25+	24.1	30.7	34.2	33.6	31.0
Females					
<15	46.2	37.6	34.7	33.8	35.0
15–24	40.8	43.4	42.0	45.6	42.0
25+	13.0	19.0	23.2	20.6	23.0

SOURCE: National Health Interview Survey (1983). *Smoking and health: A national status report. A report to Congress.* (USDHHS HHS/PHS/CDC 87-8396.) Washington, DC: US Government Printing Office.

Increased levels are correlated with reduced risk of peripheral vascular disease, subarachnoid hemorrhage, and severe or malignant hypertension (see Chapter 1).[16] The risk to women of a cardiovascular event from smoking is dose related. Women who smoke more than 25 cigarettes per day have a relative risk of 5.4 for a fatal coronary event and 5.8 for nonfatal coronary disease.[18] Women have been shown to have a protective factor for heart disease before menopause; however, the mechanism by which smoking "destroys" this natural protection for women is not well understood.

Cancer

Cigarette smoking has been shown to be a major risk factor for cancers throughout the body. Specifically it is causally associated with cancer of the lung, larynx, oral cavity, and esophagus in women as well as in men. Smoking accounts for 87 percent of lung cancer deaths and 30 percent of all cancer deaths.[1] A unique feature to women is that it is also associated with kidney cancer. Both cigarette smoking and exposure to passive smoke significantly increase a woman's risk of cervical cancer.[19] Lung cancer rates for women had a 250 percent increase from 1950 to 1977 compared with a 200 percent increase for men.[20] The changing trends in women's lung cancer rates are attributed to the fact that when the male-to-female ratio was greater (before 1960), women had shorter smoking histories; they started smoking later in life; and their numbers of cigarettes smoked per day were less than in 1960. As a result of the declining prevalence of smoking among men, lung cancer death rates for men have begun to level off. Among women, however, lung cancer death rates have continued to increase and have now surpassed breast cancer as the leading cause of cancer deaths for women. Women now have an incidence rate of lung cancer nearly identical to that of men 30 years ago.[1] As current female smokers continue the cigarette habit, it has been predicted that lung cancer rates will continue to rise for both male and female smokers, and the male-to-female ratio will continue to fall. A similar trend has been noted for male-to-female laryngeal cancer ratios. The combination of addictive behaviors seems to be particularly damaging in women. Studies demonstrate that the excessive ingestion of alcohol acts synergistically with cigarette smoking to increase the incidence of oral and laryngeal cancer in women.[16]

Smoking and Pregnancy

Cigarette smoking present special risks to pregnant women and their unborn babies. It has been estimated that if all pregnant women stopped smoking, the number of fetal and infant deaths would be reduced by 10 percent.[21] Cigarette smoking during pregnancy accounts for 20 to 30 percent of low-birth-weight babies, up to 14 percent of all preterm deliveries, and about 10 percent of all infant deaths. Maternal cigarette smoking during pregnancy also retards fetal growth and is associated with miscarriage, stillbirth, sudden infant death syndrome, and infant mortality.[16] Women who smoke during pregnancy also have a greater risk for ectopic pregnancy.[22] These risks increase directly with increasing doses of smoking. Nicotine and carbon monoxide are considered the two most important components in cigarettes that constitute major hazards to the fetus. Nicotine has been shown to reduce fetal breathing movements, reduce uterine blood flow, and increase fetal heart rate. Carbon monoxide reduces the amount of oxygen available to the fetus. Quitting smoking may be one of the most significant things a pregnant woman can do to optimize the well-being of her baby. Maternal prenatal smoking is not the only detrimental smoking source for the infant. Studies suggest that paternal smoking may present a genetic risk for the baby as well. Women can continue to transmit smoking effects directly biologically after the baby is born via breast milk. Breast-fed babies whose mothers smoke show evidence of a nicotine metabolite in their urine, indicating that nicotine passes through breast milk.[23]

Other Health Consequences

Cigarette smoking severely damages the respiratory system. **Chronic obstructive lung disease** (COLD), also known as chronic obstructive pulmonary disease (COPD), is characterized by permanent airflow obstruction. This condition is also characterized by extended periods of disability and restricted activity. Cigarette smoking is the major risk factor for developing COLD, with more than 80 percent of all COLD deaths in the United States attributed to smoking.[3] COLD male-to-female mortality ratios are decreasing in a similar pattern to lung cancer ratios. Experts predict that owing to the long duration of smoking

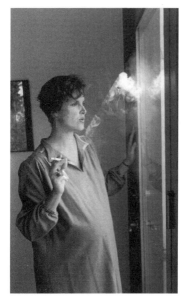

Smoking presents many risks to a mother and her unborn child.

I realized when I became pregnant that the cigarettes would have to go. All these years I haven't worried about what effect smoking had on me. But I wanted to do everything I could to ensure the health of my baby.

25-YEAR-OLD WOMAN

required to damage lungs resulting in COLD death, the next few decades will show a continued rise in mortality attributed solely to the increase in women's smoking. **Emphysema** and **chronic bronchitis** are usually included in the broad definition of COLD. With emphysema, the limitation of airflow is the result of disease changes in the lung tissue. The air sacs in the lungs become destroyed, and the lungs are compromised in bringing oxygen and removing carbon dioxide from the body. As a result, breathing becomes compromised, and there is increased demand placed on the heart. Chronic bronchitis is characterized by constant inflammation of the bronchial tubes. The inflammation thickens the walls of the bronchi, and the production of mucus increases, resulting in a constricting or narrowing of the air passages.

Cigarette smoking is also associated with many other illnesses, including stomach and duodenal ulcers and cirrhosis of the liver. Smoking appears to worsen the symptoms or complications of allergies, diabetes, hypertension, and existing disorders of the pulmonary and circulatory system. Like men, women experience these other health consequences of cigarette smoking as well as other gender-specific consequences. Women who smoke face an increased risk of osteoporosis, prematurely wrinkled skin, and urinary incontinence. Women who smoke are also less fertile than nonsmoking women. Researchers have also demonstrated an association between cigarette smoking and the age of natural menopause, with smokers reaching spontaneous menopause 1 to 2 years earlier than nonsmoking women. The age differences in menopause appear to be smoking dose dependent.

Involuntary Smoking

Involuntary smoking is also known as passive smoking or environmental tobacco smoke (ETS). It results in nonsmokers having to breathe the contaminated air from smokers. Involuntary smoking is not benign, causing disease, including lung cancer, in healthy nonsmokers and severe respiratory problems in young infants and children.[2,24] The ETS issue is of special concern for children, where the major source of smoke exposure for young children is their home. Children of parents who smoke are more likely to develop lower respiratory tract infections, be hospitalized, or see a physician for these conditions during the first year of life than children of parents who do not smoke. Parental smoking may compromise lung infection in young children and the developing lungs of the growing child.[25] Some researchers suggest that it may also contribute to the rise of chronic airflow obstruction later in life.[26] Otitis media, the most common illness requiring medical attention among children, is considerably more common among children whose parents smoke.[27]

Adults are also seriously affected by ETS. Nonsmokers who live with smokers are at a higher risk of death from cancer and heart disease than those who live with nonsmokers. For women, there is a trend of increasing mortality with increasing levels of exposure.[28] The home is not the only area of concern about ETS. Involuntary smoking has become a recent issue in the workplace. The separation of smokers and nonsmokers within the same airspace may reduce but does not eliminate the exposure of nonsmokers to ETS. Studies have shown an increased risk of lung cancer in nonsmokers chronically exposed to tobacco smoke. For adults living in households where no one smokes, the workplace is the greatest source of exposure to ETS. Although long-term studies on the effect of worksite ETS have not yet been conducted, preliminary findings suggest that employees exposed to ETS are at greater risk of developing small airways dysfunction than are nonexposed employees.[29] These findings are significant because small airway disease is also the first pathological change seen in beginning smokers, suggesting that these employees may be at increased risk of developing disabling airways obstruction.

Smoking as a Health Behavior

An understanding of smoking as a health behavior requires an understanding of cigarettes. There are literally thousands of compounds in tobacco smoke, but the most significant from a health perspective are nicotine, tar, and carbon monoxide. Nicotine is the addictive element in cigarettes. Nicotine has multiple effects on the body including increasing blood pressure, increasing heart rate, and negating hunger. Tar is a thick, sticky dark fluid produced when tobacco is burned. Tar is actually composed of hundreds of compounds, many of which are carcinogenic, capable of promoting growth of cancerous cells, in their own right. Through inhalation, tar settles and accumulates throughout the oral cavity and pulmonary system. The combination of tar and smoke further compromises the cardiopulmonary system. Carbon monoxide is another deadly byproduct of cigarettes. Carbon monoxide interferes with the ability of the blood to carry oxygen, impairs normal functioning of the nervous system, and contributes to degradation of the cardiopulmonary system.

Health risks to smokers not only depend on their smoking status, but also on their specific smoking behaviors and the duration of such behaviors. Cigarette dose is based on the age of initiation of smoking, the total number of years smoked, cigarette type (nicotine levels, tar content), and the number of cigarettes smoked per day. Inhalation patterns and puffing behavior also determine exposure to carbon monoxide and other toxic compounds. Studies have shown that nicotine-dependent smokers change their inhalation patterns to obtain varying amounts of the drug. This compensatory behavior has been observed in smokers who switch to brands with lower tar and nicotine levels, suggesting that such brand switching probably does not reduce overall health risks. Researchers have attempted to ascertain possible sex differences in smoking patterns, but to date the findings have been somewhat contradictory.

Smoking as an Addiction

Tobacco dependence is an addictive disorder affecting most smokers. Tobacco dependence disorder is recognized as a distinct clinical condition. It is defined as the inability to discontinue smoking despite the awareness of medical consequences. Addiction is defined as dependence on a drug such that stopping results in withdrawal symptoms. When measured by the percentage of users who lose control of their substance intake, nicotine is six to eight times more

I realized that I really was hooked on cigarettes when I became desperate in the middle of the night and couldn't find any in the house. I was frantic. I tried to pretend that I could get along without having a cigarette but it didn't work. We were having a terrible snowstorm, and I actually left the children alone in the house and drove to a convenience store in my bathrobe to buy a pack.

32-YEAR-OLD WOMAN

addictive than alcohol.[12] Smoking is clearly an addictive behavior, and nicotine is the addictive pharmacological component. It may be considered the ideal drug of abuse because it is easily available, can be delivered in various doses, is fast-acting, and has multiple behavioral and physiological effects. Smoking cessation results in withdrawal, an adverse reaction characterized by unpleasant symptoms and an intense psychological and physiological demand for nicotine. The symptoms usually include cigarette craving, irritability, restlessness, anxiety, difficulty concentrating, headache, drowsiness, and varied gastrointestinal disturbances such as diarrhea and constipation. To date, there have been no definitive studies on male/female differences in withdrawal symptoms or patterns. Self-Assessment 5.1 provides an opportunity to assess whether or not an individual is addicted to cigarette smoking.

Why Women Smoke

Women often initiate cigarette smoking in adolescence in the context of social interactions with peers. Cigarettes are initially found to be aversive to the beginning smoker, but peer pressure may provide the appropriate social rewards for tolerance. Studies have found smoking status of "best friends" to be a predictor of adolescent smoking status. Another important influence appears to be imitation of peers and significant adults. Adolescents are more likely to be smokers if their parents or older siblings smoke. Reasons for the current male/female differences in smoking initiation rates are not currently understood.

There is no consensus yet on why women smoke. Women often rationalize their reasons for smoking (Information Box 5.3). Perhaps there are many physiological reasons for women's smoking because an interesting effect of nicotine is that it is capable of multiple effects, acting at times as a relaxer and at other times as a stimulant. Affect regulation is an important component of

---

SELF-ASSESSMENT 5.1

Are You Addicted to Cigarettes?

Carefully read and answer each of the questions honestly.

Have you ever failed in an attempt to give up cigarettes? _____ yes _____ no

Have you ever failed in an attempt to cut back on cigarettes? _____ yes _____ no

Have you ever failed in an attempt to switch to a lower tar and nicotine cigarette? _____ yes _____ no

When you have not had a cigarette for a while, do you feel any withdrawal symptoms, such as an urge for a cigarette, irritability, anxiety, difficulty concentrating, or drowsiness? _____ yes _____ no

Have you developed any smoking-related side effects, such as a morning cough or a hoarse voice, yet continue to smoke? _____ yes _____ no

If you answered "yes" to any of these questions, you are probably hooked on cigarettes and have an addiction to tobacco. It is time to quit cigarettes.

INFORMATION BOX 5.3

Common Rationalizations of Women Smokers

It can't be as bad as they say. The government wouldn't let them sell cigarettes if they were that harmful.

I am not worried. My aunt lived to be 80 and she smoked.

We all have to die sometime.

I have so much stress in my life. I really need cigarettes to make things better.

I don't want to gain weight.

I smoke for pleasure. I actually enjoy my cigarettes.

It is OK if I smoke because I eat well and exercise every day.

I only smoke at work, not at home.

I only smoke low-tar cigarettes.

I am too busy to eat, and smoking helps me control my hunger.

---

smoking, with many smokers reporting that their primary reason for smoking is to reduce negative affect. Male/female differences have been reported: Female smokers are more likely than males to smoke to reduce negative affect, and male smokers are more likely to smoke out of habit than female smokers.[16] Pleasure is a reason often cited by women for smoking. Nicotine does reinforce and strengthen the desire to smoke. It also may facilitate short-term memory, help in performing certain tasks, reduce anxiety, negate hunger symptoms, and increase pain tolerance.

Fear of unwanted weight gain is one reason that women report for not quitting smoking.[30] Even many pregnant women who smoke indicate that their reason for doing so is to avoid weight gain. Smokers do tend to weigh less than nonsmokers. There is no agreement of scientists yet regarding the physiological or biochemical mechanism responsible for weight regulation and smoking behavior. There is evidence that nicotine elevates the body's basal metabolic rate (BMR). Women's concerns about weight gain and the maintenance of their smoking behavior sadly reflect their preoccupation about body size and their willingness to risk long-term detrimental and potentially catastrophic consequences for body image and weight control issues.

Quitting Smoking

Quitting smoking is the most significant personal behavior in improving one's health. Seventeen percent of all adult women are now former smokers. Although the recovery from smoking takes time, cessation of smoking results in a gradual decrease in cancer and cardiovascular disease risk; for example, after 10 to 20 years of cessation, lung cancer rates for former smokers approach the rates of lifetime nonsmokers.[2,31] Unfortunately this is not true for COLD. With cessation of smoking, the rate of functional pulmonary loss declines, but lost function cannot be regained. Timely cigarette smoking cessation is the best prevention of symptomatic pulmonary disease.

Quitting smoking is not an easy process. Most smokers report that they would like to quit. Men's smoking rates have experienced a 14 percent decline in the last 20 years, whereas women's rates have declined only 5 percent in the same period. Similar numbers of male and female smokers have reported ever trying to quit, but these attempts are largely unsuccessful. Although there are numerous strategies, formal and informal in nature, for quitting smoking, most of the people who have quit smoking have done so on their own after numerous previous failures. An important determinant in smoking cessation is ascertaining what type of smoker an individual may be. Self-Assessment 5.2 assesses a person's smoker type.

For the woman who wants to quit smoking on her own, there are two options, gradual reduction and "cold turkey." Gradual reduction is a process of gently tapering not only the number of daily cigarettes by cutting back on the absolute number of cigarettes, but also the relative amount of tar and nicotine by changing brands to lower and lower levels. It is wise to set a quit date at some point in the future, usually a few weeks and aim for that day with a gradual reduction. There are many strategies that can be used in the process of gradual reduction (Information Box 5.4). All of these strategies serve to modify traditional smoking behavior and reinforce progress toward total cessation. Going cold turkey means a decisive, sudden break from cigarettes. Some people find that they are able to go cold turkey if they do it one day at a time. They promise themselves to be smoke free for 24 hours, and at the end of that day, they reaffirm their commitment to another day. It may take several weeks or months for a former heavy smoker to become confident about the newly acquired nonsmoking status.

Smoking cessation programs have evolved since 1964 with the First Surgeon

---

INFORMATION BOX 5.4

Strategies to Quit Cigarettes Gradually

Wait 15 minutes after the initial urge for a cigarette. This gives a feeling of control and sometimes the urge will go away.

When an urge for a cigarette presents, use a distraction such as drink water, make a phone call, take a short walk, or brush the teeth.

Avoid the places where the smoking habit has thrived—a favorite chair, lingering after a meal, a coffee break.

Establish nonsmoking hours and gradually extend them.

Buy cigarettes only by the pack and never the same brand twice in a row.

Try to buy successively lower brands of tar and nicotine.

Make it harder to get your cigarettes. Keep them in a locked drawer or with a friend.

Declare old smoking areas "nonsmoking areas," such as the car, house, and office.

Don't empty ashtrays. Collect cigarette butts and take a deep breath of the collection every day as a reminder of how dirty and smelly the smoking habit is.

Keep a daily record to document and reinforce progress with quitting.

General's Report on Smoking. Although there have been many attempts to compare "success" rates of methods over the years since, numerous confounding variables make such comparisons of limited value. Many programs measure "success" at the completion of the program, not 6 months or 1 year later, when many individuals may have relapsed. Other programs "count" only the individuals present at the end of the program, dropping those from the denominator who left the program before its completion, perhaps because of their inability to quit smoking. It also can be argued that smokers today are "different" from those of previous years—with the "light" or "easy" smokers having quit in the first round of cessation programs and the heavier or more addicted smokers remaining. Self-reported "success" presents validation difficulties, although self-reported smoking status can be biologically verified by urine, blood, or saliva tests.

Intervention strategies for smoking cessation include a variety of treatment modalities. They may be individually or group based, formal or informal in design. Multicomponent behaviorally oriented programs seem to elicit the most favorable results for short-term and long-term cigarette cessation. These programs often incorporate a variety of treatment modalities, including aversive conditioning, contracting, self-control, stimulus control, group support, and cessation maintenance. Pharmacological agents such as nicotine gum are often used with multicomponent treatment programs. Although not all studies of nicotine gum have produced consistent results, a number have shown that use of the gum—not by itself but in conjunction with sessions of counseling to deal with psychological issues—can help some people stop smoking.

Some people have found that nicotine gum has a disagreeable taste or upsets the stomach. A recent addition to the smoking cessation strategy arena is the nicotine patch. The transdermal nicotine patch is proving to be a more effective alternative to the gum. A piece of fabric is impregnated with nicotine and is worn on the skin and changed daily. By providing a steady dose of nicotine through the skin, the patch relieves withdrawal symptoms of smoking cessation. The patch is not to be used longer than 3 months, and the dose of nicotine delivered is slowly reduced over that time period. In its first 6 months on the market, the patch had more than $300 million in sales.[32] The patch delivers a steady low dose of nicotine through the skin. Studies have found that smokers who used the patch, in conjunction with a comprehensive smoking cessation program, were able to stop smoking more easily than those who simply relied on counseling.[33] The patch must be worn correctly. Overdosing on the patch can result in abdominal pain, vomiting, and mental confusion, and severe overdoses can cause respiratory problems. It is also important that the user not continue to smoke while wearing the patch. Smoking while wearing a patch can lead to low blood pressure and respiratory failure. Nicotine patches are not inexpensive, but they do not cost more than a two-pack per day cigarette habit, either.

Cigarette smoking cessation may be accompanied by a wide range of withdrawal symptoms that show considerable variability in their duration and intensity. For heavy smokers, withdrawal symptoms may occur within 2 hours of the last cigarette. The peak period of physiological symptoms from smoking cessation is usually 24 to 48 hours into abstinence, but many smokers report "craving" cigarettes for as long as a year.

Why Do I Smoke?

This activity will help you identify smoking behaviors that, if recognized and controlled, could help you kick the habit. It will also advance your understanding of smoking behavior. If you do not smoke, have a friend who does smoke respond to these questions and discuss the results.

Directions: Respond to each question by circling one of the choices: 5 = Always, 4 = Frequently, 3 = Occasionally, 2 = Seldom, 1 = Never. Important: *Answer every question.*

		Always	Frequently	Occasionally	Seldom	Never
A.	I smoke cigarettes to keep myself from slowing down.	5	4	3	2	1
B.	Handling a cigarette is part of the enjoyment of smoking it.	5	4	3	2	1
C.	Smoking cigarettes is pleasant and relaxing.	5	4	3	2	1
D.	I light a cigarette when I feel angry about something.	5	4	3	2	1
E.	When I run out of cigarettes, I find it almost unbearable until I can get more.	5	4	3	2	1
F.	I smoke automatically, without even being aware of it.	5	4	3	2	1
G.	I smoke to stimulate myself, to perk myself up.	5	4	3	2	1
H.	Part of the enjoyment of smoking a cigarette comes from the steps I take to light it.	5	4	3	2	1
I.	I find cigarettes pleasurable.	5	4	3	2	1
J.	When I feel uncomfortable or upset about something, I light a cigarette.	5	4	3	2	1
K.	When I am not smoking a cigarette, I am very much aware of that fact.	5	4	3	2	1
L.	I light a cigarette without realizing I still have one burning in the ashtray.	5	4	3	2	1
M.	I smoke cigarettes to give me a lift.	5	4	3	2	1
N.	When I smoke a cigarette, part of the enjoyment is watching the smoke as I exhale it.	5	4	3	2	1
O.	I want a cigarette most when I am relaxed and comfortable.	5	4	3	2	1
P.	When I feel blue or want to take my mind off cares and worries, I smoke.	5	4	3	2	1
Q.	I get a real gnawing hunger for a cigarette when I haven't smoked for a while.	5	4	3	2	1
R.	I've found a cigarette in my mouth and didn't remember putting it there.	5	4	3	2	1

Scoring

1. In the spaces that follow, enter the number you have circled for each question, putting the number you have circled for question A over line A, for question B over line B, and so on.
2. Add the three scores on each line to get your totals. For example, the sum of your scores over lines A, G, and M gives you your score on Stimulation; lines B, H and N give the score on Handling; and so on.

_____ + _____ + _____ = _____
  A   G   M   Stimulation

_____ + _____ + _____ = _____
  B   H   N   Handling

_____ + _____ + _____ = _____
  C   I   O   Pleasurable relaxation

_____	+	_____	+	_____	=	_____	
D		J		P			Crutch: tension reduction
_____	+	_____	+	_____	=	_____	
E		K		Q			Craving: signs of addiction
_____	+	_____	+	_____	=	_____	
F		L		R			Habit

Your total score in each category gives a rough indication of how important each factor is to you:

11–15 Highly important   7–10 Somewhat important   3–6 Not important

If you scored below 7 in every one of the six categories, it should be easy for you to quit smoking. If you scored higher in two or more, and particularly if you scored high in the "craving" and "habit" categories, you may have to use multiple strategies to counteract the reward that smoking currently gives you.

A score of 11 or above on any item indicates that this factor is an important source of satisfaction for you. The higher your score (15 is the highest), the more important a particular factor is in your smoking and the more useful the discussion of that factor can be in your efforts to quit.

Explanation of Factors

1. *Stimulation.* If you scored high on this factor, it means that you are one of those who is stimulated by the cigarette—that is, you feel that it helps you wake up, organize your energies, and keep you going. If you try to give up smoking, you may want a safe substitute—a brisk walk or moderate exercise, for example—whenever you feel the urge to smoke.
2. *Handling.* Handling things can be satisfying, but there are many ways to keep your hands busy without lighting up or playing with a cigarette. Why not toy with a pen or pencil? Try doodling, or play with a coin, a piece of jewelry, or some other harmless object.
3. *Accentuation of pleasure—pleasurable relaxation.* It is not always easy to find out whether you use the cigarette to feel good—that is, to get real pleasure out of smoking (factor 3)—or to keep from feeling so bad (factor 4). Those who do get real pleasure out of smoking often find that an honest consideration of the harmful effects is enough to help them quit. They substitute eating, drinking, social activities, and physical activities—within reasonable bounds—and find they do not seriously miss their cigarettes.
4. *Reduction of negative feelings or crutch.* Many smokers use the cigarette as a kind of crutch in moments of stress or discomfort, and on occasion it may work; the cigarette is sometimes used as a tranquilizer. However, those who smoke heavily, people who try to handle severe personal problems by smoking many times a day, are apt to discover that cigarettes do not help them deal effectively with problems.

   When it comes to quitting, this kind of smoker may find it easy to stop when everything is going well but may be tempted to start again in times of crisis. Again, physical exertion, eating, drinking, or social activity—in moderation—may serve as useful substitutes for cigarettes, even in times of tension.
5. *Craving or psychological addiction.* Quitting smoking is difficult for people who score high on the factor of psychological addiction. For them, craving for the next cigarette begins to build up the moment they put one out; so tapering off is not likely to work. They must go cold turkey. It may be helpful for these smokers to smoke more than usual for a day or two, so that the taste for cigarettes is spoiled, and then isolate themselves completely from cigarettes until the craving is gone. Giving up cigarettes may be so difficult and cause so much discomfort that once they do quit, they will find it easy to resist the temptation to go back to smoking.
6. *Habit.* This kind of smoker is no longer getting much satisfaction from cigarettes. Those who smoke from habit frequently light cigarettes without even realizing they are doing so. They may find it easy to quit and stay off them if they can break the habit patterns they have built up. Cutting down gradually may be quite effective if there is a change in the way cigarettes are smoked and in the conditions under which they are smoked. The key to success is becoming aware of each cigarette you smoke.

SOURCE: Adapted from Test III of the *Smoker's Self-Testing Kit,* which was developed by Dr. Daniel H. Horn and originally printed by the National Clearinghouse for Smoking and Health, Department of Health, Education, and Welfare, 1980.

Many women are afraid to quit cigarettes for fear of gaining weight. Nicotine intake does seem to decrease the consumption of sweet foods. Women quitting cigarettes seem to want to eat more than usual and gain weight more than their male counterparts.[30] Because teenage girls are so weight conscious, this may be one of the reasons that they are the fastest-growing group of smokers. It should be remembered that smoking is far more detrimental to health and longevity than a few extra pounds, and it is far less appealing. The American Cancer Society reports that smokers who develop a fitness program in conjunction with their cessation efforts stay at the same weight or lose weight.[34] When quitting smoking, it may be the perfect time to think about total health and fitness by selecting foods carefully and incorporating an exercise program in the new nonsmoking lifestyle (see Chapters 1 and 2). The benefits from this combination of activities are far more important than the weight control subject.

It is difficult to draw specific conclusions on smoking cessation programs and women. Studies are not available that conclude that male and female quit rates are different when history and method of cessation are controlled. Current research is deficient in program development and evaluation of cessation treatment strategies for women.

Informed Decision Making for Women

Smoking is a major risk to all facets of women's health. Smokers face disproportionate risks of morbidity and mortality, but nonsmokers are not exempt or immune because of society's tolerance of tobacco. Informed consumers are aware of the multidimensional and interdependent issues of smoking and realize that there is no immediate or simple solution to the problem. What can the informed woman do regarding smoking? If a woman is a smoker, the single most significant step she can take to improve her chances of well-being is to quit smoking. Regardless of the difficulty, and there is no denying that breaking any addictive behavior is difficult, there are no excuses or rationalizations that suffice or compare to the devastating consequences of smoking. If a woman is a nonsmoker, she should avoid involuntary smoking.

Tobacco can be considered to be a drug. When two drugs are taken together, they can interact to produce side effects that do not occur or that may be more tolerable if the drug is taken alone. For that reason, it is important that physicians know which drugs a patient is taking. Women often fail to consider tobacco as a drug. Information Box 5.5 presents a summary of common drugs with which tobacco interacts. Sample representative brand names are included. Tobacco should be identified as a drug when health care providers inquire about medications or drug use. It may also be helpful to advise friends who smoke that there are potential interactive effects of tobacco with pharmacological preparations.

The avoidance of involuntary smoking is not as simple as it sounds. Although legislation is restricting smoking areas, smoking still occurs in public transportation, worksites, and shopping facilities. Nonsmokers' desire for a "smoke-free"

Common Drugs with Which Tobacco Interacts

Tobacco Smoking interacts with	Adverse Effects
Acetaminophen (Anacin-3, Tylenol, Valadol)	Decreases effect
Antidepressants, tricyclic (Elavil, Norpramin, Tofranil)	Decreases effect
Benzodiazeprines (Dalmane, Halcion, Valium, Xanax)	May decrease sedative effect
Cimetidine (Tagamet)	Slows ulcer healing
Contraceptives, oral (Norinyl, Ovral, Triphasil)	Increases risk of heart and blood vessel disease
Estrogens (Estraderm, Estratab, Premarin)	May decrease effect of estrogen; increases risk of heart and blood vessel disease
Insulin (Humulin, Novolin, Velosulin)	Decreases effect
Mexiletine (Mexitil)	May decrease effect
Nifedipine (Adalat, Procardia)	Decreases effect
Propranolol (Inderol)	Decreases beta-blocking effect
Theophylline (Slo-Phyllin, Theo-Dur)	Decreases effect

SOURCE: "Alcohol, caffeine, and tobacco are drugs, too." Copyright 1991 by Consumers Union of U.S., Inc., Yonkers, NY 10703-1057. Reprinted by permission from CONSUMER REPORTS ON HEALTH, February (1991).

environment presents a potential threat to smokers, who feel that their rights to smoke are violated. Is it possible for both nonsmokers and smokers to coexist in "separate but equal" environments? This question and others are currently being pursued in legal and legislative debate. The challenge for nonsmokers is to assert their right for a smoke-free environment in a nonviolent but assertive manner. Much of the resistance by smokers is defensive, further reminders of their own awareness of the need to quit and their fear of failure and frustration with the process.

Summary

A woman's decision to smoke is generally made during her early teen years. Despite the overwhelming evidence of the detrimental effects of smoking, many adult women continue to smoke and risk further harm to themselves, their children, and others in their environment. The single most healthy decision a woman can make is not to smoke and to quit if she does. Nonsmokers can help smokers through the difficult quitting process with encouragement and patience. The elimination of smoking behavior is a cornerstone to the improvement of women's health in the United States.

"Poison at Home and at Work"

Newsweek, June 28, 1992

The Environmental Protection Agency (EPA) has released a draft form of a new report that links Environmental Tobacco Smoke (ETS) with a range of respiratory diseases. ETS is referred to as a "human carcinogen." This is a significant designation of ETS, for if the EPA adopts this designation, ETS would have the same status as arsenic and asbestos. Although the findings in the report are not new, the conclusions reached by the report are generally stronger than previous reports. The current report states that ETS causes thousands of annual lung cancer deaths, contributes to hundreds of thousands of respiratory infections in babies, triggers new cases of asthma, and exacerbates symptoms of asthmatic children. Women are not immune from the effects of ETS. In a review of over 30 worldwide studies comparing lung cancer rates for two classes of nonsmoking women, those living with smokers and those living with nonsmokers, smokers' spouses had significantly greater prevalence of lung cancer. The women breathing the most smoke, suffered the greatest increase in risk. Americans who live or work among smokers experience a 20 to 30 percent increase in lung-cancer risk.

Philosophical Dimensions: Smoking and Women's Health

1. Cigarette manufacturers have increased their advertising and promotional efforts in recent years by targeting teens, young women, and minorities, groups which may be less aware of the detrimental effects of smoking. Should the government restrict advertising to these groups? Why or why not?

2. Can smokers' rights and nonsmokers both be protected at the same time?

3. How can young girls be inoculated to resist peer pressure and advertising pressure to initiate cigarette smoking?

4. What are the benefits and risks of women's groups accepting monies from the tobacco industry?

5. If a woman does not need a medical prescription to purchase cigarettes, why should she need a prescription for a nicotine patch to quit cigarettes?

References

1. USDHHS (1987). *Smoking and health: A national status report. A report to Congress.* (USDHHS HHS/PHS/CDC 87-8396.) Washington, DC: US Government Printing Office.

2. USDHHS (1990). *Healthy People 2000: National health promotion and disease prevention objectives.* (USDHHS HHS/PHS/CDC 91-50212.) Washington, DC: US Government Printing Office.

3. Escobedo, L.G., and Remington, P.L. (1989). Birth cohort analysis of prevalence of cigarette smoking among Hispanics in the United States. *Journal of the American Medical Association, 261*(1), 66–69.

4. Prager, K., Malin, H., Spiegler, D., VanNatta, P., and Placek, P.J. (1984). Smoking and drinking behavior before and after pregnancy of married mothers of live born infants and still born infants. *Public Health Reports, 99,* 117–127.

5. Schoenborn, C.A. (1988). Health promotion and disease prevention: United States: 1985. *Vital and Health Statistics.* (Series 10, No. 155. DHHS Pub. No. (PHS)88-1591.) Washington, DC: US Government Printing Office.

6. Fingerhut, L.A., Klineman, J.C., and Kendrick, J.S. (1990). Smoking before, during, and after pregnancy. *American Journal of Public Health, 80*(5), 541–544.

7. Pierce, J., Fiore, M., Novotny, T., Hatzaindreu, E., and Davis, R. (1989). Trends in cigarette smoking in the United States: educational differences are increasing. *Journal of the American Medical Association, 261*(1), 56–60.

8. USDHHS (1989). National Institute on Drug Abuse. *Illicit drug use, smoking, and drinking by American high school students, college students, and young adults, 1975–1987.* (DHHS Pub. No. (ADM) 92-1887.) Washington, DC: US Government Printing Office.

9. Davis, R.M. (1987). Current trends in tobacco advertising and marketing. *New England Journal of Medicine, 316,* 725–732.

10. Centers for Disease Control. (1990). Cigarette advertising—United States, 1988. *Morbidity and Mortality Weekly Report, 39,* 261–265.

11. Warner, K.H., Goldenhar, L.M., and McLaughlin, C.G. (1992). Cigarette advertising and magazine coverage of the hazards of smoking. *New England Journal of Medicine, 326*(5), 305–309.

12. Pollin, W. (1984). The role of the addictive process as a key step in causation of all tobacco-related diseases. *Journal of the American Medical Association, 252*(20), 2874.

13. USDHHS (1989). *Reducing the health consequences of smoking: 25 years of progress. A report of the Surgeon General.* (DHHS Pub. No. (CDC) 89-8411.) Washington, DC: US Government Printing Office.

14. Rice, D.P., and Hodgson, T.A. (1983). *Economic costs of smoking: an analysis of data for the United States.* Paper presented at Allied Social Science Association Annual Meeting. San Francisco, CA.

15. Williams, M. (1991, November). Tobacco's hold on women's groups. *The Washington Post,* p. A1.

16. USDHHS (1983). *Health consequences of smoking for women: a report of the Surgeon General.* Washington, DC: US Government Printing Office.

17. Colditz, G.A., Bonita, R., Stampfer, M.J., Willett, W.C., Rosner, B., Speizer, F.E., and Hennekens, C.H. (1988). Cigarette smoking and risk of stroke in middle-aged women. *New England Journal of Medicine, 318*(15), 937–941.

18. Cyr, M., and Moulton, A. (1990). Substance abuse in women. *Obstetrics and Gynecology Clinics of North America, 17*(4), 905–924.

19. Slattery, M.L., Robison, L.M., Schuman, K.L., French, T.K., Abbott, T.M., Overall, J.C., and Gardner, J.W. (1989). Cigarette smoking and exposure to passive smoke are risk factors for cervical cancer. *Journal of the American Medical Association, 261*(11), 1593–1598.

20. USDHHS (1990). *Cancer Statistics Review.* (NIH Pub. No. 90-2789.) Bethesda, MD: Division of Cancer Prevention and Control, National Cancer Institute.

21. Kleinman, J.C., Pierre, M.B., Madans, J.H., Land, G.H., and Schramn, W.F. (1988). The effects of maternal smoking on fetal and infant mortality. *American Journal of Epidemiology, 127*(2), 274–282.

22. Handler, A., Davis, F., Ferre, C., and Yeko, T. (1989). The relationship of smoking and ectopic pregnancy. *American Journal of Public Health, 79*(9), 1239–1242.

23. Labrecque, M., Marcoux, S., Weber, J.P., Fabia, J., and Ferron, L. (1989). Feeding and urine cotinine values in babies whose mothers smoke. *Pediatrics, 83*(1), 93–97.

24. Martin, T.R., and Bracken, M.B. (1986). Association of low birth weight with passive smoke exposure in pregnancy. *American Journal of Epidemiology, 124,* 633–642.

25. Neuspiel, D.R., Rush, D., Butler, N.R, Golding, J., Bijur, P.E. and Kurzon, M. (1989). Parental smoking and post-infancy wheezing in children: a prospective cohort study. *American Journal of Public Health, 79,*(2) 168–171.

26. Overpeck, M.D., and Moss, A.J. (1991). Children's exposure to environmental tobacco smoke before and after birth: health of our nation's children, 1988. *Advance Data. Vital and Health Statistics of the National Center for Health Statistics, 202.*

27. Rush, D., and Callahan, K.R. (1989). Exposure to passive cigarette smoking and child development: a critical review. *New York Academy of Sciences, 562,* 74–100.

28. Helsing, K.J., Sandler, D.P., Comstock, G.W., and Chee, E. (1988). Heart disease mortality in nonsmokers living with smokers. *American Journal of Epidemiology, 127*(5), 915–922.

29. White, J.R., and Froeb, H.F. (1980). Small-airways dysfunction in nonsmokers chronically exposed to tobacco smoke. *New England Journal of Medicine, 302,* 720–723.

30. Pirie, P.L., Murray, D.M., and Leupker, R.V. (1991). Gender differences in cigarette smoking and quitting in a cohort of young adults. *American Journal of Public Health, 81*(3), 324–327.

31. USDHHS (1990). Office of the Surgeon General. *Health benefits of smoking cessation.* A report of the Surgeon General. Washington, DC: US Government Printing Office.

32. Public Citizen Health Research Group (1992). The Patch. *Health Letter, 8*(7), 5.

33. Rose, J., Levin, E., Behm, F., Adivi, C., and Schur, C. (1990). Transdermal nicotine facilitates smoking cessation. *Clinical Pharmacology Therapy, 47,* 323–330.

34. American Cancer Society (1987). *General facts on smoking and health.* New York: American Cancer Society.

Resources

AMERICAN CANCER SOCIETY

Provides information about quitting smoking and smoking cessation programs.

1599 Clifton Road
Atlanta, GA 30329
404-320-3333

AMERICAN HEART ASSOCIATION

Provides information about quitting smoking and smoking cessation programs.

7320 Greenville Avenue
Dallas, TX 75231
214-373-6300

AMERICAN LUNG ASSOCIATION

Provides information about quitting smoking and smoking cessation programs.

1740 Broadway
New York, NY 10019
212-315-8700

ASH (ACTION ON SMOKING AND HEALTH)

A national nonprofit organization concerned with the problems of smoking and the rights of nonsmokers; publishes a regular newsletter.

ASH
2013 H St NW
Washington, DC 20006
202-659-4310

GASP (GROUP AGAINST SMOKERS' POLLUTION)

Provides information on nonsmokers' rights and related subjects.

PO Box 632
College Park, MD 20740
301-577-6427

OFFICE ON SMOKING AND HEALTH (OSH)

This office provides information on smoking, smoking cessation, and research on smoking.

Center for Chronic Disease Prevention and Health Promotion
Mail Stop K-50
Centers for Disease Control
1600 Clifton Road NE
Atlanta, GA 30333
404-488-5705 (public information)
404-488-5708 (technical information)

STAT (STOP TEENAGE ADDICTION TO TOBACCO)

A nonprofit educational organization dedicated to reducing tobacco addiction among young people; publishes a regular newsletter.

STAT
121 Lyman St #210
Springfield, MA 01103

CHAPTER

6

Violence, Abuse, and Harassment

CHAPTER OBJECTIVES

On completion of this chapter, the student should be able to discuss:

1. The difference between criminal and intimate violence.

2. What is meant by a "just world" hypothesis.

3. The concept of "blaming the victim."

4. Rape from a historical perspective.

5. How poverty contributes to violence in the United States.

6. How pornography contributes to violence in the United States.

7. The relationship between alcohol and violence.

8. How the media contributes to violence in the United States.

9. Definitions of forcible rape and acquaintance rape.

10. Prevalence of rape in the United States.

11. The discrepancy between actual rapes and the number of reported rapes.

12. At what age a woman is at greatest risk for rape.

13. Rape myths.

14. Posttraumatic stress disorder.

15. Rape trauma syndrome.

16. How rape can affect health and sexual intimacy.

17. Healthy and unhealthy rape displacement activities.

18. Issues with resistance in a rape situation.

19. Essential components of a rape prevention program.

20. Distinction between physical violence, sexual violence, property violence, and psychological and social violence.

21. Relationship violence.

22. The special considerations regarding violence in lesbian relationships.

23. Concerns with battering during pregnancy.

24. Concepts and issues of child abuse.

25. Concepts and issues of elder abuse.

26. Sexual harassment and how it operates as a form of social control.

27. Issues in relationship communication about intimacy.

28. How sexual harassment affects women in the workplace.

29. Strategies for effectively dealing with sexual harassment.

Introduction

Violence takes place throughout modern society and it occurs in many forms. Violence is the leading killer of young people in the United States. Domestic violence, including relationship abuse, child abuse, and elder abuse, is one facet of the violence epidemic. Sexual harassment must also be considered a form of violence for it, too, is an unjust use of power. Women are disproportionately victims of violence. This chapter provides an overview of violence and the issues that contribute to the violence and victimization in the United States and reviews informed decision-making criteria for women.

Overview of Violence

The reduction of violent and abusive behavior has been identified as a major focus of the Year 2000 National Health Objectives.[1] At least 2.2 million people are victims of violent injury each year. The United States ranks first among industrialized nations in violent death rates.[1] Violence is not limited to death rates for in its broadest sense, **violence** refers to the unjust use of force and power. This definition implies much more than the physical forms of violence and includes social norms, values, and political and economic policies. Violence often results in death or long-term disability. Interpersonal violence can exist in both **criminal** and **intimate** forms. Criminal violence includes robbery, burglary, aggravated assault, forcible rape, and homicide. Intimate violence includes child abuse, incest, courtship violence, date rape, battering, marital rape, and elder abuse. Although most intimate violence qualifies as a crime, a historical tradition to a large extent has condoned violence within the family setting.

Sociocultural Dimensions of Violence

Cultural differences in values, attitudes, and behavioral norms across ethnic and racial groups must be considered in any examination of violence. Unfortunately, data are scarce in this area. It has been difficult to assess attitudes toward rape and other violent crimes. Some studies indicate that the public tend to blame victims of rape, rather than those who commit the behavior. To explain this phenomenon, a "just world" hypothesis has been proposed that essentially states that "good things happen to good people, and bad things happen to bad people . . . so if something bad, like rape, happens to a woman, then she must be bad." Studies have shown that the more an individual believes in a "just world," the more likely he or she is to blame the victim.[2]

Cultural attitudes about rape may be based on societal acceptance of male dominance and false beliefs regarding women and rape. Stereotypical beliefs about women have also been shown to influence victim blaming. Women holding traditional beliefs regarding roles for women were more likely to blame the victim than less traditional women.[3] Studies have found that both judges and juries hold stereotypes about women and are willing to attribute blame if the woman is viewed as contributing, even if it is "unwittingly," to her victimization.[4] These perspectives continue to influence attitudes about rape, as revealed in a recent Time/CNN survey (Information Box 6.1). A critical concept revealed in the survey is the ambiguity over the definition of rape. If rape is defined as sex without consent, clearly, what "consent" is needs to be carefully defined and communicated in a relationship.

Society's tolerance of rape is an important dimension. Some studies suggest that individuals are becoming more tolerant of rape. There is variability in the degree to which individuals disapprove or condemn rape. Factors such as the victim's marital status, style of dress, her relationship with the assailant, evidence of resistance, the extent of her injuries, psychological attributes, and sociodemographic characteristics may all contribute to attitudes toward rape victims.[5] Some individuals may disapprove of rape under all circumstances whereas others may believe that in certain circumstances, rape is actually excusable or understandable (Information Box 6.1). Tolerance of rape may include denial that rape ever occurred, claiming that the accusations are false; excusing rapists and blaming rape victims for provoking or precipitating the rape, i.e., "she led him on;" or denying the seriousness of rape and the injury inflicted on the victim, i.e., "when rape is inevitable, relax and enjoy it." The consequences of society's tolerance for rape are severe. Convictions for rape may be more difficult to attain when judges, attorneys, and jury members are predisposed to blame the victim or to believe that the rape was really consensual. Social tolerance of rape may also impede the adjustment and psychological recovery of the rape victim, who may not be able to elicit reliable support and sympathy from others.

Another key concept in relationship violence from a women's health perspective is "blaming the victim," which occurs when women are labeled as being at fault for the psychological and physical degradation they experience and for remaining in the relationship.[6] Cultural differences regarding the role of women and victim attribution may account for these differences, but data are scarce and limited in quality. Research generally indicates that victims' reactions to rape by race and ethnicity are fairly consistent. No differences in reactions have been found between African-American and white women victims; however, Asian-American women have been noted to have more severe reactions to rape.[7] When women are involved in a relationship that results in their abuse, they are trapped between the proverbial "rock and a hard place." Women are socialized to nurture their family members, to care for the sick, and to make personal

---

Time/CNN *Rape Attitude Survey*

Would you classify the following as rape or not?

		Rape	Not Rape
A man has sex with a woman who has passed out after drinking too much	Female	88%	9%
	Male	77%	17%
A married man has sex with his wife even though she does not want him to	Female	61%	30%
	Male	56%	38%
A man argues with a woman who does not want to have sex until she agrees to have sex	Female	42%	53%
	Male	33%	59%
A man uses emotional pressure, but no physical force, to get a woman to have sex	Female	39%	55%
	Male	33%	59%

		Yes	No
Do you believe that some women like to be talked into having sex?	Female	54%	33%
	Male	69%	20%

From a telephone poll of 500 American adults taken for TIME/CNN on May 8 by Yankslovich Clancy Shulman. Sampling error is plus or minus 4.5%. "Not sures" omitted.

Do you believe a woman who is raped is partly to blame if:

	Age	Yes	No
She is under the influence of drugs or alcohol	18–34	31%	66%
	35–49	35%	58%
	50+	57%	36%
She initially says yes to having sex and then changes her mind	18–34	34%	60%
	35–49	43%	53%
	50+	43%	46%
She dresses provocatively	18–34	28%	70%
	35–49	31%	67%
	50+	53%	42%
She agrees to go to the man's room or home	18–34	20%	76%
	35–49	29%	70%
	50+	53%	41%

		Yes	No
Have you ever been in a situation with a man in which you said no but ended up having sex anyway?	Asked of females	18%	80%

Reported in *Time*, June 3, 1991. Copyright 1991, Time, Inc. Reprinted by permission.

---

sacrifices for their relationships,[6,8] yet women who exhibit this behavior in relationships, particularly in alcohol-dependent or drug-dependent relationships, are held responsible for another adult's acts of neglect and abuse. Women who leave or avoid such relationships have been accused of being self-centered, uncaring, and doomed to life "without a man."[6,8,9] A woman can play a role in changing the dynamics of a dysfunctional relationship, but this individual change is of limited impact when society tolerates—through omission or commission—the broad spectrum of emotional, verbal, physical, and sexual abuse experienced by women.

Historical Influences

Rape has been documented in American history since the arrival of the Europeans. Spanish explorers believed that female Native-American captives were inferior and were used for sexual services. They also felt free to rape Indian women whose tribes they conquered. Native-American cultures, however, prohibited rape, and it had rarely occurred until the arrival of the explorers. Fear of brutal rapes by Indians was found to be unsubstantiated during colonial-era Indian wars. English women who had been held captive reported no such treatment.[10] In seventeenth century New England, female servants were at high risk of rape and sexual harassment. It is estimated that during that era, one-third of rape victims were female servants, a group that constituted only 10 percent of the population.[10] Later in the South, where slave labor was increasingly used instead of indentured servants, African female servants found themselves victimized by white owners and overseers who viewed them as property—available for service of their sexual needs. Other historians note how rape was used to dominate female slaves in a system that otherwise treated them as equals to male slaves.[11] It has also been noted that the fear of rape and the myth of the African-American male rapist were used as political tools both to control and to intimidate African-American men as they migrated north after 1940 as well as to instill "fear into white women who moved too freely in the public world."[10]

Poverty Influences

Poverty has devastating impact on all facets of health, including healthy lifestyle and access to health care services. Poverty has also been identified as an extremely important factor in violence, particularly homicides. Homicides are disproportionately present among African Americans and minorities, as is poverty. The **feminization of poverty** refers to the fact that women and children are overwhelmingly the victims of poverty. Women often remain trapped in abusive relationships because of simple economics. Poverty and joblessness contribute substantially to family violence as well. The majority of reported cases of child neglect and abuse involve families from lower socioeconomic backgrounds,[12] and estranged, unemployed husbands or boyfriends are more likely to react with acts of violence against the woman.[13]

There are myriad economic dimensions associated with rape. One variable, lost income due to criminal victimization, is calculated by the Department of Justice. For the rapes reported in 1991, 15 percent involved economic loss.[14] Medical treatment and counseling costs are another economic variable associated with rape. Some victims may not submit bills for reimbursement to third-party insurers owing to issues of confidentiality or embarrassment. Depending on the woman's choice and the availability of services, counseling can be a costly medical expense. The cost, if no free services are available, may be a barrier to someone seeking these services.

Pornography Influences

> Pornography is an expression, always, of disrespect and even hatred for women. Furthermore, it is one of the important mechanisms for the social control of women by men. It teaches girls and boys, women and men, something about their reciprocal unequal roles and legitimizes the power differential in both groups. It teaches and reinforces low self worth in females and some of it threatens them if they step out of line. It instructs males in modes and methods of domination and grants them permission to use these methods.
>
> WHEELER, H. (1985). PORNOGRAPHY AND RAPE: A FEMINIST PERSPECTIVE. IN A.W. BURGESS (ED.), *Rape and sexual assault, a research handbook*, (PP. 374–391). NEW YORK: GARLAND PUBLISHING.

Pornography is an example of media violence against women. **Pornography** is generally understood to be sexually arousing images in film, print, or electronic media. Much of this sexually arousing material depicts unjust use of force against women in the expression of sexuality. Violent pornography, a multimillion dollar subset of the entertainment industry, is perhaps the most blatant example of media representation of both physical and psychological abuse of women. It has been hypothesized that a society can become insensitive to violence when it is repeatedly exposed to film violence.[15] A 1985 Federal Commission examined the effects of violent pornography and tried to identify possible links between exposure to sexually violent media images and sexually violent behaviors. The Commission concluded that substantial exposure to sexually violent material was causally related to antisocial acts of sexual violence and, for some subgroups, possibly to unlawful acts of sexual violence.[16] Feminists have argued that pornography is but one element in a system of violence against women that promotes male dominance and female subordination.

Alcohol and Drug Influences

Alcohol and other drug intoxication have consistently been found to be associated with all forms of relationship violence. It is unclear if there is a direct cause-and-effect relationship between alcohol and violence or if it is a situation of two overlapping social epidemics. Efforts to link alcohol abuse and domestic violence may reflect a tendency to view battering as an individual deviant behavior rather than a pervasive social problem that knows no sociodemographic limits. Data on the concurrence of domestic violence and alcohol abuse vary widely, from 25 to 80 percent.[17] Heavy drinking is strongly associated with acts of violence; 80 to 90 percent of those arrested for crime are men, and approximately half of all convicted criminals were drunk at the time of their offense.[18] Heavy drinkers are typically male, and the non-chemically dependent victim is usually a woman.[18,19,20] Although female problem drinkers certainly exist, such women are usually abandoned by their male partners. Women in relationships with male problem drinkers, however, tend to remain in the relationship. Women who are romantically involved with problem drinkers have been characterized as having emotional dependency problems of their own. Increasingly scholars in the field of addiction research and the psychology of women are calling for men to be held socially accountable for their role in perpetuating the more subtle aspects of female subordination as well as acts of violence against women.[6,8,9,12]

Media Influences

> We begin to believe that violence is a socially acceptable and credible way of responding to frustration or insult or some other direct, personal hurt. . . . Children especially become "desensitized" to violent interpersonal conflict and, when seeing another child being hurt, will tend not to do the thing that civilization requires be done—step in and protect the victim. Instead, they will watch, as if this too, were dramatized entertainment.
>
> FORMER US SURGEON GENERAL, EVERETT C. KOOP

It is difficult to measure the exact influence that violence in media has on society. Beatings, rapes, and murders are common themes in popular television, cinema, and music. In both print and electronic media, women are disproportionately represented as victims of violence. Advertising is another media form that may portray women as victims. Demeaning images of women who are obsessed with the cleanliness of their toilet bowls or the nutrition in their morning cereal are often used to sell products. These images contribute to the perpetuation of inappropriate gender stereotypes.

Rape

Rape is a crime of aggression. Although men can certainly be victims, most of the cases are women. Recently prominent figures such as William Kennedy Smith and boxer Mike Tyson have been tried as rapists. National attention to these events has served to heighten awareness of the issue. Discussion of these trials and the myths and issues surrounding acquaintance rape have been openly addressed in the workplace, on campuses, on television, and in popular print.

Overview

Rape is forced sex. Acquaintance rape, or **date rape**, is defined as rape in which the victim and rapist were previously known to each other and may have interacted in some socially appropriate manner.[21] Prevalence rates of date rape vary among studies. Despite the differences, researchers generally agree that the prevalence of rape, especially date rape, which is rarely reported, has become a serious problem on college campuses. Many researchers believe that the prevalence has reached epidemic proportions.[22] Studies generally indicate that 50 percent or more of rapes occur in the social context of dating.[23] Several studies have examined self-reported incidents of aggressive sexual behaviors in male college students, generally indicating that 25 percent of males surveyed admitted performing at least one act of sexual aggression since beginning their college experience.[24,25] In another study, male college undergraduates rated the justifiability of date rape under various circumstances. The circumstances surrounding the act of rape, such as whether a couple went to the man's apartment rather than to a religious function or if the man paid all the dating expenses rather than splitting them with the woman, were found to play an important role in predicting student attitudes toward the rape victim and the rapist.[26] Rape can also happen in a marriage and during a legal separation. Rape may be committed by ex-spouses. Rape in marriage is often called spousal rape or marital rape, but it, along with rape by an ex-spouse, also meets the criteria of acquaintance rape. The concept of marital rape is not recognized in all states. Rape by a co-worker, teacher, professor, a husband's friend, or boss—*anyone* the individual knows—can be considered acquaintance rape.

Epidemiology

Rape in America, a national report released in 1992, is the first national empirical data set about forcible rape in the United States.[27] Before this report, national information about rape was limited to data on reported rapes from Federal Bureau of Investigation (FBI) reports or data from crime statistics. The FBI defines rape as carnal knowledge of a female forcibly and against her consent. Nearly 700,000 forcible rapes are estimated to occur annually (Fig. 6.1). African-American females have a greater statistical risk of rape than white or Hispanic-American females (Information Box 6.2). Government estimates suggest that for every rape reported, three to ten rapes are committed but not reported.[25]

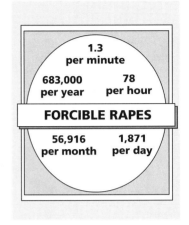

FIGURE 6.1

Estimated occurrence of forcible rapes.

SOURCE: National Victim Center (1992). *Rape in America.* Arlington, VA. Reprinted with permission from the National Victim Center and Crime Victims Research and Treatment Center.

INFORMATION BOX 6.2

Rape Rates by Race/Ethnicity

Race/Ethnicity	Rate for 1,000 Persons
African-American females	1.7
White females	1.1
Hispanic-American females	0.8
Non-Hispanic females	1.2

SOURCE: US Department of Justice (1991). *Criminal victimization in the United States, 1989: A national crime survey report.* Washington, DC: Bureau of Justice Statistics.

FIGURE 6.2

Comparison of rape data sources, 1990.

SOURCE: National Victim Center (1992). *Rape in America—A report to the Nation.* Arlington, VA. Reprinted with permission from the National Victim Center and Crime Victims Research and Treatment Center.

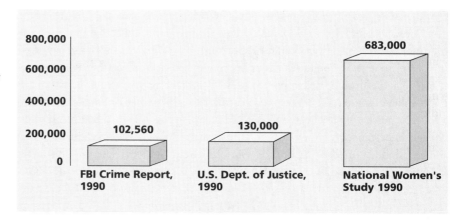

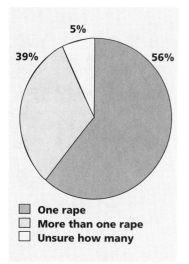

FIGURE 6.3

Number of times raped in lifetime. An estimated 12.1 million women have been raped.

SOURCE: National Victim Center (1992). *Rape in America—A report to the Nation.* Arlington, VA. Reprinted with permission from the National Victim Center and Crime Victims Research and Treatment Center.

Fig. 6.2 provides a graphic comparison of current national estimates of forcible rapes from these data sources. **Forcible rape** in this report was defined as an event that occurs without a woman's consent and involves the use of force or threat of force and involves sexual penetration of the victim's vagina, mouth, or rectum. Thirteen percent of women surveyed reported having been victims of at least one completed rape in their lifetimes. Based on US Census estimates of the number of adult women in the United States, one out of every eight adult women, or at least 12.2 million American women, has been the victim of forcible rape in her lifetime. Many women were raped more than once[27] (Fig. 6.3).

The survey also found that rape in the United States is a tragedy of youth. Most rape occurred between childhood and adolescence. Twenty-nine percent of all forcible rapes occurred when the victim was less than 11 years old, and 32 percent occurred between the ages of 11 and 17 (Fig. 6.4). Most rape victims were assaulted by someone they knew (Fig. 6.5). Almost half of all rape victims described being fearful of serious injury or death during the rape experience. Rape victims, all and those within the last 5 years, were questioned about the extent to which they were concerned about issues specific to their personal rape experiences. These concerns are summarized in Fig. 6.6. The concerns indicate that rape victims are afraid that other people will find out about the rape and find reasons to blame them for the rape. It is apparent that the stigma of rape is a real concern for rape victims. The study also documented that very few rapes (16 percent) were reported to the police.[27]

The National Women's Study also produced dramatic confirmation of the mental health impact of rape by comparing rape victims with nonvictims of crime. As seen in Fig. 6.7, 31 percent of all rape victims developed posttraumatic stress disorder (PTSD) sometime during their lifetimes. Rape victims were 6.2 times more likely to develop PTSD than nonvictims. Major depressive episodes were three times more prevalent among rape victims than nonvictims. Rape victims were 4.1 times more likely to have contemplated suicide and 13 times more likely to have attempted suicide.[27]

Rape as a Crime

Rape is a difficult crime to assess. Many societal pressures and norms have reinforced beliefs that rape is sometimes justifiable, depending on the circumstances. Rape is not a "clear-cut" crime such as murder. Although national crime statistics indicate that rape has increased, as the *Rape in America Report* indicated, most rapes are not reported. These unreported rapes may be perceived as a threat to public safety because if the rapists are not dealt with in the criminal justice system, the opportunity clearly presents for the violent behavior to continue. The underreporting of rape is due to a number of factors, including "victim blaming." Many women fear publicity of the event, and others distrust hospital and law enforcement agencies. In reality, 84 percent of all rape victims *do not* report the crime to the police.[27] If the rapist is an acquaintance or employer, the victim may fear reprisal or punishment for reporting. Other

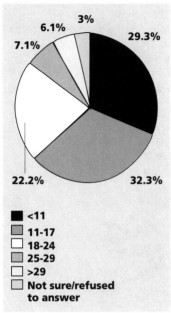

FIGURE 6.4

Age of victim at time of rape.

SOURCE: National Victim Center (1992). *Rape in America—A report to the Nation.* Arlington, VA. Reprinted with permission from the National Victim Center and Crime Victims Research and Treatment Center.

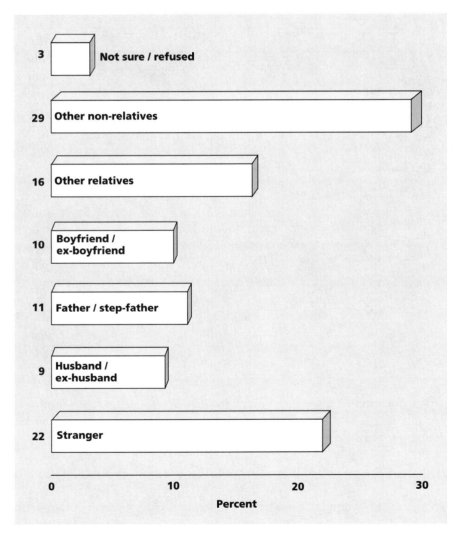

FIGURE 6.5

Relationship between rape victim and perpetrator.

SOURCE: National Victim Center (1992). *Rape in America—A report to the Nation.* Arlington, VA. Reprinted with permission from the National Victim Center and Crime Victims Research and Treatment Center.

FIGURE 6.6

Identified important concerns of rape victims: recent rapes versus all rapes.

SOURCE: National Victim Center (1992). *Rape in America—A report to the Nation.* Arlington, VA. Reprinted with permission from the National Victim Center and Crime Victims Research and Treatment Center.

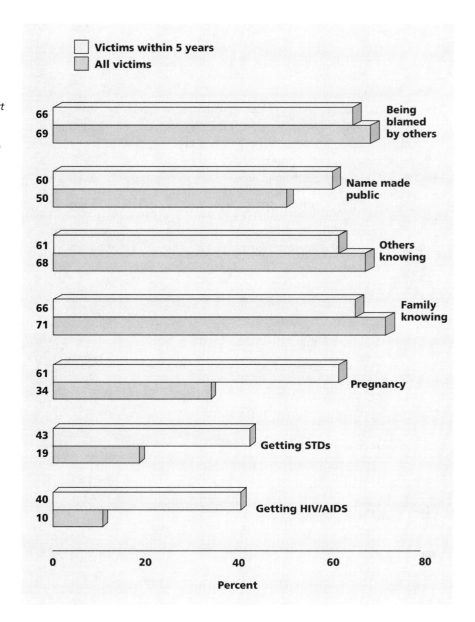

reasons for women not reporting rape include feelings of shame or guilt and fear that they would not be believed. Clearly the issues of rape as a crime are multifaceted and diversified.

Rape Myths

There are many myths about rape, rapists, and rape victims (Information Box 6.3). Unfortunately, the common theme of all these myths is that the

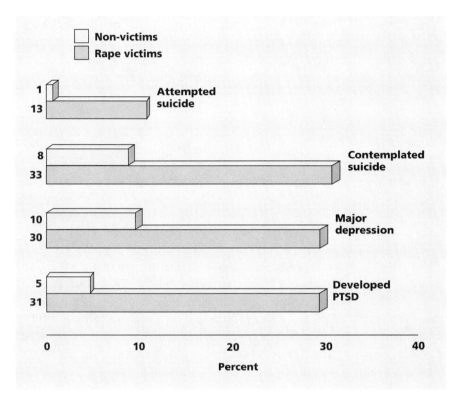

FIGURE 6.7

Comparison of mental health problems among rape victims and nonvictims of crime.

SOURCE: National Victim Center (1992). *Rape in America—A report to the Nation.* Arlington, VA. Reprinted with permission from the National Victim Center and Crime Victims Research and Treatment Center.

INFORMATION BOX 6.3

Myths About Rape

Rape

Rape only occurs in the "bad part of town," not nice neighborhoods.

Rape only occurs late at night, in the dark.

Rape cannot occur unless a woman "gives up."

If a male pays for a date, he has the right to expect something back, that is, sex.

Rapists

Men who commit rapes are unable to control their sexual urges.

A rape is a one-time event, representing a temporary lapse in reasoning and judgment.

Rapists are always strangers to the victim.

All rapists are African-American men who rape white women.

All rapists are mentally ill.

Rape Victims

Women "ask" for rape if they wear certain types of clothing.

Only promiscuous women are victims of rape.

Victims are usually out alone when the rape occurs.

I cannot describe how I felt when it was over. I was wondering if it would have been better if I had died. I was humiliated, angry, hurt, and so violated. He had been someone I had trusted—I thought that he was a friend. Looking back, though, there were clues to his violent nature. I had ignored them. It was a mistake that I paid dearly for.

18-YEAR-OLD STUDENT

victim is blamed for the event. This is inconsistent with other acts of violent crime such as murder or assault. As indicated earlier, these widespread myths have contributed to the high lack of nonreporting of rape by victims and the fear that others might learn of the event. These myths also contribute to the recovery of victims from a rape experience.

Resisting Rape

Many strategies such as physically hitting, kicking, screaming, scratching, and biting as well as martial arts, have been suggested as tactics for resisting rape. Proponents of such strategies argue that rape continues because women have been socialized to be passive and nonresistant, particularly in sexual matters. If women were to be more reactive and forceful in response to rape, the prevalence of rape would decrease. Others disagree, noting that violence promotes additional violence, and increased physical response by women increases their risk for further injury and harm. In addition, it compounds the existing problem of further blaming the victim. Not only does society see her as inciting the event, but when she does not effectively resist, she fails again. Opponents of resistance further argue that this approach fails to deal with the essence of the problem—those social structures, values, and attitudes that permit rape to occur in the first place.

In studies to determine which avoidance strategies are most successful in rape situations, results indicate that avoiders of rape used more strategies than women who were raped, and, in addition, these strategies differed. Avoiders more often tried to flee or scream or speak loudly or used physical force. Rape victims, however, either used no strategy or attempted only ineffective verbal strategies, such as begging or pleading.[28,29] Cognitive verbal strategies, such as reasoning, verbally refusing, threatening, and conning, which have been frequently recommended by "experts" in the past, were not effective in preventing rape when used alone. If these strategies were followed with physical force, however, the chance of rape decreased.

Another significant finding is that rape victims who physically resisted the attack were found to be less depressed after the experience than those who did not offer physical resistance.[28–30] Researchers have found no link between fighting back and severe injury. Some researchers have concluded that by fighting back a woman significantly increases her chances of rape avoidance but only somewhat increases her chance of rough treatment. Not resisting, however, is no guarantee of humane treatment. Considering the long-term negative impact that rape has on a victim's mental health, fighting back may decrease the likelihood of becoming a victim; if not, it may still increase the victim's ability to adapt to the traumatic event and continue on with her life.

The circumstances and characteristics of each rape and each victim are unique, and it is not practical or realistic to imagine that one specific strategy would be effective in preventing sexual violation or harm. Prevention is perhaps the best, albeit limited, tool currently available to women.

Recovery from Rape

Reactions and recovery to rape show considerable variability among individuals. Most reactions may be classified as a PTSD, an event that is outside the range of usual human experience and would be markedly distressing to almost anyone. To be diagnosed with PTSD, an individual must experience for at least 1 month's duration, (1) at least one persistent reexperience of the event, (2) at least three of the avoidance or numbing behaviors, and (3) at least two of the arousal symptoms. A delayed-onset PTSD is diagnosed if the symptoms do not begin until at least 6 months after the traumatic event.

Rape traumatic syndrome has also been defined to explain the recovery process of rape victims, as the acute and long-term reorganization process that occurs as a result of forcible rape or attempted forcible rape.[31] This syndrome is usually described as having two or three phases. The first phase includes the immediate emotions following the event. These emotions can vary and include but are not limited to shock, anger, numbness, guilt, disbelief, embarrassment, shame, feelings of being unclean, anxiety, denial, fear, self-blame, or restlessness. The second phase of rape traumatic syndrome includes attempts at reorganizing one's life and lifestyle, beginning 2 or 3 weeks after the event. The phase is often characterized by significant disruption in daily routines. Victims may decide to change schools, jobs, or routes to school or work in an attempt to remove reminders of the event from their daily lives. Overwhelming feelings often develop that the victim may not directly link to the rape. Often the rape is repressed and not acknowledged (sometimes for years), but the feelings do not disappear. A third phase, the final stage of dealing with rape trauma, occurs over a long period of time. Victims may perceive themselves as changed by the rape either because they feel differently about themselves or because they believe that others see them as changed. Not all victims experience all possible emotions, reactions, and behaviors associated with rape.

Being a victim of rape can also have a significantly negative impact on a woman's sexual health and intimacy and places her at risk for depression and physical illness. Physical ailments, such as headaches, skeletal muscle tensions, fatigue, startle reactions, gastrointestinal irritability, severe colds, dysmenorrhea, and stiff muscles and joints, commonly can be experienced weeks, months, or even years after the event.[32] These experiences may be more severe in those women who do not seek counseling or delay counseling. Mediating factors that may influence how a woman reacts to a rape experience include individual coping and reaction patterns, demographic variables, characteristics of the assault, historical variables, and social supports.

Displacement activities by victims following the rape event may be described as either healthy or destructive in nature. The more healthy displacement activities would include immersion in work, school, or leisure pursuits. These activities, however, may be insufficient and possibly destructive if not combined with active counseling. The activities could be considered healthy if they serve to displace anxiety and stress until the counseling process is undertaken and completed. Research has found that women who had actively engaged in leisure

I reported the rape to the police. In a way, it was like being raped twice. I felt that I had to prove that it had happened and that I had resisted. The medical exam took a long time. I so desperately wanted a long shower to literally and figuratively cleanse myself but I had to answer hours of questions and repeatedly relive the experience. They never found him. I am still afraid. I often wonder if it was worth the effort to make the report.

20-YEAR-OLD WOMAN

pursuits before becoming a victim of sexual assault were more successful in adapting to the event. Reengaging in these leisure activities appeared to promote successful reorganization. Unhealthy displacement activities by women following rape would include drug and alcohol abuse, limited social interaction, and "promiscuous" or nondiscriminatory behavior that is in sharp contrast to pre-rape behavior and lifestyle.[7,33]

Preventing Rape

If prevention is the best tool currently available to women, it is important to clarify this concept. Prevention of rape refers to those actions that women and society can take to eliminate this inappropriate use of physical and sexual force. These strategies include taking measures to reduce the susceptibility of physical assault (Information Box 6.4). This does not mean that women are "at fault" if communication attempts fail and a rape subsequently occurs; it does mean that women owe it to themselves to communicate explicitly their intent, or lack thereof, in sexual matters.

An important concept in rape prevention is formalized preparation and training. Four critical components should be included in any rape prevention program:

1. Understanding and dispelling all the myths of rape.

2. Skills training in developing honest and direct communication about dating and sexual needs and desires.

3. Practical interventions (combination of audiovisual presentations and group discussions, role playing, group discussions).

INFORMATION BOX 6.4

How to Prevent Date Rape

Be wary of a relationship that is operating along classic stereotypes of dominant male and submissive, passive female. The dominance in ordinary activities may extend to the sexual arena.

Be wary when a date tries to control behavior or pressure others in any way.

Be explicit with communication. Don't say "no" in a way that could be interpreted in any way as a "maybe" or "yes."

Avoid ambiguous messages with both verbal and non-verbal behavior. Saying "no" and permitting heavy petting implies confusion or ambiguity.

First dates with a unknown companion may be safer in a group.

Avoid remote or isolated spots where help is not available.

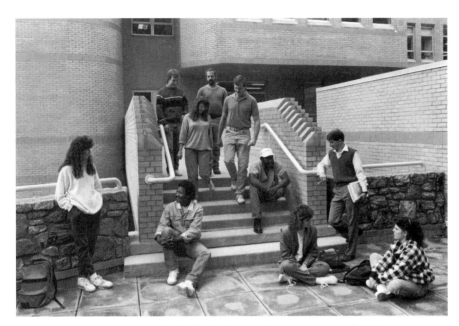

There are no stereotypes for both victims and perpetrators of violence.

4. What to do if they or someone they know becomes a rape victim with an emphasis on early support and counseling.

These measures are valuable in improving a woman's self-esteem and self-confidence as well as providing practical rape intervention strategies and a heightened awareness of local supportive resources and services.

Helping a Victim

When interacting with a victim or survivor of acquaintance rape, it is critical not to pass judgment or imply that she is responsible for the attack in any way. Encourage victims to seek counseling and offer to go with them. Encourage victims to prosecute but respect their wishes if they decline. If support is promised to provide assistance or accompany the victim through the process, it is important to follow through. Work to enlighten the political system by becoming politically proactive.

Homicide

Homicide is defined as death due to injuries purposely inflicted by another person. Homicide is the 11th leading cause of death in the United States.[1] One in six homicides involves family members, and half of these murders are committed by spouses. Women are 1.3 times more likely to be victims in these circumstances than men.[34] The FBI Reports indicate that among all female victims of murders in 1989, 28% were believed to have been killed by their husband or boyfriend.[35] Homicide seems to be the result of repeated violence. In most cases of spousal homicide, police have been repeatedly called to the home previously for domestic violence events.[36] The media has had a focus on the reversal of this picture, that is, women who kill their spouses. Data indicate that frequently women who kill their spouses have been victims of repeated, escalating levels of abuse, in terms of both frequency and severity.[37]

Relationship Abuse

Overview

Battering has been defined as repeatedly subjecting a woman to forceful physical, social, and psychological behavior in order to coerce her, without regard to her rights. Battering includes five types of interpersonal violence: physical, sexual, property, psychological, and social. **Physical violence** includes slapping, choking, punching, kicking, pushing, and the use of objects as weapons. Forced sexual activity constitutes **sexual violence.** Property violence denotes threatened or actual destruction of property. **Psychological and social violence** include threats of harm, physical isolation of the woman, extreme jealousy, mental degradation, and threats of harm to children.

Relationship Violence

Relationship violence refers to domestic violence between individuals in a significant relationship. Previously referred to as "wife abuse," or "spouse abuse," the term "relationship violence" acknowledges that a couple need not be married for violence to occur and that violence is not necessarily limited to traditional heterosexual relationships. Battering of women is a major health problem (Information Box 6.5). It occurs in families of all racial, economic, educational, and religious backgrounds. It is reported that violence against wives will occur at least once in two-thirds of all marriages, and once the battering begins, escalation in severity and frequency usually follows. Studies suggest that 2 to 4 million women are physically battered each year by partners, including husbands, former husbands, boyfriends, and lovers. Often violence in a home involves more than the adult couple. It has been estimated that in homes where the mother is beaten, 30 to 70 percent of the children are also abused.[38]

Battering of women occurs at all sociodemographic levels of society. Spouse abuse perhaps appears more frequently under economically disadvantaged conditions because educated, middle-class and affluent women tend to have more resources to avoid or leave violent relationships. More affluent women may seek confidential professional help and not use residential shelters. Regardless

---

Facts on Battering

Battering of women is the most unreported crime in the United States.

3–4 million American women are battered each year.

95 percent of all spouse abuse cases are women who are hurt by men.

Battering occurs among people of all races.

A battering incident is rarely an isolated event.

Battering tends to increase and become more violent over time.

Many batterers learned violent behavior growing up in an abusive family.

SOURCE: Helton, A.S. (1987). *Prevention of battering during pregnancy.* March of Dimes Foundation. White Plains, N.Y.

---

of socioeconomic status, battered women face numerous obstacles in breaking away from violent situations. Battering may be a major cause of injury to women in the United States. In one study, battering accounted for almost one in five visits to emergency rooms by women.[39] Battering is often under-identified because both the patient and the health care provider may be reluctant to initiate or discuss the topic. Although most states have mandated reporting requirements for child abuse or elder abuse, there is no corresponding requirement for health care providers to report battering of women.[40]

Violence in Lesbian Relationships

Although research on domestic violence has grown considerably in the last two decades, very little attention has been given to the problem of partner abuse among homosexual couples. Research in this area is especially difficult. Lesbian victims of partner abuse are doubly stigmatized because of their victimization and because of their sexual orientation. The problem is perhaps compounded by reluctance within the lesbian community to address issues openly that could be used to fuel heterosexist stereotypes and antilesbian sentiment.[41] Studies indicate that a history of aggression, whether the person is a target or observer of aggression, is a risk factor for subsequent experiences with aggression. Traditional perpetrator/victim models in heterosexual conflicts may be inappropriate for characterizing aggression in intimate female relationships, in which aggression tends to be reciprocal, with many women who reported experiencing aggression reporting having used it as well. In addition, this use of aggression was less often in self-defense alone than it was mutual aggression or self-defense combined with mutual aggression.[42] A preliminary research study with lesbian victims of psychological and physical abuse indicates a need for further research and the development of supportive resources and services for victims.[43]

Battering During Pregnancy

Women are not immune to battering during pregnancy (Information Box 6.6). Some studies have reported that 8 to 36 percent of women are battered during pregnancy.[39,44] Battering in a relationship may start or become worse during pregnancy. Estimates are that 25 to 45 percent of battered women continue to be battered during pregnancy. In addition to inflicting physical and psychological damage to the mother, battering during pregnancy may lead to miscarriage, and pregnant women in battering relationships have an increased risk of delivering low-birth-weight infants.

Child Abuse

Child abuse is another tragic form of violence. Defined by the 1988 Child Abuse Prevention, Adoption, and Family Services Act of 1988, **child abuse and neglect** is physical or mental injury, sexual abuse or exploitation, negligent treatment, or maltreatment of a child by a person who is responsible for the child's welfare, under circumstances that indicate that the child's health or welfare is harmed or threatened. An estimated 1.6 million children in the United States experience some form of abuse or neglect annually.[1] The numbers of cases of child abuse have been steadily rising. It is not known if the rise reflects an actual increase in the prevalence of the problem or if newer programs have generated greater awareness, identification, and reporting of the problem. An axiom of child abuse is especially tragic. Almost without exception, abusive parents were themselves abused or neglected as children. This cycle of abuse is obvious: battered children grow up to become battering adults. Child abuse is often a symptom of family violence—45 percent of the mothers of abused children are themselves battered women.[1]

INFORMATION BOX 6.6

Facts on Battering and Pregnancy

Battering may start or become worse during pregnancy.

Battering may result in miscarriage.

Battering may lead to alcohol or drug abuse—a form of abuse to the child.

25–45 percent of all women who are battered are battered during pregnancy.

Battering during pregnancy may be an indication of what life holds in store for the unborn child.

Pregnant women in battering relationships have an increased risk of delivering low-birth-weight infants.

SOURCE: Helton, A.S. (1987). *Prevention of battering during pregnancy.* March of Dimes Foundation. White Plains, N.Y.

Several psychological traits have been associated with child abusers. These traits include immaturity and dependency, a sense of personal incompetence, difficulty in seeking pleasure and finding satisfaction as an adult, social isolation, a reluctance to admit the problem and seek help, fear of spoiling children, a strong belief in the value of punishment, unreasonable and age-inappropriate expectations of children, and low personal self-esteem. Any combination of these traits results in an inability to cope and problem solve effectively when a problem or crisis evolves, and the outcome is abuse.

Although physical abuse and neglect account for the greatest portion of abuse incidents, child sexual abuse is another tragic dimension. Childhood sexual abuse is estimated to occur in about 40 percent of girls before the age of 17. Of this 40 percent, many have experienced ongoing repetitive abuse spanning many years. Studies indicate that a history of child abuse predisposes adolescents to high-risk health behaviors, including increased substance abuse, smoking, self-mutilation, suicidal behavior, aggression toward others, laxative abuse, promiscuity, and running away.[45]

Elder Abuse

Elder abuse is a term that denotes a variety of activities. Elder abuse is a serious problem for women because they generally live longer than men and in their later years are increasingly dependent on others for their care. The prevalence of elder abuse is difficult to ascertain accurately, although estimates are from 1 to 4 percent.[46–48] **Physical elder abuse** is defined as any activity that causes pain or injury to an older person. **Psychological elder abuse** is defined as inflicting a person with mental anguish. **Material elder abuse** or exploitation occurs when the financial resources of a person are misused or misappropriated by another.[49] The laws of many states specifically name these types of abuse as being criminal and reportable offenses. Neglect is often considered a form of abuse. Some state laws treat neglect and psychological abuse as if they were equivalent terms.[50] Neglect has also been specifically identified as a separate entity as the intentional failure or refusal to acknowledge an obligation to care for an older person (**active neglect**) or an intentional failure to fulfill an obligation to care for an elder (**passive neglect.**) These definitions can encompass a spectrum of acts and attitudes. The commonalities of neglect and psychological abuse are that the actions of the abuser or the failure of the abuser to act result in mental distress for the elderly dependent person.

Elder abuse is often seen as a manifestation of modern violent contemporary society. Prevalence estimates of elder abuse are difficult to calculate, but between 500,000 and 1,500,000 cases were reported yearly in the 1980s.[51,52] Elder abuse can occur in a private home or in a supervised living situation, such as a nursing home. The phenomenon of elder abuse in institutionalized settings is much less studied and much less reported than in private homes. The numbers are believed to be underreported. Several states require nursing homes to post prominent notices of patient and resident rights, including the right to report abuse to authorities. Although anonymity of reporting is guaranteed by law,

My stepfather started fondling me when I was 6. It evolved into sex by the time I was 12. I think my mother knew, but she had so many other problems to deal with. I had three younger sisters and I was so afraid for them. He said that he wouldn't touch them if I wouldn't tell "the secret." I was trapped. Eventually I found out that he was telling them the same thing. I have been in therapy for a year. I am still so hurt and so angry. The feelings and memories just won't go away.

21-YEAR-OLD WOMAN

many residents of nursing homes are either unable to comprehend the notices or intimidated by fear of possible reporting consequences.

Elder abuse has been discovered in people of all racial, ethnic, and economic backgrounds in the United States. Most victims have at least one physical or mental impairment.[51] The abused may have behavioral problems or place physical or psychological demands on the caregiver, who may lack the capacity to deal effectively with the situation. The abused person may deny being abused or may minimize complaints when confronted by health care professionals. The older abused person may seem fearful of the caregiver or seem overly compliant with the caregiver or health care professional. The elder may often deny abuse and try to attribute injuries to an unlikely cause. Necessary assistive or adaptive devices such as proper glasses, dentures, hearing aids, or a walker may be lacking. Medication compliance may seem poor owing to a lack of attention by the caregiver. The elder person may be lacking adequate nutrition or may need immediate medical attention that the caregiver has not been willing to make available.[53] Abuse of the elderly is also likely to be recurrent in 80 percent of the cases.[51]

Researchers have compiled a profile of the person most vulnerable to abuse.[53] A white woman between the ages of 66 and 83 who is living with her spouse is most likely to be the abuse victim. The woman is not severely ill, and the family income is very low. This person is most likely to experience physical, psychological, or multiple forms of abuse.

Studies have also compiled the characteristics of the elderly abuser. Researchers have found that 68 percent of elderly abusers were spouses, sons, and daughters of the victim. Another 6.8 percent were grandchildren of the victim.[54] Another major study found that in 86 percent of elder abuse cases, the abuser is a relative, and in 75 percent of cases, the relative lives with the victim.[51] They also noted that 40 percent of the abusers were spouses, and 50 percent were grandchildren. The abuser had been the abused person's caregiver for an average of 9.5 years.

Several factors have been identified that contribute to a high stress level for relatives of a dependent older person and therefore may contribute to elder abuse. These factors include resentment of dependency, especially as the level of dependency increases. Elder abuse is also related to emotional problems, such as alcohol or drug use by the abuser. Social isolation of the abuser and the abused is a risk factor for elder abuse. Lack of community support may also contribute to elder abuse because few communities have resources and facilities to provide respite care, adult care, or shelters for the abused older person. Other non-caregiving relatives of the abuser and the victim may create additional stress for the family of the dependent person. It has also been hypothesized that the abuser may be repeating a cycle of violence, such as has been identified in cases of child abuse and neglect. The abuser of an elderly parent may have been abused by the parent in childhood, or the abuser may have been witness to the same type of elder abuse by the parent against the abuser's grandparent.

Dealing with Relationship Violence

Knowing the facts about violence can lead to a certain level of paranoia and anger, two unhealthy conditions. Instead, identifying the factors that contribute to violence and working to eliminate them are constructive reactions. Although miscommunication is clearly not the only or major cause of rape, it is often a factor. Misinterpretation of communication is frequently a reason cited for the high prevalence of date rape and courtship violence. In a study to determine how men and women perceive friendliness, results indicated that men tend to view friendliness as sexual intent.[55] Men were found to perceive more sexuality in their own and in others' behaviors than women. These findings indicate a need for clearer communication between men and women on these issues. Women and men need to communicate more effectively, both in terms of their feelings and in explicitly stating their personal preferences and wishes about sexual behavior. Many people still believe that men should be aggressive, and women should be passive, compliant, please others, and give in. When people, male or female, buy into these stereotypes, the stage is set for problems. Men and women may act the way they think that they are "supposed to act" and expect their partners to act the way they are "supposed to act" as well. For example, women who have been socialized to be passive may not think that they have a right to express their opinions openly and freely. Men who have

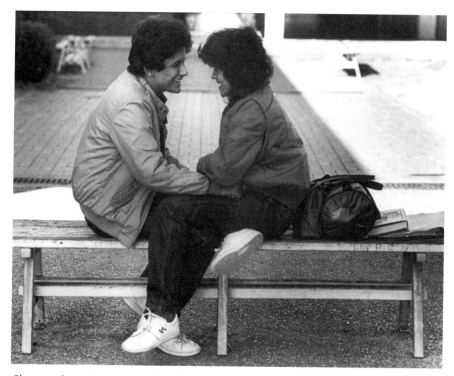

Clear and concise communication about expectations for the relationship and sexual behavior is essential.

been socialized that they need to live up to a "macho" image may think that they need to "score" with women in order to be a "real" man. They may expect women to go along with their need to prove themselves or believe that a woman means "yes" when she says "no." To address these stereotypes, a woman must:

■ Recognize the inherent limitations in these stereotypes.

■ Be open in discussing values with respect to relationships and sexuality.

■ Decide for herself and be explicit about when she will or will not have sex.

Many women find it difficult to talk openly about relationships and sexuality. Instead of using clear communication, they rely on assumptions, hints, innuendoes, and considerable hope that their partner understands. Unfortunately, such telepathic communication is highly unreliable. Expectations and values about relationships and sexuality should be explicitly expressed. Communication is bidirectional: In a relationship, each person must carefully listen to the other and confirm what has been said or not said. Finally, "no" means "no" (Fig. 6.8). When a woman says "no" but really means "yes" or "maybe," she is perpetuating a vicious cycle of miscommunication.

Women in dysfunctional relationships first need to identify and acknowledge the presence of the problem. Denial, avoidance, and protection of the dysfunctional partner often prevent or delay such acknowledgment. This is particularly true for women who may have grown up in a dysfunctional family situation. Professional assistance is needed in the form of counseling and support when the problem has been identified. Most cities have shelters for battered women that provide both physical safety and psychological counseling and referral services.

Sources of Help

Most communities have services and facilities to support female victims of violence, including local crisis hotlines. Hotline counselors are able to provide callers with phone numbers of facilities that provide counseling, supportive services, and emergency shelter. Many local organizations have been organized by women who have been battered themselves and realize the need for sensitive and protected outreach services. Support groups provide the opportunity for women to share common concerns, fears, and information. For many women, the most important step in taking control of a violent situation—admitting there is a problem and reaching out for help.

Sexual Harassment

In a society where the sexual victimization of women is so widespread as to have been effectively invisible, sexual harassment remains the last great open secret. Although all women know of it and most will experience it, until

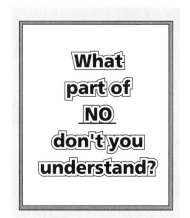

FIGURE 6.8

Communication issues are an important dimension of personal violence.

recently it had no name or legal existence. Even now, there are no official statistics or national surveys; its existence is ignored in studies of both sexual victimization and workplace behavior, and women's stories of their experiences are routinely disbelieved.

THE LAST GREAT OPEN SECRET, THE SEXUAL HARASSMENT OF WOMEN
IN THE WORKPLACE AND ACADEMIA. *Federation News,* AMERICAN
PSYCHOLOGICAL ASSOCIATION. 5/92, P. 10.

Sexual Harassment Defined

Sexual harassment may also be considered a form of violence. Although sexual harassment can occur in any setting, it has been most commonly reported in the workplace. Women at most risk for sexual harassment are those in careers traditionally considered to be male occupations. A worksite definition of **sexual harassment** includes any unsolicited nonreciprocal male behavior that asserts a woman's sex role over her function as a worker. It can include any of the following behaviors: staring, commenting, touching, requests for sexual favors, repeated requests for dates or sexual intercourse, or rape. Sexual harassment can be initiated by anyone, but it is more likely to be used by someone with more power or authority than the recipient. In addition to the physical and emotional victimization, there is an additional threat of economic vulnerability, leaving the victim with few real options in the situation. Sexual harassment is often trivialized and not taken as a violation of rights or personal dignity. Excuses are often encountered with sexual harassment (Information Box 6.7), but these excuses serve to perpetuate power disparity and further dehumanize

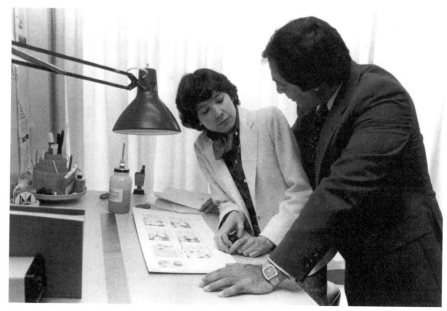

Sexual harassment is most common in the workplace.

Common Excuses for Sexual Harassment

"Sexual harassment is a trivial distraction from the real work."
Sexual harassment can have long-term emotional impact on the victim. The emotional and economic impact of sexual harassment are not trivial in nature or form.

"I didn't mean any harm. I was just having fun."
Sexual harassment is similar to poking someone with a stick. The fun is one-sided and unfair.

"She should take it as a compliment that we like her when we say things like that."
Unwanted and unsolicited sexual advances and innuendoes, particularly from others in positions of power, can be frightening. The victim can hardly feel "complimented" when she feels threatened and put down.

"She just wanted to make trouble here with a complaint."
Women are caught between the proverbial rock and a hard place. If they accept the harassment, they perpetuate the behavior and risk further, and perhaps worse, harassment. If they file a complaint, they are labeled as troublemakers, with no guarantees that the situation will be corrected. Filing a complaint may also place a woman's job security or career in jeopardy.

women. Like other forms of sexual victimization, harassment operates as an instrument of social control.

Effects on Women in the Workplace

Many working women are subjected to sexual harassment on the job. Although some may consider sexual harassment to be trivial, the reality is that harassment is widespread. Employers are becoming increasingly sensitive to the issue, perhaps motivated in part by a number of court decisions that have awarded large payments to victims.

Sexual harassment on the job can appear in many forms, and the ramifications can be devastating. A common situation involves a boss or supervisor who requires sexual services from an employee as a condition for keeping a job or promotion. Less blatant forms of workplace sexual harassment include being subjected to obscenities or being made the target of sexual jokes and innuendoes. Personal humiliation and degradation are ramifications of workplace sexual harassment, and the financial consequences of not complying with sexual coercion on the job may be devastating, especially for people in lower level positions such as clerical and blue-collar workers. Many victims, especially if they are supporting families, cannot afford to be unemployed. Many find it difficult to seek other work while they are employed. If they are fired for refusing to be victimized, unemployment compensation is not always available. When it is available, it is usually at a fraction of the regular salary. Thus, a person who quits or is fired as a result of sexual harassment faces the prospect of severe financial difficulties.

Victims of sexual harassment may experience a range of adverse emotional and physical effects, including anger, humiliation, shame, embarrassment, nervousness, irritability, and lack of motivation. Guilt is another common feeling, as if the victim had done something wrong to encourage the harassment. The sense of alienation and helplessness reported by many victims of sexual harassment is similar to that experienced by many rape victims. Psychosomatic effects may also be experienced by sexual harassment victims. These symptoms may include headaches, stomach ailments, back and neck pain, and a variety of other stress-related ailments.

Dealing Effectively with Harassment

A number of options are available to the individual who experiences sexual harassment. It is important to know that criminal charges can be filed against the perpetrator. If the coercion is short of attempted rape or assault, it is often wise to confront the person doing the harassment. The confrontation should be stated in clear terms, and the specific behaviors should be identified as sexual harassment. The victim should make it clear that the behavior will not be tolerated and that if it continues charges will be filed through appropriate channels. Some victims carefully document what has occurred and provide written confrontation rather than verbal discussion. If the behavior does not stop, the next step is to discuss it with the supervisor of the person responsible for the harassment. It is often helpful to talk to other employees—many times there is more than one victim. Discussing with other employees provides peer support and pressure for behavior to stop. Official complaints can be filed with local or state Human Rights Commissions or Fair Employment Practice Agencies. If legal action is necessary, lawsuits can be filed in federal courts under the Civil Rights Act. They can also be filed under city or state laws prohibiting employment discrimination. One lawsuit can be filed in a number of jurisdictions. A person who has been the victim of sexual harassment is more likely to receive a favorable court ruling if attempts were made to resolve the problem within the organization before taking the issue to court.

Summary

Violence is harmful to individuals, families, and society, but women bear a disproportionate burden as victims of violence. Violence against women takes many forms, and over time, women victims may experience isolation from others, lowered self-esteem, depression, increased alcohol or drug use, emotional problems, illness, denial, pain and injuries, and possible permanent physical damage and even death. Children in battering households may also experience illness, emotional problems, increased fears, increased risk of abuse, injuries, and death. They may also learn to role model abusive behavior. Societal costs with battering are high as well, with increased crime; legal, medical, and counseling costs; and an overall decrease in quality of life. Efforts are urgently needed to address and reduce the full spectrum of violence against women.

Violence

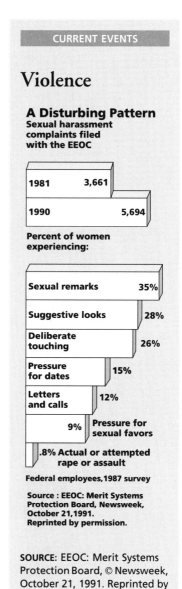

A Disturbing Pattern
Sexual harassment
complaints filed
with the EEOC

1981	3,661
1990	5,694

Percent of women experiencing:

Sexual remarks	35%
Suggestive looks	28%
Deliberate touching	26%
Pressure for dates	15%
Letters and calls	12%
9% Pressure for sexual favors	
.8% Actual or attempted rape or assault	

Federal employees,1987 survey

Source : EEOC: Merit Systems
Protection Board, Newsweek,
October 21,1991.
Reprinted by permission.

SOURCE: EEOC: Merit Systems
Protection Board, © Newsweek,
October 21, 1991. Reprinted by
permission.

Philosophical Dimensions: Violence, Abuse, and Harassment

1. How does style of dress serve as a form of nonverbal communication? How can this communication be interpreted or misinterpreted?

2. How do socio-cultural values and attitudes contribute to the continuing victimization of women?

3. How can the media contribute to violence in contemporary society?

4. How should society deal with the subject of pornography?

5. What can a woman do to reduce her risk of assault?

References

1. USDHHS (1991). *Healthy people 2000: National health promotion and disease prevention objectives.* (DHHS Pub. No. (PHS) 91-50212.) Washington, DC: US Government Printing Office.

2. Chen, J.M., and Lin, P.L. (1988). American college student's attitudes toward rape victims and beliefs in a just world. Indianapolis, IN: University of Indianapolis, Department of Behavioral Sciences. (ERIC Document Reproduction Service No. ED 305-290.)

3. Coller, S.A., and Resick, P.A. (1987). Women's attributions of responsibility for date rape: The influence of empathy and sex-role stereotyping. *Violence and Victims, 2*(2), 115–125.

4. Kanin, E. (1984). Date rape: Unofficial criminals and victims. *Victimology, 9*(1), 95–108.

5. Alexander, C.S. (1980). The responsible victim: Nurses' perceptions of victims of rape. *Journal of Health and Social Behavior, 21:* 22–33.

6. Johnson, K., and Ferguson, T. (1990). *Trusting ourselves.* New York: Atlantic Monthly Press.

7. Calhoun, K.S., and Atkeson, B.M. (1991). *Treatment of rape victims: Facilitating psychosocial adjustment.* New York: Pergamon Press.

8. Unger, R., and Crawford, M. (1992). *Women and gender.* New York: McGraw-Hill.

9. Faludi, S. (1991). *Backlash.* New York: Crown Publishers.

10. D'Emilio, J., and Freedman, E.B. (1988). *Intimate matters.* New York: Harper & Row.

11. Davis, A.Y. (1983). *Women, race and class.* New York: Vintage Books.

12. Peele, S. (1985). *The diseasing of America.* Lexington, MA: Lexington Books.

13. Walker, L. (1989). Psychology and violence against women. *American Psychologist, 44,* 695–702.

14. United States Department of Justice (1991, June). *Criminal victimization in the United States, 1989: A National Crime Survey Report.* Washington, DC: Bureau of Justice Statistics.

15. Donnerstein, E., Linz, D., and Penrod, S. (1987). *The question of pornography: Research findings and policy implications.* New York: The Free Press.

16. Attorney General's Commission on Pornography (1986). *Final report of the attorney general's commission on pornography.* Washington, DC: US Department of Justice.

17. National Woman Abuse Prevention Project. (1990). *Domestic violence fact sheets.* Washington, D.C.: Office for Victims of Crime, U.S. Department of Justice.

18. USDHHS (1987). *Alcohol and health.* (DHHS Pub. No. (ADM) 87-1519.) Washington, DC: US Government Printing Office.

19. Fingarete, H. (1988). *Heavy drinking.* Berkeley: University of California Press.

20. Cahalan, D. (1987). *Understanding America's drinking problem.* San Francisco: Jossey-Bass Publishers.

21. Johnson, J.D., and Jackson, L.A. (1988). Assessing the effects of factors that might underlie the differential perception of acquaintance and stranger rape. *Sex Roles, 19:*37–45.

22. Buhrke, R., and Lustgraaf, M. (1988). Date rape awareness program: A model for education and consciousness raising. *Journal of College Student Development, 29,* 478–479.

23. Russell, D. (1984). *Sexual exploitation: Rape, child sexual abuse, and workplace harassment.* Beverly Hills, CA: Sage Publications.

24. Koss, M.P., Gidycz, C.A., and Wisniewski, N. (1987). The scope of rape: incidence and prevalence of sexual aggression and victimization in a national sample of higher education students. *Journal of Consulting and Clinical Psychology, 55,* 162–170.

25. Kanin, E. (1969). Selected dyadic aspects of male sex aggression. *Journal of Sex Research, 5,* 12–28.

26. Muehlenhard, C.L., Friedman, D.E., and Thomas, C.M. (1985). Is date rape justifiable? The effects of dating activity, who initiated, who paid, and men's attitudes towards women. *Psychology of Women Quarterly, 9,* 297–310.

27. National Victim Center (1992). *Rape in America—a report to the nation.* Arlington, VA.

28. Bart, P., and O'Brien, P. (1984). Stopping rape: Effective avoidance strategies. *Signs: Journal of Women in Culture and Society, 10,* 83–101.

29. Bart, P., and O'Brien, P. (1985). *Stopping rape: Successful survival strategies.* New York: Pergamon.

30. Siegel, J.M., Sorenson, S.B., Golding, J.M., Burnam, M.A., and Stein, J.A. (1989). Resistance to sexual assault: Who resists and what happens? *American Journal of Public Health, 79,* 27–31.

31. Burgess, A.W., and Holstrom, L.L. (1974). Rape trauma syndrome. *American Journal of Psychiatry, 131,* 981–986.

32. Eyman, J.S. (1980). *How to convict a rapist.* New York: Stein & Day.

33. Parrot, A. (1990, April.) Date rape. *Medical aspects of sexuality,* 28–31.

34. Mercy, J.A., and Saltzman, L.E. (1989). Fatal violence among spouses in the United States, 1976–1985. *American Journal of Public Health, 79,* 595–599.

35. Federal Bureau of Investigation. (1990). *Crime in the United States: uniform crime reports for the United States, 1989.* (Pub. No. 90-477-P.) Washington, DC: US Government Printing Office.

36. Margolin, G., Sibner, L.G., and Glebermau, L. (1988). Wife battering. In V.B. van Hasselt, R.L. Morrison, A.S. Bellack, and M. Herson (Eds.), *Handbook of family violence,* pp. 88–117. New York: Plenum Press.

37. Browne, A. (1988). Family violence: When victimized women kill. In V.B. van Hasselt, R.L. Morrison, A.S. Bellack, and M. Herson (Eds.), *Handbook of family violence,* pp. 271–289. New York: Plenum Press.

38. Stacey, W.A. and Shupe, A. (1983). *The Family Secret: Domestic Violence in America.* Boston: Beacon Press.

39. Stark, E., and Flitcraft, A. (1982). Medical therapy as repression; the case of the battered woman. *Health and Medicine, 1,* 29–32.

40. Chez, R.A. (1988). Women battering. *American Journal of Obstetrics and Gynecology, 158,* 1–4.

41. Lobel, K. (1986.) *Naming the violence: Speaking out about lesbian battering.* National Coalition against Domestic Violence. Seattle: Seal Press.

42. Lie, G.Y., Schiit, R., Bush, J., Montagne, M., and Reyes, L. (1991). Lesbians in currently aggressive relationships: How frequently do they report aggressive past relationships? *Violence and Victims, 6*(2), 121–135.

43. Renzetti, C.M. (1988). Violence in lesbian relationships; a preliminary analysis of causal factors. *Journal of International Violence, 3,* 381–399.

44. Hillard, P.J.A. (1985). Physical abuse in pregnancy. *Obstetrics and Gynecology, 66,* 185–190.

45. Childhood sexual abuse and the consequences in adult women. (1988). *Obstetrics and Gynecology, 71,* 631–642.

46. Block, M., and Sinnott, J. (1979). *The battered elder syndrome study.* College Park, MD: Center on Aging.

47. van Hasselt, V.B., Morrison, R.L., Bellack, A.S., and Herson, M. (Eds.) (1988). *Handbook of family violence,* pp. 247–269. New York: Plenum Press.

48. Straus, M.A., and Gelles, R.J. (1986). Societal change and change in family violence from 1975 to 1985 as revealed by two national surveys. *Journal of Marriage and Family, 48,* 465–479.

49. Circirelli, V.G. (1986). The helping relationship and family neglect in later life. In K.S. Pillemer and R.S. Wolf (Eds.), *Elder abuse: Conflict in the family,* pp. 49–66. Dover, MA: Auburn House.

50. Salend, E., Kane, R.A., Satz, M., and Pynoos, J. (1984). Elder abuse reporting: limitations of statutes. *Gerontologist, 24,* 61–69.

51. Council on Scientific Affairs (1987). Elder abuse and neglect. *Journal of the American Medical Association, 257,* 966–971.

52. Crystal, S. (1987). Elder abuse: The latest "crisis." *Public Interest. 88,* 56–66.

53. Ebersole, P., and Hess, P. (1985). *Toward healthy aging: Human needs and nursing response.* St. Louis: C.V. Mosby.

54. Walker, J.C., and Potter, D.E. (1983). Analysis of elder abuse in a state-wide reporting system. *Gerontologist, 23,* 151.

55. Abbey, A. (1982). Sex differences in attributions for friendly behavior: Do males misperceive females' friendliness? *Journal of Personality and Social Psychology, 42,* 830–838.

Resources

NATIONAL COALITION AGAINST DOMESTIC VIOLENCE

2401 Virginia Avenue NW, Suite 306
Washington, DC 20037
202-293-8860

NATIONAL ORGANIZATION FOR VICTIM ASSISTANCE

Dept P
717 D Street NW
Washington, DC 20004
202-232-6682

NATIONAL VICTIM CENTER

309 W 7th Street, Suite 705
Fort Worth, TX
817-877-3355

An advocacy and resource center founded in honor of Sunny von Bulow to help spearhead the fight for rights for the victims of violent crime. The Center connects victims with providers of care, service, and assistance and helps grass roots organizations develop quality programs to help victims.

NATIONAL WOMAN ABUSE PREVENTION PROJECT

2000 P Street NW #508
Washington, DC 20036
202-857-0216

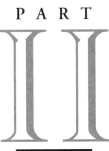

PART

II

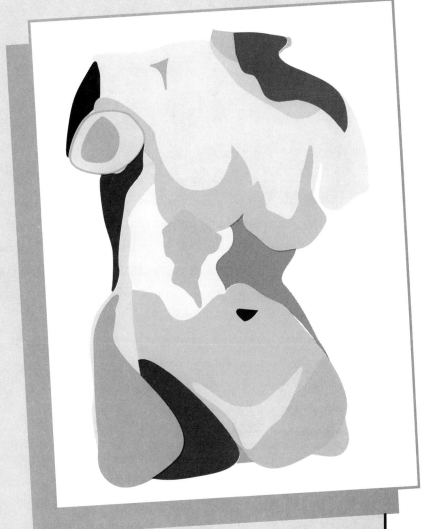

Personal and

Sexual

Dimensions

in Women's

Health

Sexual Health

CHAPTER OBJECTIVES

On completion of this chapter, the student should be able to discuss:

1. How cultural values may define sexual behavior.
2. The difference between male circumcision and female clitoridectomy.
3. How stereotypes influence the sexual health and behavior of women.
4. How socialization influences sexual behavior.
5. Why research on sexual behavior is difficult.
6. How definitions affect the interpretation of sexual research.
7. The significance of Kinsey's research.
8. The significance of the work by Masters and Johnson.
9. What is meant by gender identity and gender role.
10. The implications of androgyny for sexual behavior.
11. Homosexual, heterosexual, and bisexual orientations.
12. The range of activities associated with homophobia.
13. The location and function of major external female genital structures.
14. The location and function of major internal female genital structures.
15. The three phases of the menstrual cycle.
16. The four basic phases of the female sexual response cycle.
17. Several examples of sexual expression.
18. How sexuality is expressed in childhood.
19. How sexuality is expressed in adolescence.
20. The myths of sexuality and aging.
21. How hormonal changes of menopause affect sexual response.
22. The significance of the gynecological examination.
23. The three phases of the gynecological examination.

24. **The four major areas of sexual dysfunction in women.**

25. **The significance of communication in intimate relationships.**

26. **The significance of communication in the relationship with a health care provider.**

Introduction

Sexual health is a nebulous term to define because it can refer to physical, psychological, social, cultural, and emotional facets of human interactions. Sexual health is not limited to an individual's being but also extends into the relationship with another. The need for intimacy and physical sharing is a lifelong biological and social theme. Understanding sexual health requires a multifaceted examination on both scientific and psychosocial perspectives.

Perspectives on Sexual Health and Sexuality

Overview

An underlying assumption throughout history and throughout cultures has been that little boys grow up to be men and do what men do, while little girls grow up to be women and do what women do. Yet when cultures are examined, it is readily apparent that a universal standard is not applicable. That naturally leads to the question of what programs people to assume specific roles and specific identities. The biological hypothesis that sexual behavior is simply a reproductive function is not substantiated across generations or across cultures.

Cultural Dimensions

Sexual behavior is often defined by cultural values. The tremendous cultural diversity throughout the world creates considerable diversity regarding sexual norms. This diversity represents a wide spectrum of sexuality issues, including what is considered arousing, types of sexual activity, and sanctions and prohibitions on sexual behavior. This diversity of sexual expression does have one consistent theme, though, that of "marriage" in some form or another. Within all cultures, marriage provides sanctioned sexual privileges and obligations. Social scientists have recognized that every society shapes, structures, or constrains the development and expression of sexuality in all its members.[1]

Circumcision is an example of cultural sexual tradition. The practice of male **circumcision,** the removal of the **prepuce,** foreskin or fold of skin over the glans penis, can be traced back to Egyptian times. Biblical accounts of the procedure and religious as well as social traditions have perpetuated the practice

I used to feel confused about what was feminine or what was masculine. I finally decided that it didn't matter what I called a behavior. What mattered is what I wanted to do. I really enjoy nontraditional activities. That really does not make me less of a woman.

18-YEAR-OLD STUDENT

into modern times. In the United States, almost all circumcisions of newborns are done for religious or hygienic reasons. It is estimated that only 15 percent of the world's population currently practices circumcision.[2] "Female circumcision" is a term used to describe **clitoridectomy,** a procedure in which the entire clitoris is removed. This practice is now generally limited to some countries in Africa and to a lesser extent other regions of the world. Each country or culture uses its own technique for the procedure according to religious, cultural, or folklore background. Often the procedure involves mutilation of other vaginal structures and is performed by nonmedical individuals. Short-term and long-term consequences include a spectrum of conditions from infection to death. Many organizations, including the World Health Organization, oppose female circumcision, but cultural change is a slow process.

Other cultural influences, not as severe as circumcision, extend into gender role expectations. In many European and Middle Eastern societies, for example, a brief kiss on the cheek is considered appropriate masculine behavior. In American society, such behavior by men is considered inappropriate. Cultural expectations or acceptance of masculine and feminine behaviors evolve over time. In post–World War II America, men exclusively used the services of a barber shop. It was unheard of them to go to a hair "stylist" or a "beauty shop." Today hair stylists and customers don't blink at the mixed male-female clientele who present for service.

Gender-Role Dimensions

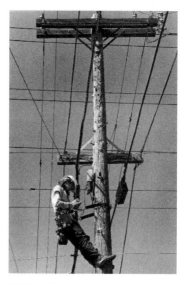

Cultural expectations or acceptance of masculine or feminine behaviors evolve over time.

The issue of gender goes beyond the processes of a subjective sense of maleness or femaleness. A set of behaviors that are considered "normal" and appropriate for the sex are ascribed by society. The ascribing of gender roles leads to assumptions about how people will behave. Once these assumptions or expectations are widely accepted, they may begin to function as **stereotypes.** A stereotype is a generalized notion of what a person is like based only on characteristics such as sex, race, religion, ethnicity, or social background. For example, in Western culture, men have been expected to behave independently, aggressively, and nonemotionally. Women have been expected to be passive, submissive, and dependent.

Stereotyping has clearly influenced the ability of women to succeed in traditional male arenas such as sports and professional careers. Stereotyping also influences the sexual health and behavior of women, who naturally find conflict with assumptions and expectations that they be passive, submissive, dependent, emotional, and subordinate. Despite the limiting impact of rigid, stereotypical gender roles, many men and women behave in a manner remarkably consistent with the norms that these roles establish. **Socialization** refers to the process whereby society conveys behavioral expectations to the individual. These expectations are reinforced by parents, peers, schools, textbooks, and the media.

Epidemiology—Sex Research

Researchers attempting to understand sexual behavior face many of the same problems that handicap all research into human social behavior. Human subjects cannot be placed in a laboratory-type setting where variables that influence outcome measures can be controlled. Human behavior is also infinitely more complex, and studies, particularly on human behavior, are prone to many types of contamination and bias. Sex is considered a private arena and as such is even more limited than other arenas of behavioral research. Clearly many problematic issues occur in an attempt to understand the prevalence and nature of contemporary sexual behavior.

I like to think that I don't stereotype people, but when I really reflect on my thoughts or comments, I realize that I do. It is one of the things that I am trying hard to work on. I don't want to be stereotyped and it is not fair to others when I do it.

21-YEAR-OLD WOMAN

Research Issues

Sexual behavior may be the most important of all human activities. It is the process by which the species is reproduced, it is the central behavior around which families are formed, and it is a key component in the emotional lives of individuals. Sexual behavior is also central to a number of social and medical problems: marital difficulties and divorce; incest and child molestation; the reproductive issues of infertility, sterility, contraception, unwanted pregnancy, and abortion; and sexually transmitted diseases. Yet there has been less systematic, scientific research on the sexual behavior of Americans than on any other topic of importance. The acquired immunodeficiency syndrome (AIDS) epidemic currently makes accurate information on sexual behavior of immediate concern, but the collection of scientific information on sexual matters continues to face much political opposition.

There are a number of ways to study sexual behavior. These strategies include case studies, direct observation, experimental laboratory research, and surveys. Each of these methods is obviously limited. What to measure is another difficulty of sexual research. Sexual research could be addressed directly, as in determining the actual prevalence of certain sexual behaviors such as oral-genital sex or types of sexual activity such as the prevalence of homosexual activity. Indirect assessments, such as adolescent pregnancy rates or sexually transmitted disease rates, provide insight into the consequences of sexual behavior. Definitions are another "technical difficulty" in research. For example, a frequently quoted statistic in sex research is the number of people in a given category who have engaged in premarital sex. Premarital sex has been traditionally defined as penile-vaginal intercourse that takes place before a couple is married. This definition is misleading because it excludes a broad array of noncoital heterosexual and homosexual activities. Heavy petting can include extensive noncoital types of sexual contact, often resulting in orgasm. "Virginity" may not reflect a lack of sexual activity. The term "premarital" has inherent connotations that may be inappropriate to some individuals. Not all couples who engage in sexual activity have marital intentions with that partner. Any review of sex studies must take into consideration the inherent limitations of such research.

Well-Known Studies

Several important studies on sexual behavior have been conducted, and each has its own inherent limitations. In 1948 and 1953, Kinsey conducted the most comprehensive taxonomic survey of human sexual behavior to date.[3,4] The sample was large but overrepresented certain population segments. The researchers interviewed thousands of people of various socioeconomic status, educational level, marital status, and sex education experiences. Masters and Johnson are perhaps the best known of sex researchers. In 1966, through direct observation techniques, they observed and recorded more than 10,000 completed sexual response cycles.[5] Like Kinsey, their work has been criticized for not having a randomly selected representative population. The *Redbook Survey* was a questionnaire survey of more than 100,000 women.[6] The report examined sexual behavior and attitudes of American women. The study sample was criticized also because *Redbook* readers were not a true cross section of American women. Likewise in 1976, *The Hite Report*, a questionnaire survey on female sexuality, provided extensive narrative answers to several important questions about the sexual practices of American women.[7] It has been criticized because the sample was thought to overrepresent young liberal women. Blumstein and Schwartz (1983) elicited excellent information about a variety of sexual and nonsexual components of relationships from a large national sample, but the sample underrepresented certain low socioeconomic and minority groups.[8] Despite the apparent limitations, these studies have all provided valuable information and insight into sexual behavior and attitudes. They demonstrate, however, that in evaluating any study of sexual behavior, it is important to consider the quality of the method and sampling techniques used.

Despite the limitations in conducting research on sexual behavior, several of these studies provided some insight into important issues. The prevalence of premarital sex is one of these issues. Fig. 7.1 compares 1982 and 1988 data about women who have ever had intercourse by marital status and age group. This table shows a slight increase in the proportion of all women who had ever had sexual intercourse. Fig. 7.2 from the same study reveals that the increases

FIGURE 7.1

Percentage of women who had ever had intercourse by marital status and age group, 1982 and 1988.

SOURCE: Reproduced with the permission of The Alan Guttmacher Institute from Jacqueline Darroch Forrest and Susheela Singh, "The Sexual and Reproductive Behavior of American Women, 1982–1988," *Family Planning Perspectives,* Vol. 22, No. 5, September/October 1990.

Age Group	All Women			
	Ever Had Intercourse		Never Married	
	1982	1988	1982	1988
15–44	**86.4**	**88.5**	**59.3**	**65.5**
15–19	47.1	53.2	42.1	49.5
20–24	85.7	86.4	72.3	74.8
25–29	96.7	94.8	83.8	79.9
30–34	98.0	98.0	81.3	84.8
35–39	97.9	97.9	67.5	78.1
40–44	98.2	98.9	63.0	84.5

Race/Ethnicity	15–19 years		15–17 years		18–19 years	
	1982	1988	1982	1988	1982	1988
Non-Hispanic white	44.5	52.4	29.8	36.2	60.8	74.3
Non-Hispanic black	59.0	60.8	44.4	50.5	79.1	78.0
Hispanic	50.6	48.5	35.6	36.1	70.1	70.0

FIGURE 7.2

Percentage of women aged 15 to 19 who had ever had sexual intercourse, by race/ethnicity, 1982 and 1988.

SOURCE: Reproduced with the permission of The Alan Guttmacher Institute from Jacqueline Darroch Forrest and Susheela Singh, "The Sexual and Reproductive Behavior of American Women, 1982–1988," *Family Planning Perspectives,* Vol. 22, No. 5, September/October 1990.

in the percentage of young women who have had sexual intercourse are not consistent along racial and ethnic lines, with lowest prevalence rates among female Hispanic-American teens. The distribution of sexual orientation is another research question. An analysis of data collected from the National Opinion Research Center, University of Chicago, found that nearly 91 percent of US adults self-identify as heterosexual (Fig. 7.3). Despite researchers' efforts to ensure subjects' anonymity and confidentiality, limitations to this type of information include biases of self-reporting and social desirability. Nevertheless, these studies provide some limited valuable insight into contemporary sexual behavior trends and issues.

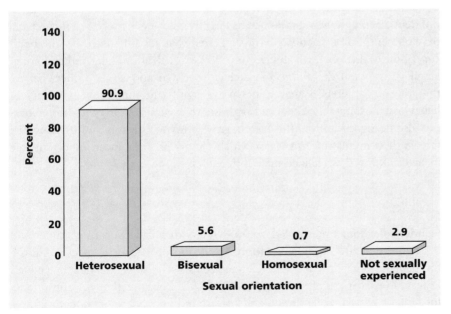

FIGURE 7.3

Percentage distribution of US adults, by sexual orientation.

SOURCE: Reproduced with the permission of The Alan Guttmacher Institute from Tom W. Smith, "Adult Sexual Behavior in 1989: Number of Partners, Frequency of Intercourse and Risk of AIDS," *Family Planning Perspectives,* Vol. 23, No. 3, May/June 1991.

Gender Identity

Gender identity refers to an individual's personal subjective sense of being a male or female, although a person's gender identity is not necessarily consistent with his or her biological sex. Some individuals experience considerable confusion and stress in their efforts to establish their gender identity. Both biological (sex) and social-learning factors (identity and roles) are involved in the determination of gender identity.

Gender and Sex

Gender identity is clearly influenced by biological sex, which is determined by a complex set of variables. The genetic material in a fertilized egg is organized in structures known as **chromosomes.** Chromosomes give rise to the process of sexual **differentiation**, whereby the individual develops physical characteristics distinct from those of the other sex. The physical femaleness or maleness is not simply a result of this chromosome mix but rather the result of processes that occur at various levels of sexual differentiation. Under normal conditions, the prenatal differentiation processes interact to determine biological sex and later gender identity. In early prenatal development, male and female external genitalia are undifferentiated. Through a series of complex interactions involving gonadal sex hormones, both the internal and the external sex structures differentiate into male or female genitalia. Because the external genitals, gonads, and some of the internal structures of males and females originate from the same embryonic tissues, it is not surprising that they have **homologous,** or corresponding, parts (Fig. 7.4).

Scientists have determined that some important structural and functional differences exist in the brains of males and females and that the process of sex differentiation of human brains occurs largely, if not exclusively, during prenatal development. Some scientists have suggested that sex differences in the brain contribute to differences in abilities or processes, such as thinking, remembering, language use, and the ability to perceive spatial relationships. Others believe that the sex differences may also have a significant impact on a variety of behaviors, most notably sexual and aggressive behaviors. Clearly these differences can also be significantly influenced by environmental factors and psychosocial factors. It is premature to suggest which factors play the most important role in determining these female-male differences.

Identity and Roles

Gender role, sometimes called sex role, refers to a collection of attitudes and behaviors that are considered normal and appropriate in a specific culture for people of a particular sex. Gender roles establish sex-related behavioral expectations that people are expected to fulfill. Behavior thought appropriate for females is termed **feminine,** and correspondingly behavior thought appropriate for males is termed **masculine.** Gender-role expectations are culturally

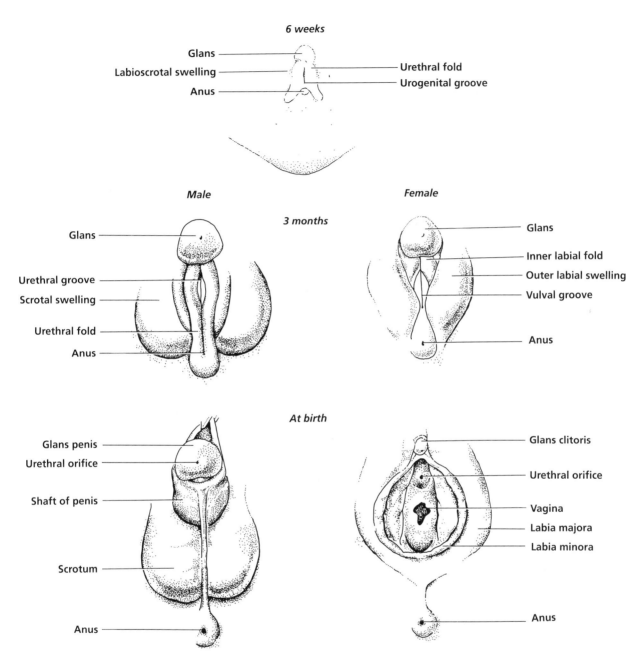

FIGURE 7.4
External genital differentiation—male and female.

defined and vary from society to society. Besides being culturally dependent, notions of masculinity and femininity may be era dependent. Social-learning theory suggests that the identification with either feminine or masculine roles or a combination (**androgyny**) results primarily from the social and cultural models and influences to which individuals are exposed since birth. Parents

I find that I am most comfortable with others who are not hung up on being "macho" or being "feminine." Those concepts really can interfere with sharing real feelings and doing what needs to be done.

25-YEAR-OLD WOMAN

typically dress boys and girls differently. Children grow up with "girls' toys" or "boys' toys" and receive reinforcement for gender-expected behaviors. At some point, children develop a firm sense of being a girl or boy and a strong desire to adopt behaviors appropriate for their sex. With the socialization process, society conveys behavioral expectations to an individual. Parents, peer groups, schools, textbooks, and the media frequently help develop and reinforce traditional gender-role assumptions and behaviors. Gender-role conditioning has an impact on all facets of an individual's life, perhaps most importantly in influencing sexuality.

Gender-role expectations exert a profound influence on sexuality. Beliefs about females and males, together with assumptions about what constitutes appropriate behaviors for each, affect many aspects of sexual sharing. These aspects include personal expectations for intimate relationships, perceptions of quality with such relationships, and the responses of others to an individual's sexuality. Stereotypical expectations of men and women are examples that clearly influence gender-role expectations (Information Box 7.1). These stereotype expectations actually hinder both men and women in maximizing their individual capabilities and in establishing fulfilling relationships.

Androgyny refers to having characteristics of both sexes. The term is often used to describe flexibility in gender role. Androgynous individuals are those who have integrated aspects of traditional masculinity and femininity into their lifestyles. Androgyny offers the option of expressing whatever behavior seems appropriate in a given situation instead of limiting responses to those traditionally considered gender appropriate. Androgynous individuals of both sexes are more likely to engage in behavior typically ascribed to the other sex than are gender-typed individuals. The implications of androgyny for sexual behavior are that both women and men can have more positive attitudes toward sexual behavior, be more tolerant and less likely to judge or criticize the sexual behavior of others, and be more communicative and responsive in sexual relationships and sexual intimacy.[9–11]

INFORMATION BOX 7.1

Sexual Stereotypes of Women and Men

Women are undersexed, and men are oversexed.

Women are inexperienced, and men are experts.

Women are recipients, and men are initiators.

Women are controllers, and men are movers.

Women are nurturing and supportive, and men are strong and unemotional.

Women are sensitive, and men are insensitive.

Women are dependent, and men are independent.

Women are passive, and men are aggressive.

Homosexuality

Homosexuality, bisexuality, and heterosexuality are terms to define an individual's sexual orientation. **Homosexual** orientation is the attraction to same-sex partners, and **heterosexual** orientation is attraction to other-sex partners. A **bisexual** person is attracted to both same-sex and other-sex partners. Although these concepts imply clear distinction between the terms, the actual delineation is not precise. Kinsey described a seven-point continuum that ranged from exclusive contact with and attraction to the other sex to degrees of heterosexual and homosexual orientation.[3,4] Although Kinsey's work has been criticized in terms of his methodology and conclusions, the continuum of orientation provides a conceptual model for understanding the variance of sexual orientation in society. The presumption that most people are heterosexual and the idea that heterosexuality and homosexuality represent sharply distinct behaviors are inconsistent with the complex, often unpredictable arena of human behavior.

The issue of homosexuality has been highlighted in association with the AIDS epidemic. Unfortunately, this association has fueled many misconceptions and furthered traditional misunderstandings about homosexuality. A homosexual is often defined as a person whose primary erotic, psychological, emotional, and social interest is in a member of the same sex. **Gay** is another word often used to describe homosexual men or women as well as social and political concerns related to homosexual orientation. Homosexual women are often referred to as **lesbians.**

Many misconceptions exist about lesbian sexual expression and lifestyles.

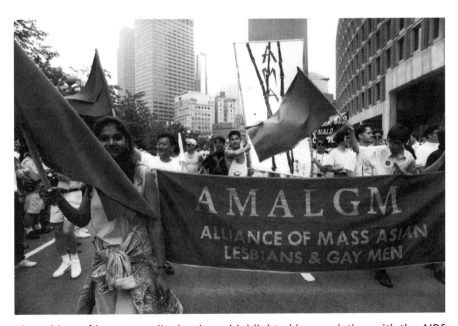

The subject of homosexuality has been highlighted in association with the AIDS epidemic. Unfortunately, this association has fueled many misconceptions and furthered traditional misunderstandings about homosexuality.

I am a lesbian. I am still in "the closet." I would like to be more open about my identity but I am afraid. I hear jokes and comments about homosexuals that really hurt me. I am continually confronted with misunderstandings and fear about homosexuality. If I could erase anything in this world, it would be homophobia.

27-YEAR-OLD WOMAN

The extent to which a lesbian decides to be secretive or open about her sexual orientation has a significant effect on her lifestyle. There are various degrees of being "in the closet" and several steps in the process of "coming out." These steps are usually incremental and include self-acknowledgment, self-acceptance, and disclosure. These steps are particularly difficult because of **homophobia**, irrational fears of homosexuality, displayed by some societal members. Homophobia usually stems from ignorance and popular myths that promote homosexual prejudice. Homophobia may result in a range of activities from overt acts of aggression, violence, to more subtle activities, such as verbal assault. Homophobia may also present in attempts to avoid any behavior that might be interpreted as homosexual. It may influence how a woman behaves or responds in lovemaking, what she chooses to wear or not wear, how she embraces other women, or whether she participates in a cause that she may otherwise believe in but does not want to be labeled as a lesbian.

Transsexuality

A **transsexual*** is a person whose gender identity is opposite to her or his biological sex. **Gender dysphoria** is a term used to describe a person who feels trapped in a body of the opposite sex. A vast array of literature has accumulated on the characteristics, causes, and treatment of transsexualism. No clear understanding of the nature and cause of transsexualism has yet emerged.[12] Explanations for transsexuality include both biological and social-learning hypotheses. Surgical procedures that change anatomical sexual structures are sometimes performed. These procedures usually involve considerable psychological therapy, personal adjustment, and some legal difficulties.

Biological Basis of Sexual Health

Female Sexual Anatomy and Physiology

External Structures

Unfortunately, many women not only harbor misconceptions about their bodies, but also they are unfamiliar with their own genitalia. Gaining knowledge and understanding of how her body functions and performs is an important aspect of a woman's sexual health and well-being. One way to begin an understanding of female sexual anatomy is to examine the vaginal area with a mirror. Some women are afraid to touch themselves. This fear may be an indication of misinformation or insecurity about oneself in a sexual sense.

AUTHOR'S NOTE: The term "transsexual" should not be confused with the term "transvestism," a term applied to the behavior of an individual who obtains sexual excitement from putting on clothes of the opposite sex.

All women have the same genital structures, but there are individual variances in terms of color, shapes, and textures (Fig. 7.5). The **vulva** encompasses all the female external genital structures, including the pubic hair, folds of skin, and the urinary and vaginal openings. The **mons veneris** refers to "the mound of Venus" and is the area covering the pubic bone. It consists of pads of fatty tissue between the bone and the skin. Numerous nerve endings in the area are responsible for the pleasure sensations from touch and pressure. At puberty, the mons becomes covered with pubic hair that varies in color, texture, and thickness. The **labia majora** consists of the outer lips that extend downward from the mons and extend toward each side of the vulva. The skin color of the labia majora is usually darker than the skin of the thighs. The nerve endings and underlying fatty tissue are similar to those in the mons. The **labia minora,** or inner lips, are located within the outer lips and often protrude between them. The **clitoris** consists of an external **shaft** and **glans** and the internal **crura.** The only function of the clitoris is sexual arousal. The shaft and glans of the clitoris are located just below the mons area, where the inner lips converge. They are covered by the clitoral hood, or prepuce. Initially it may be easier for a woman to locate her clitoris by touch rather than sight or location because of its sensitive nerve endings and small size. The external part of the clitoris, although tiny, has about the same number of nerve endings as the head of the penis. The **vestibule** is the area of the vulva inside the labia minora. It is rich in blood vessels and nerve endings. Its tissues are also sensitive to touch. Both the urinary and the vaginal openings are located within the vestibule.

The urinary opening is also called the urethral opening. Urine collected in the bladder passes out through the body via this opening. The **urethra** is the short

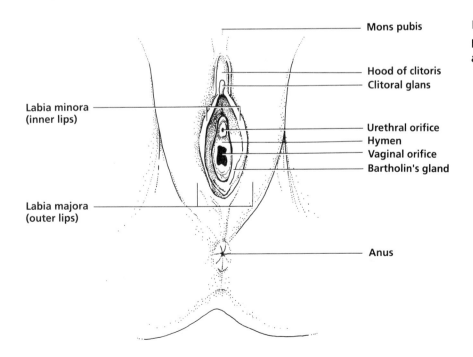

FIGURE 7.5

External female sexual anatomy.

tube connecting the bladder to the urinary opening located between the clitoris and the vaginal opening. The opening of the vagina is known as the **introitus.** It is located between the urinary opening and the anus. The **hymen** is a bit of tissue partially covering the introitus. It is typically present at birth and usually remains intact until first penetration, although the vaginal opening is partially open and flexible enough to insert tampons before the hymen has been broken. Although the hymen may serve to protect the vaginal tissues early in life, it has no other known function. Nevertheless, many cultures have traditionally placed great significance on its presence or absence. A common misconception is that a woman's virginity can be proved or disproved by the pain or bleeding that may occur with initial coitus. Although discomfort and spotting sometimes occur with first coitus, the hymen can be partial, flexible, or thin enough for there to be no discomfort or bleeding.

The **perineum** refers to the area of smooth skin between the vaginal opening and the anus. This tissue is rich with nerve endings and very sensitive to touch. During childbirth, an incision called an **episiotomy** is sometimes made in the perineum to prevent ragged tearing of tissues during delivery. This procedure, once routine with vaginal deliveries, has been seriously questioned as to its necessity and benefits.

Internal Structures

Several structures lie along the vaginal opening. The **vestibule** refers to the area of the vulva inside the labia minora. The vaginal walls are lined with a vast network of bulbs and vessels that engorge with blood during sexual arousal. The **vestibular bulbs** alongside the vagina also fill with blood during sexual excitement, causing the vagina to increase in length and the vulvar area to become swollen. These bulbs are similar in structure and function to the tissue in the penis that engorges with blood during male sexual arousal and causes penile erection. The **Bartholin's glands** are located on each side of the vaginal opening. They were once believed to be a source of lubrication during sexual arousal. This lubrication role is now questioned because they typically produce only a drop or two of fluid just before orgasm. The glands are usually not noticeable. Occasionally the duct from the gland becomes blocked and enlargement results. Medical intervention may be indicated if the condition does not subside within a few days. In addition to the glands, a complex musculature underlies the genital area. The pelvic floor muscles (see Chapter 2) have a multidirectional design (Fig. 7.6) that permit the vaginal opening to expand during childbirth and to contract after delivery. The pelvic floor muscles can lose muscle tone during childbirth or over time. A series of exercises, known as Kegel exercises (see Chapter 2), can help restore the muscular tone, reduce involuntary urinary incontinence, and enhance sexual sensations.

Internal female sexual anatomy consists of the vagina, cervix, uterus, and ovaries (Fig. 7.7). The vagina opens between the labia minora and extends upward into the body, angling toward the lower back. The nonaroused vagina

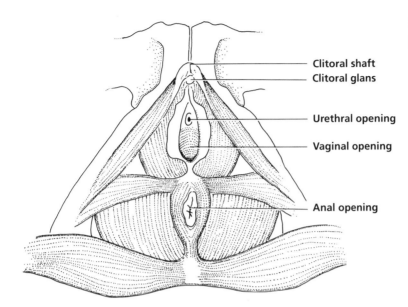

FIGURE 7.6

Pelvic floor muscles.

Clitoral shaft
Clitoral glans

Urethral opening

Vaginal opening

Anal opening

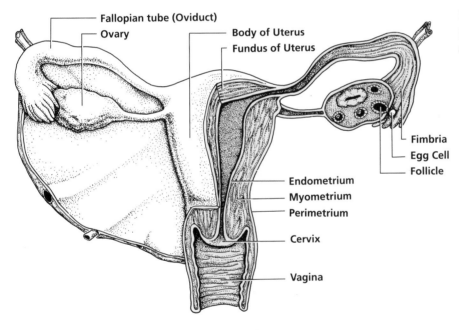

FIGURE 7.7

Internal female sexual anatomy.

Fallopian tube (Oviduct)
Ovary
Body of Uterus
Fundus of Uterus

Fimbria
Egg Cell
Follicle

Endometrium
Myometrium
Perimetrium

Cervix

Vagina

is approximately 3 to 5 inches in length. The walls are like a flat tube. The ability of the vagina to expand during sexual arousal and during childbirth is truly amazing. The vagina consists of three layers of tissue—mucous, muscle, and fibrous tissue—all of which are richly endowed with blood vessels. The **mucosa** is a layer of moist membrane inside the vagina. The folded walls are known as **rugae**. These walls are warm, soft, and moist, and they normally produce secretions that help maintain the chemical balance of the vagina. During sexual arousal, lubricating fluid exudes through the mucosa. The muscular tissue is concentrated around the vaginal opening. Fibrous tissue surrounds the muscular layer. This layer aids in vaginal contraction and expansion and also serves as connective tissue to other structures in the pelvic cavity.

The **cervix** is the mouth of the uterus, located at the back of the vagina. The cervix contains mucous-secreting glands. The cervix actually looks like a small, pink, glazed doughnut. The opening in the middle of the cervix, the *os,* connects the vagina with the uterine cavity. After childbirth, the os becomes less round and assumes a more horizontal slit position. The cervix is composed of fibrous tissue which is capable of dramatic stretching. During childbirth, the cervical canal is fifty or more times its normal width. Glands line the cervical canal and produce a constant downward flow of mucous to protect the uterine cavity from bacterial invasion.

The uterus is also known as the womb. It is a thick, pear-shaped organ, approximately 3 inches long and 2 inches wide in a woman who has never had a child. It is somewhat larger after a pregnancy. The top part of the uterus is known as the **fundus.** The walls of the fundus are especially thick. The **myometrium** consists of the longitudinal and circular muscle fibers of the uterus that are interwoven and enable the uterus to expand during pregnancy and contract during labor and childbirth. The myometrium is covered by a thin membrane that is known as the **perimetrium.** The perimetrium also functions as the external surface of the uterus. The uterus is suspended within the pelvic cavity by a series of six ligaments. The alignment of the ligaments permits some movement of the uterus within the cavity. The **endometrium** is the lining of the uterus, which in preparation for fertilization thickens in response to hormone changes during the monthly menstrual cycle. The endometrium is also a source of hormone production.

The **fallopian tubes** are thin pale pink filaments that extend from the uterus to the ovaries. The outside end of each tube is like a funnel, with fingerlike projections called **fimbriae** that draw the egg from the ovary into the tube. The ovaries are almond-shaped structures located at the end of the fallopian tubes. They are connected to the pelvic wall and the uterus by ligaments. The **ovaries** are endocrine glands that produce two classes of sex hormones. The **estrogens** influence the development of female physical sex characteristics and help regulate the menstrual cycle. The **progesterones** help regulate the menstrual cycle and stimulate development of the uterine lining in preparation for pregnancy. During puberty, these hormones play a critical role in the maturation of the reproductive organs and the development of secondary sex characteristics, such as pubic hair and breasts.

Menstruation

Women usually begin to menstruate in their early teen years. During the menstrual cycle, the uterine lining is prepared for implantation of a fertilized egg. If conception does not occur, the lining sloughs off and is discharged as menstrual flow. The menstrual discharge consists of blood, mucus, and endometrial membranes that sometimes present as small clots. The amount of menstrual flow varies but is usually 6 to 8 ounces in volume per cycle. The cycle length is often 28 days in length but can vary from 21 to 40 days.

The menstrual cycle (Fig. 7.8) is regulated by a complex relationship between the hypothalamus and the pituitary gland, the adrenal glands, and the ovaries and the uterus. The hypothalmus produces and secretes hormones and releasing factors that act directly on the pituitary gland. The releasing factor responsible for reproductive hormone control is GnRH, gonadotropin-releasing hormone. GnRH releases vary in amount and frequency during each menstrual cycle. GnRH is believed to play a role in the timing of puberty. Alterations in the GnRH pulse release may be the mechanism by which stressors such as athletic training or dieting influence menstrual cycles.

The menstrual cycle is a self-regulating and dynamic process in which the level of a particular hormone retards or increases the production of the same and other hormones. The hypothalamus monitors the hormone levels in the bloodstream throughout the cycle. It sends chemical messages to the pituitary gland, which in turn releases hormones to stimulate the ovaries. These hormones have the general name of **gonadotropins** because they stimulate the gonads but specifically are known as **follicle stimulating hormone** (FSH) or **luteinizing hormone** (LH). FSH stimulates ovarian production of estrogen and the maturation of the ova and follicles. LH induces the mature ovum to burst from the ovary, and it stimulates the development of the **corpus luteum,** the portion of the follicle that remains after the egg has matured. The corpus luteum is responsible for producing the hormone progesterone.

These sequenced events are not continuous in nature. The endometrial menstrual cycle is divided into three stages or phases. In the **proliferation phase,** the pituitary gland increases production of FSH, which stimulates the developing follicles to mature and to produce several types of estrogen. Estrogen, in turn, causes the endometrium to thicken. When the level of ovarian estrogen circulating in the bloodstream reaches a peak, the pituitary gland depresses the release of FSH and stimulates LH production. Approximately 14 days before the onset of the next menstrual cycle, **ovulation,** the release of the ova, occurs. The ova travels into the fallopian tube. Around the time of ovulation, there is an increase and a change in cervical mucous secretions owing to the increased levels of estrogen. The cervical environment becomes more alkaline, contributing to a greater likelihood of conception.

During the second phase, the **secretory phase,** or **progestational** phase, continued pituitary secretions of LH cause the cells of the ruptured follicle to develop into the corpus luteum, which secretes progesterone. Progesterone inhibits the production of cervical mucosa. Progesterone, together with estrogen produced by the ovaries, causes the endometrium to thicken and engorge with blood in preparation for implantation. If this does not occur, the pituitary gland, in response to high estrogen and progesterone levels, halts the production

FIGURE 7.8

Female Menstrual Cycle.

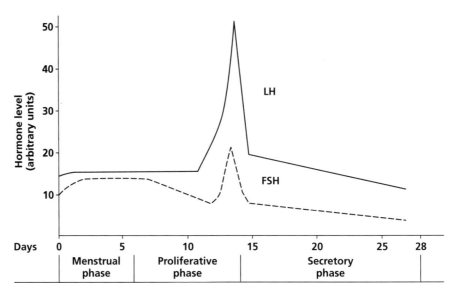

(A) Fluctuation of gonadotropin levels.

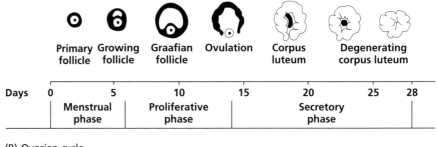

(B) Ovarian cycle.

of LH and FSH. This action deprives the corpus luteum of the necessary chemical stimulation to produce hormones. It disintegrates, and estrogen and progesterone production decrease.

The estrogen and progesterone drop-off triggers endometrial sloughing during the third phase of the cycle, the **menstrual phase.** The menstrual phase consists of the discharge of the thickened inner layer of the endometrium through the cervix and vagina. As the hormonal levels continue to fall, the hypothalamus responds to the reduction by stimulating the pituitary to release FSH. The release of the FSH initiates the maturation process of several follicles, and the entire cycle begins again.

For most women, menstruation creates no medical problems. Yet menstruation can create certain physical and emotional problems. **Dysmenorrhea,** meaning painful menstrual flow, is a term for what most women call "cramps." **Premenstrual syndrome** (PMS) is a term referring to a varied set of symptoms that present in some women before the menstrual flow, which may include

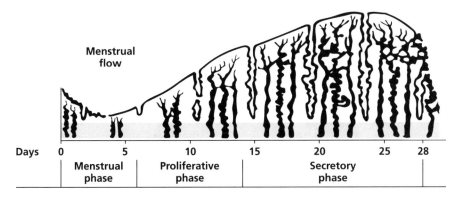

(C) Uterine cycle.

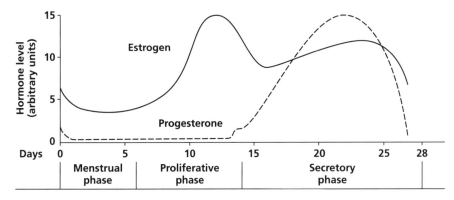

(D) Fluctuation of ovarian hormone levels.

tension, increased irritability, water retention, headaches, fatigue, breast tenderness, and cravings for certain foods. The causes of PMS are unknown, but fluctuations in sex steroids and their effects on various organ systems are believed to be involved. Research about the nature, cause and treatment of PMS lacks consistency and often has contradictory findings.

Sexual Arousal and Sexual Response

Sexual arousal and response are highly individualized physical, emotional, and mental processes. The female sexual response is not a geographically isolated phenomenon of the vaginal area. The brain, hormones, and senses all play an integrated role in the response cycle. Hormones also play a role in sexual response, in addition to their primary responsibility of regulating the menstrual cycle. Their exact role, however, is rather unclear. It is known that estrogens help to maintain the elasticity and lubricate the vagina, but their role in sexual motivation and arousal is not known. Contradictory findings from studies of postmenopausal or surgically induced menopausal (hysterectomy with bilateral oophorectomy) women have failed to answer the question. Studies have shown that circulating levels of androgens are associated with sexual interest and activity.[13] Further research is indicated to understand better the relationship between sex hormones and female sexual behavior and interest. The brain plays an important role in sexual arousal by mediating thoughts, emotions, and fantasies, which provide the psychological "stage" for the sexual experience. The senses of touch, smell, and sight provide stimuli that also can significantly influence the level of sexual arousal.

The sexual response cycle has been described in several ways, most notably by researchers Masters and Johnson, who identified three basic patterns[5] (Fig. 7.9). Each pattern distinguishes four phases: excitement, plateau, orgasm, and resolution. These models are only a framework for describing physiological sexual response patterns. Tremendous variability and differences are characteristic of sexual response, and these patterns represent only a composite of the physiological reactions. Pattern #1 most closely resembles the male pattern except that a woman is often able to have one or more orgasms without dropping below the plateau level of sexual arousal. Pattern #2 is a variation of this response that includes an extended plateau with no orgasm. A rapid rise to orgasm with no definitive plateau and a quick resolution pattern is described with Pattern #3.

In the **excitement phase** of the sexual response cycle, the clitoris swells with blood engorgement. This change ranges from very slight to quite noticeable. The clitoral glans is highly sensitive. Some women find that the entire sexual response cycle can be set into motion and maintained to orgasm by light

FIGURE 7.9

Female sexual response cycle.

SOURCE: Masters, W., and Johnson, V. (1966). *Human sexual response.* Boston: Little, Brown.

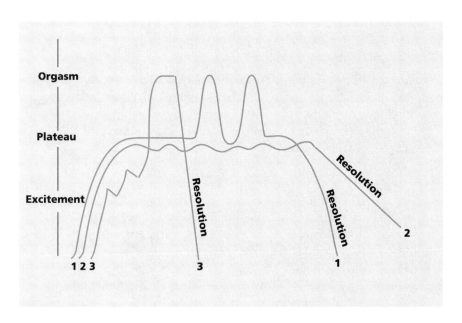

stimulation of the glans alone. The glans is so sensitive that women usually stimulate the area with the hood covering the clitoris to avoid direct stimulation. In addition to clitoral swelling, the labia majora flatten and separate. The labia minora increase in size, and lubrication begins. Lubrication is a unique feature of the vagina and an important aspect of sexual arousal. It is often the first physiological sign of sexual arousal in women. During arousal, a clear, slippery fluid appears on the vaginal mucosa. The lubrication is a result of **vasocongestion,** the pooling of blood in the pelvic area. During vasocongestion, the extensive network of blood vessels in the tissues surrounding the vagina engorge with blood. Clear fluid seeps from the congested tissues to the inside of the vaginal walls to form the slippery coating of the vagina. Vaginal lubrication serves two primary functions. It enhances the possibility of conception by helping to alkalinize the normally acidic vaginal chemical balance. Sperm are able to move more quickly and survive longer in an alkaline environment. Vaginal lubrication also helps to increase sexual pleasure. Also during the excitement phase, the uterus elevates and becomes engorged with blood, and the breasts enlarge. Superficial veins in breast tissues may become more visible during this time.

During the **plateau phase** of the female sexual response cycle, the clitoris withdraws under its hood and shortens in length. The labia majora remains unchanged from the excitement phase, while the labia minora intensifies in color. An orgasmic platform develops from further vasocongestion of the outer one-third of the vagina. Lubrication from the vagina slows, and the uterus is fully elevated in position. Breast tissue remains swollen.

As effective stimulation occurs, many women move from the plateau phase to the **orgasmic phase** of the sexual response cycle. In contrast to men, who almost always experience orgasm after reaching the plateau level, women may obtain plateau levels without the orgasmic release. Orgasm is the shortest phase of the sexual response cycle, although female orgasms often last slightly longer than male orgasms. It is important to note that there is considerable variation in orgasmic experiences, in terms of intensity, frequency, and duration, among both men and women. The female physiological responses in the orgasmic phase include an elevated blood pressure, heart rate, and breathing pattern. Orgasmic platform contractions are rhythmical, which begin at high intensity and then become weaker and slower. The uterus usually contracts at orgasm. These physiological responses are consistent whether they originate from direct clitoral stimulation or from coital stimulation, although women report wide differences in subjective feelings and preferences.[5,7]

The **resolution phase** is the final phase of the sexual response cycle. During this phase, the sexual systems return to the nonexcited state. If no additional stimulation occurs, the resolution begins immediately after orgasm. Skin coloration quickly subsides, and vital signs return to normal levels. The clitoris, labia majora, and labia minora return to their unaroused size and position. A significant male-female response difference occurs in the resolution period. After orgasm, the male typically enters a refractory period—a time when no amount of additional stimulation will result in orgasm. This time period has considerable variability among men and depends on a number of physiological and psychological factors. In contrast to men, women generally experience no comparable refractory period. They are physiologically capable of returning to another orgasmic peak during the resolution phase.

The female sexual response cycle described here is only a framework for understanding the physiological events of sexual response. The model does not attempt to incorporate the emotional, cultural, psychological, and subjective dimensions of the sexual experience. These dimensions significantly influence the sexual experience in dramatically positive or negative directions. The framework is further compromised by not identifying differences between the sexes. There is considerably more variability in the female sexual response (see Fig. 7.9). As mentioned, women do not experience a period like the male refractory ("shutdown") phase, and in addition, women are more likely to experience **multiple orgasms,** the ability to have more than one orgasmic experience within a short time interval.

Forms of Sexual Expression

Society has traditionally placed restrictions on the forms of sexual expression that are considered appropriate. Missionary heterosexual sex (male on top of female) is only one of many sexual expression options. Women may elect different forms of sexual expression under different circumstances or at different times in their lives.

Masturbation (Fig. 7.10) refers to erotic self-stimulation, usually to the point of orgasm. Historical records indicate that masturbation has been practiced since ancient times. Masturbation practices begin early in life with infants exploring their genitals and receiving pleasure from touching them. Often self-stimulation continues throughout life, whether or not the individual is a partner in a permanent intimate relationship. Even though the practice of masturbation is widespread, many women feel ashamed or embarrassed of the practice. Folklore has falsely labeled masturbation as sinful, evil, and even physically or mentally harmful. Such ideas are entirely false, and many therapists and sex experts believe that masturbation can be helpful as a sexual outlet and as a means to be comfortable with one's own body.

Petting is defined as erotic stimulation of a person by a sexual partner, without actual sexual intercourse. It can include kisses, genital caresses, and oral-genital contact. Petting may culminate in orgasm. During adolescence, petting is often a way to experience intense sexual excitement without actually engaging in intercourse. Petting is carried over into adult sexual experiences as foreplay or for sexual variety.

Oral-genital stimulation takes two basic forms. **Cunnilingus** is the act of sucking or licking the vulva, particularly the clitoris. **Fellatio** is the act of sucking or licking the penis and scrotum. The prevalence of oral-genital stimulation

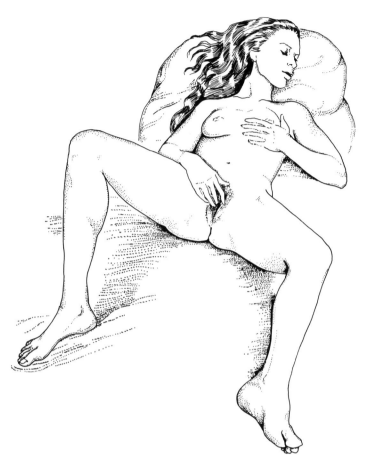

FIGURE 7.10
Female masturbation.

appears to be widespread, with one study finding 80 percent of college students and nearly 100 percent of adults having experienced oral-genital sex.[14,15]

Anal intercourse is another form of sexual expression. Because the anal opening is richly endowed with nerves, the area can be very sensitive and sexually arousing. A couple needs to be careful, however, in performing anal intercourse for many reasons. The anal sphincter tends to be tight and when stimulated can tighten even more, resulting in pain on penetration. The anal region has no natural lubrication of its own, which increases the possibility of both pain and injury. Usually anal intercourse can be accomplished without discomfort if precautions are taken. A lubricant such as K-Y Jelly (not petroleum-based products, which weaken condoms) should be used. Care should be taken to avoid contamination of the vaginal area once anal penetration has occurred. It must be emphasized that anal intercourse is not without risks. Anal intercourse has been associated with the transmission of both the hepatitis B and AIDS (HIV) viruses. Anyone engaging in anal intercourse should use a latex condom and never use a petroleum-based lubricant. In addition, after anal penetration, the genitals should be washed thoroughly before resuming vaginal or oral sex.

Sexuality Through the Life Span

In many Western societies, it has been traditional to view childhood as a time of unexpressed sexuality and behavior, and adolescence has been viewed as a time to restrain immature sexual drives. The opinion that adolescent sexual behavior should be curtailed or restricted receives considerable support from multiple sectors of American society. There is also consensus that sexuality and sexual capacity are not "awakenings" that suddenly appear at a definitive time in development, but rather both male and female infants are born with the capacity for sexual pleasure and response.

Childhood

Considerable variation in sexual development presents among individuals during childhood and adolescence. The pleasures of genital stimulation are generally discovered in the first few years of life. Besides self-stimulation, prepubertal children often engage in play that may be viewed as sexual in nature. The activities may range from exhibition and inspection to simulating intercourse by rubbing genital regions together. Both natural childhood curiosity and curiosity about what is forbidden probably play a role in these behaviors. As children get older, they become more keenly aware of and interested in body changes, particularly those involving the genitals and secondary sex characteristics.

Adolescence

Adolescence is the most dramatic stage for physiological changes and social-role development. Adolescence is generally considered to span the period from age 12 to 20 years. Most of the major physical changes of adolescence actually take place in the first few years of this period, a time known as **puberty.** The onset of puberty is generally 2 years earlier in girls than in boys. **Secondary sex characteristics** appear at this time in response to higher levels of hormones. In females, estrogen levels result in pubic hair growth and breast budding. Under the influence of hormone stimulation, additional internal changes occur. Vaginal walls gradually become thicker, and the uterus becomes larger and more muscular. The vaginal pH changes from alkaline to acidic as vaginal and cervical secretions increase in response to the changing hormone status. Eventually menstruation begins. Most girls menstruate at about the age of 12 or 13, but there is considerable variation in this timing. The first menstrual period is known as **menarche.** Initial menstrual cycles may be irregular and occur without ovulation. Research has suggested that there is a relationship between a minimal amount of body fat and menstruation.[16,17]

The difficulties of adjusting to new physical characteristics pale in comparison to psychological adjustments of adolescence. It is a period characterized by evolving responsibilities and assimilation of societal expectations. In Western cultures, these expectations have inherent double standards for women, where sexual overtones are blasted through the media in everything from ads for jeans to cars. Yet the message also prevails for young women to maintain virginity, whereas the expectations for young men are more tolerant of experimentation and overt sexual behavior.

Young Adulthood

Sexual behavior in young adults is influenced by a number of personal and cultural factors. A dramatic shift has occurred with various factors contributing to the increasing numbers of single adults. These factors include marriage at a later age, an increase in those who never marry, more women placing career goals before marriage, an increase in the number of cohabiting couples, rising divorce rates, a greater emphasis on advanced education, and an increase in the number of women who no longer must depend on marriage to ensure their economic stability. Although this association appears to be decreasing, American culture has had a double standard for unmarried men and women. Single women have been traditionally referred to as "old maids" compared with single men, who had the less derogatory label of "bachelor." Single living, cohabitation, or marriage are living arrangements. It is not appropriate to assume that sexual behavior is confined to marital arrangements. Contemporary developments and changes in sexual mores and behavior of young adults are often discussed in the context of nonmarital or extramarital activities. In a 1983 study of American married couples, the frequency of marital sexual interactions was found to be strongly associated with levels of sexual satisfaction.[8] A number of factors other than frequency of sexual interaction have also been linked to satisfaction with marital sex. These factors include mutuality in initiating sex,[8] orgasm frequency among women,[18] and good communication.[19]

Extramarital relationship is the term applied for sexual interaction experienced by a married person with someone other than his or her spouse. These relationships may be further defined as **nonconsensual,** in which there is not spousal consent for the extramarital relationship, or **consensual,** in which the spouse is aware and supports the extramarital involvement. Data evaluating these arrangements are incomplete and biased at best. In the absence of data, it is difficult to draw conclusions about these arrangements. Regardless of the formal or informal living arrangements, sexual behavior is an important dimension of adult health.

Sexuality and Aging

The perception that old age and sex are incompatible terms is totally erroneous. All too often, women dismiss sexual problems as a consequence of aging. The

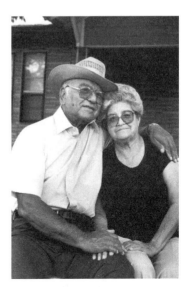

Sexuality is an important dimension of aging.

truth is, most people can enjoy an active sex life no matter how old they are. This misconception about aging may have evolved for a number of reasons. The United States is still influenced by the philosophy that equates sexuality with procreation. For older people who are neither capable nor interested in reproductive facets of life, this viewpoint offers little sensitivity or insight into personal needs. Society also sends the message via the media that love, sex, and romance are only for the young and "sexy." There is an implicit message that this scenario excludes older folks. There is also a pervasive assumption that older people do not have sexual needs. Information Box 7.2 provides a summary of stereotypes or myths about sexuality among the elderly.

The term **climacteric** refers to the physiological changes that occur during the transition period from female fertility to infertility. At about age 40, the ovaries begin to slow the production of estrogen. **Menopause,** one of the climacteric events, refers to the cessation of menstruation and generally occurs at about 45 to 55 years of age (see Chapter 13). Hormonal changes of menopause affect the sexual response of most women. In general, all phases of the response cycle continue but with somewhat decreased intensity. The depletion of estrogen associated with menopause can result in several vaginal changes, including dryness, thinning of the walls, and delayed or absent lubrication during sexual excitement. For many women, hormone replacement therapy may help. Hormone replacement therapy is not necessarily a solution for every woman. Other strategies to relieve vaginal dryness include prescription estrogen creams applied directly to the vagina that help prevent dryness and thinning. Water-soluble lubricants like K-Y Jelly and moisturizers like Replens help solve problems related to dryness. Toned pelvic muscles (see Chapter 2) with Kegel exercises can help make sex more pleasurable by toning the pelvic floor muscles that support the bladder and uterus, which tend to relax as estrogen declines.

Although the general focus on sexual response in later years tends to highlight a decline in frequency and intensity of sexual activity, it should be emphasized

INFORMATION BOX 7.2

Sexual Stereotypes and Myths of Sexuality Among the Elderly

Elderly people do not have sexual desires.

Elderly people are not able to make love, even if they want to.

Elderly people are too fragile and might hurt themselves if they attempt to engage in sexual relations.

Elderly people are physically unattractive and therefore sexually undesirable.

The whole notion of elderly people engaging in sexual activity is shameful and perverse.

SOURCE: Rienzo, B.A. (1985). The impact of aging on human sexuality. *Journal of School Health, 55,* 66–68. Reprinted with permission.

that the opportunities for sexual expression in a relationship are often increased in later years, as pressures from work, children, and fulfilling life's goals may be reduced and more time becomes available for sharing with a partner.[20] Couples may increasingly emphasize quality rather than quantity of sexual expression. Intimacy may find new and deeper dimensions in later years. One survey found that although sexual frequency declines, enjoyment of sex sometimes increases with age.[21]

Informed Decision Making

Sexual well-being is far more than sexual arousal and response. It includes effective decision making in the spectrum of issues affecting sexual health. Many of these topics are reviewed in subsequent chapters on reproductive health and personal health issues. Understanding personal feelings, thoughts, and symptoms and articulating concerns and questions are essential dimensions of effective personal communication and preventive health. Essential to female well-being are knowledge, healthy lifestyle, and preventive health practices. The gynecological examination is an opportunity to discuss general sexual health concerns and ensure that all facets of gynecological health are addressed.

Preventive Health—the Gynecological Examination

A gynecological checkup is not magic and not a guarantee, but it is an opportunity for preventive health screening and guidance in reproductive and sexual health matters. A woman can maximize the benefits of a gynecological examination by taking the time to select carefully a clinician who is sensitive to her needs. Often that means changing clinicians until the "right" one is found, but it is better to "shop" while feeling well than to wait until there is a pressing medical problem. Once a clinician is selected, a woman has a few responsibilities to make sure that the appointment is beneficial. It is important that women be explicit about what is wanted with the visit. It is critical to articulate the nature of the visit and to address questions or concerns specifically. It cannot be assumed that there is a standard list of questions that the clinician will ask or that the clinician can ascertain by examination the nature of a sexual concern or automatically detect an underlying fear or anxiety. By being explicit and honest, a woman can facilitate the clinician's efforts to help her. Insisting that all questions be answered and persisting when answers are not clear are equally important avenues for maximizing the effectiveness of the visit. Women are often eager to please their health care providers and will nod as if understanding when in actuality they do not. This behavior results in more confusion and an increased likelihood of problems. Many women find it helpful to write down their questions and concerns and deal with them one by one with the clinician in the office before clothes are removed and the examination begins.

The pelvic examination provides the woman and her clinician with essential basic information about her gynecological health. The pelvic examination should be timed to avoid the menstrual period. It is also advisable to avoid douching at least 24 hours before an examination and some clinicians recommend avoiding vaginal intercourse for at least 48 hours before the examination. These precautions ensure a more accurate visualization of the cervix and greater likelihood of diagnosing an infection if it is present.

A gynecological examination begins with a medical history and a general physical examination, including breast examination. The pelvic examination is usually conducted in the **dorsal lithotomy position.** In this position, the woman lies on her back with her bottom at the very end of the examining table and her legs supported in foot stirrups. Some clinicians and their patients prefer pelvic examination with the woman in a semirecumbent position. This position relaxes the thick sheath of abdominal muscle that covers the pelvis. The uterus and other pelvic organs are easier to palpate, and the woman is able to maintain eye contact with her clinician.

The pelvic examination consists of three phases. The first phase is the external examination, which enables the clinician to inspect the vulva and perineum visually for any evidence of infection or injury. The second phase involves the use of a speculum, a device that holds the vaginal walls apart to permit visual inspection of the cervix. The speculum is inserted with the blade closed. Once inside the vagina, the blades are opened and locked into place at the correct width. With the speculum open, the clinician inspects the vaginal walls and cervix for any redness, irritation, unusual discharge, or lesions. Specimens for laboratory tests are collected while the speculum is in place. After the specimens are collected, the speculum is removed. The third phase of the examination is the bimanual examination, which involves the insertion of two gloved fingers of one hand into the vagina while the other hand presses downward on the abdomen. The purpose of this activity is to locate and feel the size, consistency, and shape of the uterus and ovaries and to check for any abdominal masses or tender areas. A rectal examination may also be performed to evaluate the muscular wall separating the rectum and vagina, the position of the uterus, and any possible masses or tenderness in the area.

A pelvic examination takes but a few minutes, and it provides a starting point to ascertain any gynecological or sexual health concerns. Pelvic examinations should be arranged at regular intervals throughout a woman's adult life. Information Box 7.3 provides a listing of critical times for scheduling a pelvic examination.

Dealing with Sexual Problems

The private and personal nature of sex coupled with sociocultural influences and language limitations make it difficult for women to acknowledge sexual concerns or problems. Professional help may be indicated in those cases in which individualized efforts, couple efforts, or both do not produce the desired effects. Sex therapy has evolved as a legitimate method for understanding sexual problems and increasing sexual satisfaction. Communication about sexual issues

Gynecological Examination

A woman should plan to see her clinician for a pelvic examination under the following conditions:

Before first coitus

If menarche has not occurred by age 16

At age 20 or earlier for first coitus

Heavy menstrual flow

Menstrual period lasting longer than 10 days

If risk for sexually transmitted diseases is present or if there is a history of abnormal Pap smears, once a year exams

Any time there is vaginal itching, redness, sores, swelling, unusual odor, or unusual discharge

Painful intercourse

Missed menstrual period if there is a chance of pregnancy

Missed three menstrual periods if there is no chance of pregnancy

Burning or frequency of urination

Sexual partner has a genital infection or sore

Rape

Vaginal or rectal injury

and finding ways to solve problems are critical but often difficult steps toward satisfying sex life. Sex therapy can often make communication easier. Strategies with a therapist may range from expanding self-knowledge to sharing more effectively with a partner. There are many approaches to sex therapy, and many approaches share common goals.

These common goals often include permission. A therapist can play an important role in reassuring clients that thoughts, feelings, fantasies, desires, and behaviors that enhance their satisfaction and do not have potentially negative consequences are normal. Often all that is needed is reassurance that clients can appreciate their unique patterns and desires instead of comparing themselves with friends or national averages. A therapist can also be helpful in giving clients permission not to engage in certain behaviors unless they want to. Information is another common activity of therapy. By providing specific accurate and reassuring information, therapists are often able to address thoughts and feelings that may be interfering with the person's ability to enjoy or respond to sexual activity. A therapist is also able to provide specific activities or home-work "assignments" that enable the client to reduce anxiety, enhance communication, and learn new sexually enhancing behavioral techniques. Intensive therapy may be indicated in some situations in which personal emotional difficulties or significant relationship problems interfere with sexual expression.

Sexual dysfunction is defined as the inability of an individual to function adequately in terms of sexual arousal, orgasm, or in coital situations. Until recently, the sexual problems of women were classified under the general label

I used to fake orgasms. I am not sure why, but somehow I felt it was necessary. My current partner figured it out and we have spent a lot of time talking about this. I am seeing a therapist. With a few sessions, I was able to climax with masturbation, and I know that I am much more comfortable with my sexuality. I know that "faking" it was not fair to me or my partner.

35-YEAR-OLD WOMAN

of "frigidity." These problems were severely misunderstood and thought to be symptomatic of a neurosis or some other psychological disorder that required long-term psychiatric therapy. This traditional approach persisted despite the absence of a demonstrated relationship between the treatment and the alleviation of the sexual problem. Today four major areas of sexual dysfunction are defined for women. They include inhibited sexual desire, general sexual dysfunction, orgasmic dysfunction, and vaginismus.

Inhibited sexual desire (ISD) appears to be the most common of the sexual dysfunctions. Women experiencing ISD have a persistent lack of interest in or desire for sex. ISD most commonly reflects relationship problems but may also be caused by other physical or personal difficulties. ISD can also be characterized by an aversion to all sexual activity. Women with ISD often experience physical symptoms of anxiety when they attempt to engage in sexual activity. ISD treatment is often difficult because the woman may lack insight into the basic motivations of avoidance and hostility that underlie the disorder. The treatment approach most often used seeks to modify the woman's tendency to inhibit erotic feelings and allow them to emerge naturally. The woman learns not to fight or suppress the natural tendency to become aroused in sexual situations.

General sexual dysfunction is what has been most traditionally referred to as "frigidity." This value-laden term has generally been dropped. The woman who is generally nonresponsive describes herself as being void of sexual feelings. She experiences little or no erotic pleasure from sexual stimulation. Treatment of general sexual dysfunction is directed primarily at the creation of a nondemanding, relaxed, and sensuous atmosphere in which sexual responsiveness develops. Communication with a partner about her sexual wishes and feelings is encouraged. Other treatment activities for general sexual dysfunction focus on the reduction of sexual anxiety and the unfolding of sexual feelings with sensate focus, genital stimulation, and nondemanding coitus.

Orgasmic dysfunction refers specifically to the inability to experience the orgasmic component of the sexual response cycle. A woman with an orgasmic dysfunction may have a strong sex drive, become readily aroused, and develop vasocongestion and lubrication, but the neuromuscular discharge or orgasm is inhibited. Achieving orgasm is not a criterion of sexual competence or normality in women. Nor is orgasmic dysfunction necessarily a symptom of pathology. Orgasm is a physical response that is highly variable among women. Learning effective self-stimulation is often recommended for women who have never experienced orgasm. One advantage of self-stimulation is that a woman without a partner can learn to become orgasmic. For a woman with a sexual partner, becoming orgasmic first by masturbation may help develop a sense of sexual autonomy that can increase the likelihood of satisfaction with a partner.

Vaginismus is a relatively rare form of sexual difficulty in which a woman experiences involuntary spasmodic contractions of the muscles of the outer third of the vagina. Attempts to achieve coitus are painful and frustrating, and even physical examinations involving vaginal penetration are virtually impossible without anesthesia. Women with vaginismus are often extremely fearful of coital or other penetration and develop high levels of anxiety under such circumstances.

Treatment for vaginismus often begins during a pelvic examination, with the therapist or a consulting physician demonstrating the vaginal spasm reaction to the woman or the woman and her partner. Relaxation and self-awareness techniques are encouraged along with specific exercises to gradually relax the vaginal muscle spasms.

Dyspareunia is not a form of sexual dysfunction per se but relates to painful intercourse. It can stem from physical or physiological causes. Painful intercourse may be the result of vaginal irritation or insufficient lubrication. Dyspareunia may also result from very frequent intercourse. Psychological reasons, such as shame, embarrassment, and guilt, may also contribute to painful or uncomfortable intercourse for women.

Any form of sexual dysfunction or discomfort with intercourse should be evaluated to rule out any underlying pathology. In addition, the evaluation should include efforts, such as counseling or therapy, if needed to seek resolution of the condition.

Communication in Sexual Behavior and Sexual Health

Communication is a critical component of sexual behavior and sexual health. Being able to talk about needs, feelings, concerns, and fears is an essential component of a healthy relationship. Sexual communication can contribute greatly to the satisfaction of an intimate relationship. American language lacks a comfortable sexual vocabulary. Available language seems to be either "clinical" or "medical" in nature or "street language," which may be perceived as too crass or juvenile. Beyond the handicaps imposed by socialization and language limitations, difficulties in sexual communication may also be rooted in fears of too much self-exposure. Any sexual communication involves a degree of risk and vulnerability to judgment, criticism, or rejection. The willingness to take risks may be related to the amount of trust that exists within a relationship.

As in an intimate relationship, communication with a health care provider about sexual concerns is essential. Health care providers are not equipped with telepathic sensors to ascertain specific questions or concerns. Although it may be awkward to feel that the chosen words are appropriate or adequate, it is important to feel confident enough about oneself to persist with the communication effort. Other specific dimensions of sexual health and communication with health care providers are discussed throughout the reproductive health chapters of this text.

Summary

Few topics generate as much interest in people of all ages as human sexuality. Sexuality pervades every aspect of a person's life. Sexual health is an important dimension of women's health. Self-Assessment 7.1 is s a questionnaire women

---

SELF-ASSESSMENT 7.1

Assessing Sexual Practices—Safety First for Sexual Health

Answer each of the following questions:

1. I avoid having multiple sex partners. ____ yes ____ no
2. I avoid having anonymous sex partners. ____ yes ____ no
3. I avoid having sex with someone who has symptoms of AIDS, is infected with HIV, or is at high risk of HIV. ____ yes ____ no
4. I avoid having sex with someone who has had sex with people who are at risk of getting HIV. ____ yes ____ no
5. I avoid exchanging sex for money or drugs. ____ yes ____ no
6. Male partners use a latex condom with a spermicide. ____ yes ____ no
7. I avoid anal sex. ____ yes ____ no
8. I avoid sex with someone that I don't know well. ____ yes ____ no
9. I avoid shooting drugs. ____ yes ____ no
10. I avoid sex with anyone who has genital sores or lesions. ____ yes ____ no
11. I take precautions to prevent unwanted pregnancy. ____ yes ____ no

If any of these questions are answered with a "no" it is important to reconsider the risks involved with your personal sex behaviors.

---

can use to determine if they have healthy sexual practices. Women are capable of experiencing sexual arousal and response throughout their lives. Understanding the biological, psychological, and sociological dimensions of sexual health enhances total wellness. Incorporating these dimensions in personal relationships, informed decision making, and preventive health care can enhance a woman's sexual health throughout her life span.

Philosophical Dimensions: Sexual Health

1. How do the sexual norms of a society restrict individuals? How do they benefit society?

2. Which gender-role assumptions have the greatest impact on the sexuality of female adolescents? Which have the least impact?

3. What are the advantages and disadvantages to early and late physical maturation for women?

4. What are the negative and positive attitudes in modern society about menstruation?

5. A paradox is that women appear to have a greater capacity for orgasm, to experience orgasm from a wider range of stimulation, and yet seem to have more difficulty experiencing orgasm than men. Is this true? If so, what factors may be contributing to this paradox?

6. How is homophobia displayed in modern society?

7. It has been claimed that rearing children in an androgynous fashion fosters uncertainty and confusion about proper roles in society. Evaluate this claim from a personal and societal perspective.

8. How can traditional gender roles affect a woman's attitude toward her own gynecological health and her utilization of a health care system?

References

1. Beach, F. (1978). *Human sexuality in four perspectives.* Baltimore: Johns Hopkins University Press.

2. Denney, N.W., and Quadagno, D. (1992). *Human sexuality* (2nd ed.). St. Louis: Mosby-Year Book.

3. Kinsey, A., Pomeroy, W., and Martin, C. (1948). *Sexual behavior in the human male.* Philadelphia: Saunders Publishing.

4. Kinsey, A., Pomeroy, W., Martin, C., and Gebhard, P. (1953). *Sexual behavior in the human female.* Philadelphia: Saunders Publishing.

5. Masters, W., and Johnson, V. (1966). Human sexual response. Boston: Little, Brown.

6. Tavris, C., and Sadd, S. (1977). *The Redbook report on female sexuality.* New York: Delacorte Press.

7. Hite, S. (1976). *The Hite report: A nationwide study of female sexuality.* New York: Dell Books.

8. Blumstein, P., and Schwartz, P. (1983). *American couples: Money, work and sex.* New York: William Morrow & Co.

9. Reinisch, J., and Rosenblum, L. (1987). *Masculinity-femininity: Basic perspectives.* New York: Oxford University Press.

10. Walfish, S., and Myerson, M. (1980). Sex role identity and attitudes towards sexuality. *Archives of Sexual Behavior, 9,* 199–203.

11. Allgeier, E. (1981). The influence of androgynous identification on heterosexual relations. *Sex Roles, 7,* 321–330.

12. Lothstein, L. (1984). Psychological testing with transsexuals: A 30 year review. *Journal of Personality Assessment, 48,* 500–507.

13. Sherwin, B., Gelfand, M., and Brender, W. (1985). Androgen enhances sexual motivation in females: A prospective crossover study of sex steroid administration in the surgical menopause. *Psychosomatic Medicine, 47,* 339–351.

14. Hunt, M. (1974). *Sexual behavior in the 1970's.* Chicago: Playboy Press.

15. Story, M.D. (1985). A comparison of university experience with various sexual outlets in 1974 and 1984. *Journal of Sex Education and Therapy, 11,* 35–41.

16. Frisch, R. (1988, March). Fatness and fertility. *Scientific American,* pp. 88–95.

17. Warren, M. (1982). Onset of puberty later in athletic girls. *Medical Aspects of Human Sexuality, 4,* 77–78.

18. Peterson, J., Kretchmer, A., Nellis, B., Lever, J., and Hertz, R. (1983). The *Playboy* readers sex survey, Part 2. *Playboy,* (March) pp. 90–92, 178–184.

19. Banmen, J., and Vogel, N. (1985). The relationship between married quality and interpersonal sexual communication. *Family Therapy, 12,* 45–58.

20. Olds, S.W. (1985). *The eternal garden: Seasons of our sexuality.* New York: Times Books.

21. Brecher, E. (1984). *Love, sex, and aging.* Boston: Little, Brown.

Resources

AMERICAN ASSOCIATION OF SEX EDUCATORS, COUNSELORS AND THERAPISTS

435 North Michigan Avenue
Suite 1717
Chicago, IL 60611
312-644-0828

AMERICAN COLLEGE OF OBSTETRICIANS AND GYNECOLOGISTS

409 12th Street SW
Washington, DC 20024
202-638-5577

FEDERATION OF PARENTS AND FRIENDS OF LESBIANS AND GAYS

PO Box 24565
Los Angeles, CA 90024
213-472-8952

NATIONAL GAY AND LESBIAN TASK FORCE

1517 U Street NW
Washington, DC 20009
202-332-6483
800-221-7044

SEX INFORMATION AND EDUCATION COUNCIL OF THE US (SIECUS)

130 West 42nd Street
Suite 2500
New York, NY 10036
212-819-9770

CHAPTER

8

Contraception and Abortion

CHAPTER OBJECTIVES

On completion of this chapter, the student should be able to discuss:

1. The difference in terminology of "birth control" and "contraception."

2. The four primary mechanisms by which birth control can be accomplished.

3. The historical overview of contraceptive efforts.

4. The significance of the efforts of Margaret Sanger and Mary Coffin Dennett.

5. How sociocultural considerations influence contraceptive decision making.

6. Limited insights into racial and ethnic differences in contraceptive practices.

7. The concept of fertility awareness.

8. Why risk assessment is an integral component of contraceptive decision making.

9. Contraindications and why they are significant in contraceptive decision making.

10. How prevalent contraceptive use is among American women today.

11. The types of contraception and their failure rates.

12. Why contraceptive decision making is compromised with adolescents.

13. The mechanism, risks, benefits, side effects, and contraindications of hormonal methods, barrier methods, and permanent methods of contraception.

14. The strategies in effective contraceptive decision making.

15. The difference between induced and spontaneous abortions.

16. Abortion from a historical perspective.

17. Abortion from an epidemiological perspective.

18. The major types of abortion procedures.

19. The perspectives on abortion from pro-life and pro-choice positions and whether or not there is a middle ground.

Introduction

Birth control is an important issue for most American women. Being able to control reproductive functioning is a necessary component of career preparation and family growth management. Many methods of contraception are available today. Of the nearly 58 million reproductive-age women in the United States in 1988, approximately 35 million (60 percent) were using some form of birth control, with the two most popular forms of birth control being sterilization and the birth control pill (Figs. 8.1 through 8.3). No one contraceptive method is perfect. Contraception is a shared responsibility. The best method is one that a woman and her partner feel comfortable using and one that they will use correctly and consistently. The risk for sexually transmitted diseases must also be assessed with contraceptive decision making.

Perspectives on Contraception

Not all forms of sexual activity require contraceptive measures. These activities include abstinence from sexual activities and sex without intercourse. Not all couples engage in sexual intercourse. For example, sexual gratification and excitement may occur with hand holding, hugging, petting, kissing, mutual masturbation, and oral-genital sex. Ejaculation on, next to, or inside the vaginal

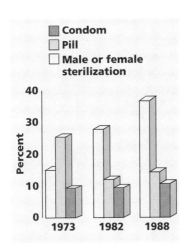

FIGURE 8.1

Percent of married couples (wives 15 to 44 years of age) using sterilization, the pill, and the condom, United States, 1973, 1982, and 1988.

SOURCE: Mosher, W.D., and Pratt, W.F. (1990). Contraceptive use in the United States, 1973–1988, National Survey of Family Growth. *Advance Data, 82*:1.

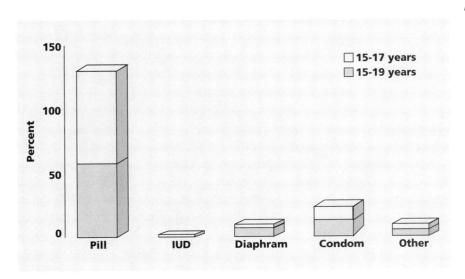

FIGURE 8.2

Contraceptive choices of unmarried, sexually active adolescents, 1982. *Note:* 67.6% of 15- to 19-year-olds and 60.0% of 15- to 17-year-olds reported using a method of contraception.

SOURCE: Adapted from Bachrach, C.A., and Mosher, W.D. Use of Contraceptives in the United States, 1982. NCHS, Advance Data, 102(4); and Bachrach, C.A. (1984). Contraceptive practice among American women, 1973–1982. *Family Planning Perspectives* (Nov/Dec), 253–259. As referenced in National Research Council. (1987). *Risking the Future: Adolescent Sexuality, Pregnancy and Childbearing.* Washington, DC: National Academy Press, p. A-52, 404.

FIGURE 8.3

Ever-married, US women aged 35 to 44 years, contraceptive users, 1988.

SOURCE: Adapted from USDHHS (1991). *Health United States, 1990.* (DHHS Pub. No. (PHS) 91-1232.) Hyattsville, MD: US Government Printing Office.

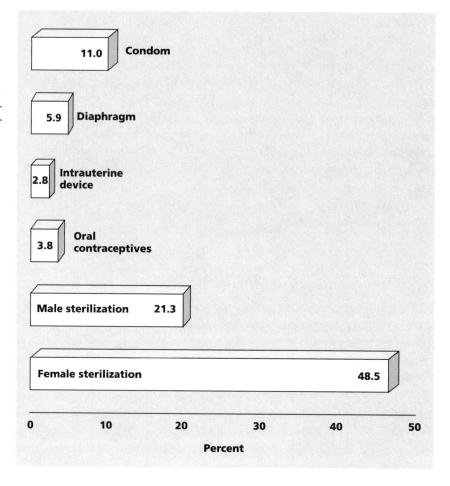

opening has inherent risks for pregnancy and a requirement for contraception if pregnancy is not desired.

Clarification of the subtle differences in terms is a necessary beginning for a discussion of contraception. Although the terms "birth control" and "contraception" are generally used interchangeably, each conveys a slightly different perspective about fertility control. **Birth control** is an umbrella term that refers to procedures that prevent the birth of a baby, so birth control would include all available contraceptive measures as well as sterilization, the intrauterine device (IUD), and abortion procedures. **Contraception** is a more specific term for any procedure used to prevent fertilization of an ovum.

Contraceptive decision making is not easy. Choices are often necessary between highly effective contraceptive methods that have some degree of risk and other methods that have few side effects but may detract from sexual enjoyment and that may have a higher failure rate. There are various mechanisms for contraception, including condoms, oral contraceptives, spermicides, diaphragms, and sponges. The four primary mechanisms by which birth control can be accomplished are:

1. Prevent sperm from entering the female reproductive system. Strategies that use this mechanism include abstinence, withdrawal, condom, and male sterilization.

2. Prevent sperm from fertilizing an ovum once it has entered the female reproductive system. Strategies that use this mechanism include diaphragm, cervical cap, contraceptive sponge, and spermicides.

3. Prevent the ovum from reaching the sperm. Strategies that use this mechanism include oral contraceptives and female sterilization.

4. Prevent progression of a fertilized egg. Strategies that use this mechanism include the IUD and abortion.

Historical Overview

Women have attempted to control their fertility status throughout history. Egyptian records indicate that women made a concoction of various compounds that was inserted into the vagina in paste form as an early diaphragm. Early Greeks followed the same plan with different recipes. Various teas and septic solutions were drunk with the hopes that they would prevent unwanted pregnancy. Early IUDs were stones that were placed in the uterus of camels to protect from pregnancy on desert treks. Women followed this example and have placed various foreign objects in the vagina over the course of history with hopes of similar results. Early attempts at spermicidal agents included various mixtures of acid, juice, honey, alcohol, opium, and vinegar.

Until the introduction of the birth control pill in 1960, diaphragms and condoms were the primary forms of contraception. Early condoms were probably made from linen sheaths. The cervical cap was introduced in the early 1800s, and the diaphragm was introduced later that century. In the mid-nineteenth century, feminists in the United States began a birth control campaign associated with the slogan "Voluntary Motherhood." This campaign advocated birth control by abstinence. Margaret Sanger (1883-1966) was an early promoter of contraceptive (sexual intercourse without pregnancy) birth control in the United States. She founded the American Birth Control League (ABCL) in 1921 (in 1942, the ABCL became Planned Parenthood Federation of America) to promote the founding of birth control clinics and the cause of fertility control. The ABCL established a clinic and dispensed diaphragms and lactic-acid jelly for contraception. Sanger also published *Family Limitation,* a pamphlet that provided clear and frank descriptions of birth control methods and devices. The distribution of diaphragms and her publication were hampered by the Comstock Laws, which had been enacted by Congress in 1873, restricting the circulation of obscene materials, specifically birth control information, in the mail.

Mary Coffin Dennett (1872-1947) was another pioneer in the birth control movement. Opposing the radical, confrontational tactics of Sanger, Dennett focused her efforts on lobbying for legislative reform that would allow for the transmission of contraceptive information. In her efforts to challenge the definition of legal obscenity, Dennett became one of the nation's most effective defenders of civil liberties. She established the Voluntary Parenthood League, and unlike Sanger, who promoted the diaphragm, which only physicians could prescribe, Dennett stressed that ordinary people should be able to get birth control information without having to rely on medical experts, so they could make their own informed decisions.

Birth control issues remained on the national front for many years. "Race-Suicide" was an antifeminist theory developed between 1905 and 1910 in reaction to the lower birth rates and changes in family structure believed to be caused by the birth control movement. Proponents of this theory, including President Theodore Roosevelt, believed that upper-class, educated women were failing by not having large families and allowing the upper classes to be overtaken by immigrants and the poor.

Although women today take for granted the availability of birth control devices and information, it has only been a few years that it has been technically legal to do so. A landmark Supreme Court decision in 1965, *Griswold v. Connecticut,* declared unconstitutional a Connecticut statute that made the use of birth control devices illegal and made it a criminal offense for anyone to give information about them or instruction on their use. Justice Douglas found the strength for the decision in the fact that the case involved "the intimate relationship of husband and wife" and contraceptives were a logical extension of the marital relationship. In 1972 in Massachusetts, the Court invalidated a law that had made it a felony to give anyone other than a married person contraceptives.

The historical and political dimensions of contraception continue to unfold. Federal restrictions on contraceptive development have resulted in the United States lagging behind many countries, with US couples having fewer contracepting options than couples in some developing nations. American women have a responsibility to become informed as contraceptive technology continues to become available and to become aware of the impact of political and economic forces that facilitate or impede the availability of these devices or agents.

Sociocultural Considerations

I am really concerned about birth control. My family expects me to be a virgin when I marry. But we aren't ready to get married yet and I am not a virgin. I am afraid that my family will not understand this problem.

20-YEAR-OLD

HISPANIC-AMERICAN WOMAN

Birth control attitudes and practices have been shown to vary among social classes. In some cultures, motherhood is the ultimate status and personal achievement. In male-dominated relationships and marriages, a woman may have considerable difficulty in expressing and asserting her concerns and needs for contraception. Religious beliefs may also play a significant role in influencing a woman's attitudes and practices with contraception. Many Protestant denominations endorse birth control as a marital option. Conservative and reform Judaism teachings are similar with couples able to limit their family size for either health or social reasons. Orthodox Jews may practice contraception under special health circumstances by consulting with medical and rabbinical authorities. The Roman Catholic Church traditionally and still officially today accepts only rhythm methods of contraception. Procreation is considered to be the primary purpose of sexual intercourse, and any interference with procreation is considered to be a violation of natural law. Various studies have shown that significant numbers of Catholics do use contraceptives, which may create emotional difficulties for contracepting Catholic women. Religion is not the only important cultural consideration, for in addition to religious beliefs about contraception, cultural groups may have values that dictate rules concerning virginity, marriage, and decision making within marriage. These factors may all contribute to cultural dimensions of contraceptive decision-making.

There is a paucity of national data examining and documenting racial/cultural differences with contraceptive practices. In a look at use of family planning services,[1] the National Survey of Family Growth conducted by the federal government has shown that African-American women were more likely to have received services in the past year than white women (39 versus 34 percent). African-American women, poor women, and teenagers were more likely to rely on clinics for their family planning services than white, higher income, and older women. Reasons for these differences are complex, but it is likely that African-American women are more likely to rely on clinics because they are less likely than white women to have health insurance coverage or sufficient monetary means to pay private practitioners. Other factors, such as the location of clinics and private practitioner's offices, may also help explain the disparity in use. Another probable explanation is that many public family planning clinics are intended specifically to serve low-income women. The same study looked at specific contraceptive behaviors by comparing white and African-American women. African-American women were less likely to be using contraception than white women (57 versus 62 percent), and African-American women were more likely than white women to have had intercourse in the last 3 months without using a contraceptive method. Overall, African-American women were less likely than white women to use a contraceptive method, but among those who did use a method, African-American women were significantly more likely to use the two most effective female methods of contraception: female sterilization (38 versus 26 percent) and the birth control pill (38 versus 30 percent). In contrast, African-American contracepting women were less likely to rely on male sterilization (1 versus 14 percent), the diaphragm (2 versus 6 percent) and the condom (10 versus 15 percent).[1] Clearly specific additional studies are needed to help to clarify and address the unique contracepting needs, clinic access, barriers, and utilization issues for all racial and ethnic groups of American women.

Contraceptive Issues

Many factors enter into the contraceptive decision-making process. These factors include fertility awareness and an understanding of risks, benefits, and complications associated with contraceptive methods.

We are happily married, and someday we wish to have children but right now our goals are to establish our careers. It would be really difficult for me to establish myself professionally if I become pregnant during the next 3 years.

26-YEAR-OLD ATTORNEY

Fertility Awareness

An understanding of the female menstrual cycle (see Chapter 7) is essential as a foundation for understanding contraceptive issues. In addition to facilitating decision making about contraceptives, knowing when she is fertile helps a woman when conception is desired, and knowing her body facilitates the recognition of any abnormal reproductive health changes that may be present.

One of the most important changes during the menstrual cycle is the fluctuation of various hormones from the anterior pituitary and the ovaries. The cyclical variations in these hormones are reflected in the biological alterations throughout the cycle. Some of the changes that occur as a result of these cyclical hormones are fluctuations in basal temperature patterns and variations in the type of cervical mucus produced. Many women are able to relate these manifestations to their fertility cycles. Methods of fertility awareness include the calendar method, basal body temperature, and cervical mucus or ovulation method. Some couples use the fertility awareness methods as contraceptive techniques, and others use them to time intercourse for pregnancy.

For a woman who absolutely does not wish to become pregnant, fertility awareness methods for contraception have inherent liabilities. The overall effectiveness of these methods will perhaps improve as technological advances evolve and have greater ovulation predictability. Timing of ovulation is not the only critical dimension of fertility awareness. Because sperm are able to survive 48 to 72 hours in the female reproductive tract, intercourse before ovulation is not necessarily free from pregnancy risk.

Risks

Women are concerned about the risks to their health that result from using contraceptives. Some experts argue that a comparison of the relative safety of different contraceptives must include a consideration of the risk of illness or death associated with any unplanned pregnancies that occur when a contraceptive method fails.[2] Risks may be direct, as in possible circulatory disorders associated with birth control pills, or indirect, as in an unwanted pregnancy. Risks vary among the various methods. Condoms and other barrier forms of contraception are unlikely to carry any long-term risks to their users. A difficulty in assessing any long-term risk associated with some methods, such as birth control pills, is that they have been in the United States only since 1960, and thus a full generation of American women have not yet used them.

Benefits

Just as there are risks associated with contraceptives, there are benefits associated with their use as well. The most obvious and direct benefit is protection from pregnancy. Birth control pills may actually protect users from ovarian cancer and cancer of the lining of the uterus. Barrier methods offer some protection from sexually transmitted diseases. In contraceptive decision making, the benefits and risks of any technique must be carefully considered within the individual unique needs of the couple making the decision.

Contraindications

A **contraindication** is a specific medical condition that renders a course of treatment inadvisable or unsafe that might otherwise be recommended. Possible contraindications for the birth control pill, for example, could be a history of thrombophlebitis (blood clots). The Food and Drug Administration (FDA) requires that birth control pill and IUD users receive an information packet that defines risks and benefits that can be expected.

Epidemiology of Contraceptives

A national survey, the National Study of Family Growth, is conducted periodically by the National Center for Health Statistics. Since 1982, all women in the sample have been interviewed regardless of marital status. Before that time, only married women or those with children in the household were included in the survey. This important difference in data gathering makes comparisons over time difficult.

Contraceptive Use

National data indicate that 60 percent of reproductive-age women (15 to 44 years) use a method of birth control. Of these methods, oral contraceptives, female sterilization, and condom use have increased in use, whereas the use of the IUD has declined[3,4] (see Fig. 8.1). The 40 percent of women not using birth control include, among others, women who are pregnant, women who are not sexually active, and women who have never had intercourse.

Contraceptive Failure

Contraceptive failure rates provide important information in the selection of a birth control method. **Failure rates** are determined by following large groups of couples who use specific methods of birth control for a specified time and then counting the number of pregnancies that occur. The larger the study that is conducted, the more reliable are the results. A failure rate of 2 percent means 2 pregnancies per 100 women per year studied. There are two types of failure rates. The lowest observed failure rate represents a method's absolute top performance, the highest efficacy ever achieved in a reputable clinical trial. The failure rate for typical users is an average rate based on an analysis of a range of reputable studies. The failure rate for typical users is usually lower than the best observed failure rates (Information Box 8.1). Age influences the efficacy of birth control method, with married older women generally being more successful contraceptors than younger women (Information Box 8.2). The reasons for this are not totally understood. It may be that younger women are

Birth Control Failure Rates

	Percent of Women Experiencing an Accidental Pregnancy in the First Year of Use		
Method	**Lowest Expected**	**Typical**	**Lowest Reported**
Chance	85	85	43.1
Spermicides	3	21	0.0
Withdrawal	4	18	6.7
Cervical cap	6	18	8.0
Sponge			
Women who have been pregnant	9	28	27.7
Women who have not been pregnant	6	18	13.9
Diaphragm	6	18	2.1
Condom	2	12	4.2
IUD			
Progestasert	2.0		1.9
Copper T 380A	0.8		0.5
Pills			
Combined	0.1		0.0
Progestogen only	0.5		1.1
Norplant implants	0.04	0.04	0.0
Female sterilization	0.2	0.4	0.0
Male sterilization	0.1	0.15	0.0

SOURCE: Reprinted and modified with the permission of the Population Council, from James Trussell et al., "Contraceptive Failure in the United States: An update," *Studies in Family Planning* 21, no. 1 (Jan/Feb 1990): 52.

*W*ell, I am proof that you need to follow directions. I thought that using a diaphragm was enough. I don't like that spermicidal stuff, and I thought a diaphragm alone was good protection. So I am pregnant. I can't believe that this is because I didn't follow directions.

21-YEAR-OLD PREGNANT WOMAN

less experienced with careful planning, they may be more fertile, they may have intercourse more often, or a combination of these reasons. At any rate, young women who wish to avoid pregnancy need to take extra care with contraception.

Several methods of contraception have demonstrated high levels of effectiveness with failure rates of 2 pregnancies per 100 couples per year or less. These methods include pills (oral contraceptives), IUDs, diaphragms, condoms (spermicidal), and sterilization. Other methods that have lower rates of effectiveness include spermicidal agents, such as foams, sponges, creams, gels, suppositories, and vaginal contraceptive film. The effectiveness of a birth control method depends in large part on how carefully and consistently it is used. The human elements of a method are important considerations because a diaphragm does not work when it is left in a drawer, pills may be forgotten, and condoms may break or leak.

Special Population—Adolescents

Teenage girls tend to rely on their male partners for contraceptive methods (withdrawal and condoms) during early sexual intercourse experiences and later

INFORMATION BOX 8.2

Percentage of Women Experiencing Contraceptive Failure During the First 12 Months of Use, by Method, According to Marital Status, Hispanic Ethnicity.*

Marital Status, Ethnicity and Race	Pill	Condom	Diaphragm
Unmarried			
Non-Hispanic White	6	16	17
Non-Hispanic Nonwhite	12	24	42
Hispanic	13	45	23
Married			
Non-Hispanic White	3	11	13
Non-Hispanic Nonwhite	8	22	43
Hispanic	4	20	9

*Numbers rounded to nearest whole integer.
SOURCE: Reproduced with the permission of The Alan Guttmacher Institute from Elise F. Jones and Jacqueline Darroch Forrest, "Contraceptive Failure in the United States: Revised Estimates from the 1982 National Survey of Family Growth," *Family Planning Perspectives,* Vol. 21, No. 3, May/June 1989.

adopt prescription methods. The average delay between first intercourse and the first visit for medical consultation is about 1 year, and then the visit is often motivated by a pregnancy scare. Among single female adolescents using contraceptives, however, the pill and condom are the most common methods (see Fig. 8.2). Adolescent sexual activity poses a risk, not only for unintended pregnancy, but also for sexually transmitted disease (see Chapter 10).

Contraceptive Methods

Hormonal Methods

Presently nearly 19 percent of women 15 to 44 years of age use **oral contraceptives** or birth control pills, making them the most commonly used nonsurgical method of birth control (see Fig. 8.2.; Fig. 8.3). Since its introduction in the United States in the 1960s, the birth control pill has been one of the most studied pharmacological preparations. The pill has changed considerably since its introduction. Although the specific hormones are the same or similar, the dosages and formulations have undergone tremendous changes. There has been considerable concern and debate over the safety of birth control pills. It is important for a woman to understand the spectrum of issues, advantages, and risks associated with birth control pill use.

With birth control pills, the woman's own reproductive hormone cycle is generally suppressed, and the synthetic estrogen and progestin of the pill produce an artificial cycle. Without the natural signals, the ovary egg follicle cannot mature, and ovulation cannot occur. The pill is responsible for other contracepting events, including the development of thick cervical mucus. This is in contrast to the profuse, slippery mucus associated with ovulation. The thick cervical mucus serves to impede sperm movement through the cervical canal and inhibits chemical changes in sperm cells that would permit the sperm to penetrate the outer layer of the egg. Another contracepting event associated with pill is that the lining of the uterus does not thicken as it normally does in the natural cycle, so even if ovulation and conception did manage to occur, successful implantation would be quite unlikely. Birth control pills are effective in preventing pregnancy. Effectiveness rates of 99 percent can be expected when they are taken properly.

Side Effects

Side effects have been associated with birth control pills. These side effects may include both negative and positive changes that are a result of taking birth control pills:

1. *Shorter and lighter menstrual periods.* The reduced amount of uterine lining results in less uterine shedding.

2. *Reduction or elimination of menstrual cramps.* Cramping is believed to be linked to ovulation, and because ovulation does not occur, cramping is reduced or eliminated. When menstrual bleeding begins, *prostaglandin* is released by the endometrial cells as they are shed from the uterine lining. Women who have severe cramps have significantly higher levels of prostaglandin in their menstrual fluid than women who do not have cramps. Steady progestin exposure with birth control pills tends to reduce or eliminate cramps.

3. *Mood changes.* Birth control pills may influence how a woman feels, or she may react to how she feels about taking the pills. A decreased fear of pregnancy and less anxiety about "getting ready" for sex may result in an increased sex drive. Other women may experience a decreased sex drive. Other reported mood changes include depression, irritability, or mood swings.

4. *Reduction or elimination of premenstrual symptoms.* **Premenstrual syndrome** (PMS) tends to be significantly reduced or eliminated with birth control pills for most women.

5. *Spotting or bleeding between periods.* The estrogen level maintained in the body by the pill is often lower than the natural level produced

by the ovaries. This lower level may trigger slight uterine bleeding, which is generally referred to as "breakthrough bleeding." This is more likely to occur when a pill is taken late or forgotten.

6. *Weight changes.* Some birth control pill users gain weight with the pill, and others lose weight.

7. *Acne improvement.* Most women who have acne notice significant improvement when they take birth control pills. Birth control pills may cause chloasma, however. **Chloasma** is the darkening of skin pigment on the upper lip, under the eyes, and on the forehead. It is not common and disappears when the birth control pills are discontinued.

Risks and Complications

Risks and complications are also associated with birth control pills. The most significant cause of serious and potentially fatal complications are circulatory disorders. The estrogen in birth control pills can alter the blood-clotting mechanisms of the body. Some women may experience abnormal clot formation. Clots are especially serious if they are in a vital organ or if they become dislodged and then travel to a critical site and impede blood circulation. An additional concern is that birth control pills may alter blood lipid levels. Elevated blood lipids, such as cholesterol, place a woman at greater risk for cardiovascular disease. In evaluating the risks associated with birth control pills, it is also important to consider lifestyle and genetic risk factors as well. The risk factors (Information Box 8.3) should be carefully evaluated before deciding to take birth control pills. Cigarette smoking is an important determinant with birth control pills. By age 35, the death risk of birth control pills is higher than the death risk of full-term pregnancy, so most clinicians will not prescribe birth control pills to women over 35 who smoke. Having more than one risk factor multiples the risk. A woman who already has had circulatory problems, such as a stroke, thrombophlebitis, a heart attack, or blood clots anywhere in her body, should never take birth control pills. For women who do not have other cardiovascular risk factors, the overall risk with birth control pills is low.

Birth control pills are responsible for changes in the surface of the cervix. These changes may make pill users more vulnerable to sexually transmitted diseases of the cervix, particularly *Chlamydia* infection. It is wise for women to consider using condoms with birth control pills, particularly if they are younger than 25, have more than one sexual partner, or both (see Chapter 10).

Some birth control users develop hypertension (elevated blood pressure). Pill-related hypertension usually is not severe and subsides when the pills are discontinued. If a woman's blood pressure is already high, birth control pills may or may not influence the problem. All women who take birth control pills should have regular blood pressure checks.

Some birth control pill users experience *post-pill amenorrhea*, a delay in the return of normal menstrual cycles after they stop the pills. This delay is more likely to occur in women who had irregular periods or long intervals between

---

INFORMATION BOX 8.3

Cardiovascular Risk Factors With Use of Birth Control Pills

Smoking

Age over 35

High blood pressure

Diabetes or family history of diabetes

Heart or circulatory disease

Heart attack in close relative <50, particularly a mother or sister

Obesity

High blood lipid levels

Sedentary lifestyle

Immobilization (after accident or injury)

periods before they started taking pills. In most cases, menstrual periods return spontaneously within 3 months. Most women do not experience this hormone suppression, however, and they conceive soon after stopping any method of birth control. If a woman does not want to become pregnant when she goes off the pill, it is important to begin an alternate form of birth control immediately.

Cancer is another area of tremendous concern and discussion with the pill. Despite considerable adverse publicity resulting in great anxiety among American women, there is no evidence today that birth control pills cause cancer. Despite this abundance of information, a 1985 Gallop Poll found American women to be misinformed about oral contraceptives. Because it takes a considerable amount of time for cancer to develop, however, continuous studies remain ongoing, and women should be alert for findings from these studies as they become available. Studies to date have shown important cancer-related benefits of the pill, however, which have significant impact on women's health. Modern birth control pills have been shown to reduce a woman's risk for uterine and ovarian cancer. Pill users have about half the rate of these cancers that would normally be expected, and protection may last as long as 10 years after the pills have been discontinued. Pill users, however, may have a somewhat higher risk for cervical cancer and for a very rare form of liver cancer. The increased risk for cervical cancer may be an effect of the pill itself or perhaps due to other variables, such as frequency of Pap testing or the number of sexual partners. The pill/breast cancer question has not yet been fully resolved, with a recent Centers for Disease Control study finding that pills neither increased nor decreased a woman's breast cancer risk, and a major report on breast cancer and oral contraceptives found that the weight of evidence still suggests no overall increased risk.[5] Regardless of the contraceptive form, an important consideration is that all potential risks with any form of contraception must always be weighed against the known health benefits and the prevention of unwanted pregnancy. Figure 8.4 provides a graphic representation of the annual number of newly diagnosed cases of ovarian, endometrial, breast, and liver cancer per 100,000 women. Drug interactions are another area of concern with birth control pills. Several drugs have been shown to reduce the contraceptive effectiveness of the pill and also contribute to bleeding between periods. These drugs include **barbiturates,** phenytoin (Dilantin), and certain antibiotics such as isoniazid, rifampin, and possibly tetracycline. It is probably wise for any woman on the birth control pill who is taking other medications to use a backup form of contraception while taking the other medication.

Advantages

Birth control pills provide the maximum protection possible with a temporary contraceptive method. They do not require any additional supplies or equipment, and they do not interfere with the spontaneity of lovemaking. They provide freedom from heavy menstrual cramps and excessive menstrual bleeding, and premenstrual symptoms are often relieved. Menstrual periods become regu-

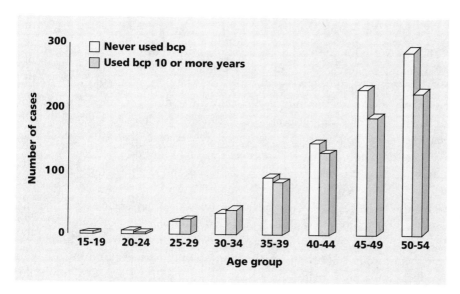

FIGURE 8.4

Estimated annual number of newly diagnosed cases of ovarian, endometrial, breast, and liver cancer per 100,000 women.

SOURCE: Reproduced with the permission of The Alan Guttmacher Institute from Susan Harlap, Kathryn Kost and Jacqueline Darroch Forrest, *Preventing Pregnancy, Protecting Health: A New Look at Birth Control Choices in the United States,* New York, 1991.

lar and predictable. Birth control pills provide benefits in addition to pregnancy prevention. As mentioned earlier, women who take birth control pills have lower prevalences of ovarian and uterine tumors. In addition, certain common benign breast tumors, fibroadenomas, and fibrocystic disease are less common in women who use birth control pills.[5] Women who take the pill also have fewer ectopic pregnancies and ovarian retention cysts as well as less risk of developing rheumatoid arthritis, pelvic inflammatory disease (PID), toxic shock syndrome, uterine fibroids, osteoporosis, and endometriosis.[5,6]

Contraindications

A contraindication is a medical condition that renders inadvisable or unsafe a treatment or procedure that otherwise might be recommended. Women who are contemplating birth control pills should carefully review and evaluate the contraindications before deciding to proceed with them. Absolute contraindications, meaning that the pills absolutely should not be taken, that have been specified by the FDA include:

- Known cardiovascular disorder, now or in the past, such as thrombophlebitis, stroke, heart attack, or coronary artery disease.
- Impaired liver function.
- Known or suspected cancer of the breast.
- Known or suspected estrogen-dependent neoplasia (abnormal tissue growth).
- Current or suspected pregnancy.
- Abnormal vaginal bleeding.

Types of Birth Control Pills

There are currently more than 30 different birth control pill brands available in monophasic (each cycle provides 21 identical hormone-containing pills), biphasic (two-phase) and triphasic (three-phase) pills. Triphasic pills are the latest of the combination pills and contain three different progestin doses for different parts of each pill cycle. The primary advantage of triphasic pills is that the overall amount of progestin in a cycle is lower than it is with regular, identical-dose pills. Estrogen dose is generally considered to be the single most important factor in selecting a pill. Side effects and complications are reduced with lower estrogen doses.

Minipills are relatively new birth control pills. They are estrogen-free and provide a continuous, low dose of progestin. Minipills are slightly less effective than the phasic pills and often cause irregular menstrual patterns. Minipills do not totally suppress hormone production. Natural estrogen and progesterone production usually remains sufficient to trigger menstrual periods. There is less margin of error with minipills. The likelihood of pregnancy increases substantially with one or two missed tablets. Although menstrual periods tend to be less predictable with the minipills, women who use them generally find fewer premenstrual symptoms.

Hormonal Implants

In late 1990, the first new approach to contraception since the birth control pill, the subdermal contraceptive implant, was approved for use in the United States. It had been studied extensively in clinical trials of more than 55,000 women in 44 countries for several years before being approved for general use in the United States. Norplant is the commercial name of the implant. The system works like the minipill. Hormonal implants consist of six 1- to 2-inch flexible rods that are filled with hormonal contraceptive, levonorgestrel, a synthetic form of progesterone, and implanted with local anesthesia just under the skin. Usually a ¼-inch incision is necessary. The hormone is gradually and constantly released into the bloodstream with no user compliance necessary after the insertion. Contraceptive protection begins within 24 hours of insertion. The system contains no estrogen and is designed to remain in place and prevent pregnancy for at least 5 years. The contraceptive mechanism is the prevention of ovulation and the thickening of cervical mucosa, impeding the passage of sperm into the uterus.

Menstrual irregularities (prolonged bleeding, spotting, amenorrhea, and an increase in spotting/bleeding days) have been the primary adverse effects reported with the implants. Headache and acne have also been reported as side effects to the implant. Cautions and contraindications for implant use are similar to the minipill. Although many women are concerned about possible pain with insertion of the implant, most women who have had the implant feel that they had either no or only slight discomfort during the insertion procedure, which includes the use of a local anesthetic. The usual site for hormonal implants is the inner aspect of the upper arm. This site is advantageous to other body sites because it is easy to expose, well protected, not highly visible, does not have significant amounts of fat tissue, and does not result in excessive bleeding. Removal of the implant takes a little longer than insertion. Again anesthetic is used, and a small dressing is applied to the site. Fertility is not affected after the implant is removed.

Women who may be candidates for hormonal implants include those women who do not desire children for at least 3 to 5 years and who do desire an effective, convenient form of birth control. Women for whom other methods may be contraindicated or who have had difficulty complying with other methods may also be candidates for implants. When total costs are considered for a 5-year period, the implant is less expensive than oral contraceptives, although the initial cost is high.

Other forms of hormonal contraceptives include injections and vaginal rings. Long-acting progestin injections, sometimes called "the shot," are used in many countries, and only recently has one been approved for use in the United States. Medroxyprogesterone (Depro-Provera) is the most common of the injectable progestins and has been approved for use. The long-acting progestin injection, which is usually given as an intramuscular injection every 3 to 4 months, has a theoretical and actual-use effectiveness of almost 100 percent. Depro-Provera was delayed for approval in the United States for several reasons, including a concern that laboratory dogs and primates developed cancers with the drug. There was also a concern that Depro-Provera might cause fetal deformities if the method failed as contraceptive.[7] Vaginal rings containing progesterone that are effective for 1 to 6 months are being tested in various countries throughout the world. The rings may be removed during intercourse if they cause discomfort.

Barrier Methods

Barrier methods of contraception were the primary forms of contraception before the pill and IUD. After the introduction of these newer and "high-tech" birth control measures, barrier methods were seen as messy, unromantic, and less sophisticated. Barrier methods have seen a resurgence in popularity. Feminists and health advocates objected to the pill on the grounds that it introduced unknown chemicals into the body and long-term effects were unknown. The condom has reemerged in the AIDS epidemic as a major form of protection, not only against AIDS, but also against other sexually transmitted diseases, such as herpes and gonorrhea. In addition, the diligent and proper use of spermicides has demonstrated pregnancy protection rates fairly comparable to the pill and IUD. In addition, a major compelling reason is that barrier methods have virtually no health risks associated with them with the exception of rare allergic responses or localized irritation.

Barrier methods, as the name implies, provide a physical or chemical barrier that prevents sperm from fertilizing eggs. All barrier methods (except plain condoms) include spermicide, chemicals that break down the cell walls of sperm. Most barrier methods are used inside the vagina to cover the cervix and prevent sperm from entering the uterus. Condoms are protective sheaths that enclose the penis during intercourse and ejaculation.

Barrier methods are very safe for the user, and problems and risks tend to be rare. One rare but important risk from barrier methods is toxic shock syndrome (TSS), which may be associated with the diaphragm, cap, and sponge. Although the TSS risk is small, it is recommended that the diaphragm, sponge, or cervical cap not be used during a menstrual period or when there is vaginal bleeding for any reason. Further recommendations include delaying using these devices 4 to 6 weeks after having a baby or until all postpartum bleeding completely stops. TSS risk can also be minimized by not leaving the devices in place in the vagina for longer than the recommended time period. TSS is not the only possible complication of vaginal birth control devices. A diaphragm, sponge, or cervical cap may cause a vaginal bacterial infection if it is left in place for more than 24 hours. A foul-smelling discharge is an indication of such an infection and should be evaluated by a clinician.

The advantages to barrier methods are diverse. Overall, barrier methods are very safe. Although the diaphragm and cervical cap require fitting by a clinician, the other barrier methods may be conveniently purchased in pharmacies. Barrier methods have an important advantage in that they help to protect users from sexually transmitted diseases. Spermicides kill the organisms that cause gonorrhea, herpes, and *Trichomonas* infections. Barrier methods may also help protect against cervical cancer. The virus, human papilloma virus (HPV), that causes genital warts is also responsible for cervical cancer, and the herpes simplex virus (HSV), is believed to be a co-factor for cervical cancer as well. Barrier methods are seen as noninvasive contraceptive measures by those women who do not want to have an IUD inside their uterus and who do not want to manipulate their hormonal system. Barrier methods may also be used as backup contraceptive measures when pills have been forgotten or during times when an IUD's effectiveness may be questioned. Some couples have intercourse sporadically or infrequently and find that barrier methods are appealing because they are effective but only have to be used when necessary. Older women and careful users find barrier methods to be more effective than younger women, women who have frequent intercourse, and those who are not careful users.

Spermicides

Spermicidal agents may be in the form of cream, foam, film, suppository, or gel (Fig. 8.5). These agents are available without prescription, and most contain detailed printed materials on their use. Spermicidal barriers work as a mechanical barrier in that they spread over the surface of the cervix and block access to the cervical opening. The more important mechanism by which they work, however, is that they inactivate the sperm by breaking down the surface of the sperm cells on contact. The spermicide should be inserted deep into the vagina. An advantage of these agents is that they are effective rather immediately upon use, but they do have time limits for their effectiveness. It is important to read the printed sheet available with each product and know the range of time for

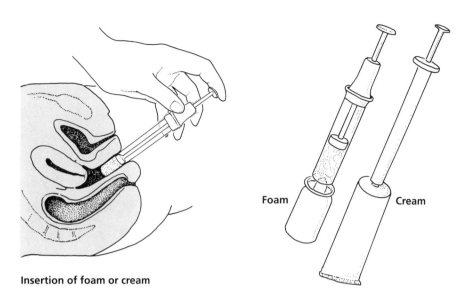

Insertion of foam or cream

Foam   Cream

FIGURE 8.5

Spermicidal agents. *Hints:* (1) Woman should lie down after insertion; spermicide will leak out and have reduced effectiveness if she is in a vertical position. (2) No douching for 8 hours. (3) Keep extra supplies available—it is not possible to measure residual amounts of foam in containers. (4) Repeat intercourse requires repeat application of spermicide. (5) Wash reusable applicators with soap and water after use. Follow directions carefully for amounts and frequency of use.

effectiveness. An additional application is needed for each round of lovemaking, and the product should be left in place, with no douching, for at least 6 hours after the last round. **Contraceptive film** is the newest form of spermicide. It is contained in a small thin sheet of glycerine, which is placed over the cervix before intercourse. Its effect is similar to that of contraceptive suppositories in that as the sheet dissolves, the spermicide is released.

Cervical Cap

Although it has not ever been widely used in the United States, the **cervical cap** (Fig. 8.6) has been a popular contraceptive in Europe. Caps are still not readily available in the United States, although they were approved by the FDA in 1988. The cervical cap looks and works much like a small deep diaphragm. It fits snugly over the cervix and is held in place by suction. Caps require a clinician's examination, fitting, and prescription. Not every woman who wants to use a cervical cap can be properly fitted, and some women find that insertion and removal of the cap are more frustrating than the diaphragm. The cap shares many characteristics of the diaphragm. It is made of latex and is used with a spermicidal agent such as cream or jelly. It also may be inserted up to 6 hours before having sex so it need not interrupt the activity.

Diaphragm

The **diaphragm** is a dome-shaped latex cup rimmed with a firm but flexible band or spring (Fig. 8.7). A diaphragm must be first coated with a spermicidal agent before being inserted into the vagina before intercourse. The spermicidal agent is important because the diaphragm does not remain fixed against the cervix, and it does not create a tight seal. It is possible for sperm to enter

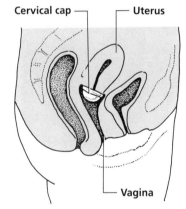

Cervical cap — — Uterus

Vagina

FIGURE 8.6

Cervical cap. *Hints:* (1) Fill cap approximately two-thirds full with spermicide. (2) Insert the cap by holding it in one hand, squeezing rim together in center. With other hand, spread labia and insert cap. Use with spermicidal agent. (3) Cap is inserted deep into the vagina. Use the index finger to press cap around the cervix until dome covers the cervix. (4) To avoid odor and reduce risk of complications, remove within recommended time. (5) To remove the cap, break the suction by placing index finger between cap and pubic bone. Grasp dome and pull down and out.

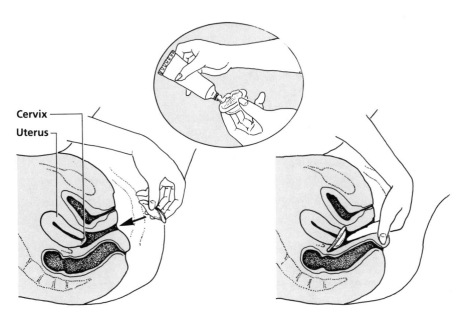

Cervix

Uterus

FIGURE 8.7

Diaphragm. *Hints:* (1) Apply 1 to 2 tsp of spermicide to diaphragm rim and inside dome. (2) Insert the diaphragm by holding it in one hand, squeezing rim together in center. With other hand, spread labia and insert diaphragm. (3) Diaphragm is inserted deep into the vagina with the anterior rim tucked into place last. (4) Check for proper placement of the diaphragm. Cervix is felt through dome—feels like tip of the nose. (5) To remove the diaphragm, assume a squatting position and break the suction by placing index finger between diaphragm and pubic bone. Hook finger behind anterior rim, bear down, and remove.

around the rim of the diaphragm and come in contact with the cervix. The primary function of the diaphragm is to hold the spermicidal agent directly against the cervix. Because the diaphragm must fit the cervix it is to cover, diaphragms require clinician examination, fitting, and prescription. During the fitting, it is important to evaluate the comfort of the diaphragm as well as practice insertion and removal of the diaphragm.

Diaphragm effectiveness depends on proper fit and diligent use. A diaphragm that is too small may not stay in place and slip off the cervix, and one that is too large may press on the urethra and cause a urinary tract infection. Application of the spermicidal cream or gel and insertion of the diaphragm can occur up to 6 hours before intercourse. If intercourse occurs more than once, it is important to use an additional application of spermicide for each event, regardless of how short a time the diaphragm has been in place. The diaphragm should not be removed or dislodged to add the cream or gel for a follow-up round of lovemaking. The diaphragm may be inserted in a standing, squatting, or lying-down position. For insertion, the diaphragm should be held with dome down (spermicide inside the dome) in one hand. The opposite sides of the rim should be pressed together so the diaphragm folds. The other hand should spread the lips of the vagina to facilitate insertion. The diaphragm should be inserted into the vagina toward the small of the back as far as it will go. A finger can tuck the rim behind the firm bulge in the roof of the vagina that covers the pubic bone. Once the diaphragm is in place, the women should not be able to feel it except with her fingers. If it is uncomfortable, it should be removed and reinserted. It is a good idea to check the position of the diaphragm before having intercourse. This can be done by the woman or her partner. The back rim should be below and behind the cervix, and the front rim should be tucked up behind the pubic bone. It should be possible to feel the cervix through the soft rubber dome of the diaphragm.

Like the cervical cap, an advantage of the diaphragm is that it may be inserted up to 6 hours before intercourse and need not interrupt or interfere with lovemaking. It should be left in place for a minimum of 6 hours after intercourse, and douching should not occur during that time. It should not remain in place longer than 24 hours. A spermicidal gel or cream must be used with the diaphragm. The gel or cream remains active for six hours. If intercourse does not occur within that time, the diaphragm can be removed and fresh gel or cream inserted. If intercourse occurs more than once, an additional applicator full of spermicide should be used each time. The diaphragm should *not* be removed or dislodged until 6 hours after the last act of intercourse. The diaphragm may be removed by reaching up inside the vagina with an index finger or thumb and grabbing the front rim of the diaphragm. It then can be pulled down and out of the vagina. A squatting position facilitates removal of the diaphragm for some women. After removal, the diaphragm should be washed with warm water and soap, rinsed, and dried with a towel. It is a good idea to inspect the diaphragm for defects or holes. Petroleum jelly should not be used with a diaphragm for lubrication because it will cause deterioration of the latex. If additional lubrication is desired, a water-soluble lubricant may be used.

Side effects with the diaphragm are infrequent. An allergic response to the latex of the diaphragm or to the spermicide is possible but rare. Symptoms of an allergic response include burning, itching, swelling, or perhaps blistering. Urinary tract infections are another possible side effect of the diaphragm. These infections may be in the form of either **cystitis,** infection of the bladder, or **urethritis,** inflammation of the urinary opening. Some diaphragm users feel bladder pressure, rectal pressure, or cramps when the diaphragm is left in place 6 hours after intercourse. A smaller diaphragm or a different rim type might help relieve this side effect.

Condom

Condoms (Fig. 8.8) have resurfaced as a popular barrier contraceptive in recent years. Women are now responsible for nearly 40 percent of total condom sales, and condoms are advertised in women's magazines. Condoms are available with lubricants and spermicides and a variety of colors and textures. An important advantage of condoms is that they are portable and disposable. They may be discreetly carried and thus available for use when necessary. Women do not experience any post-intercourse vaginal leaking, and condoms permit the male

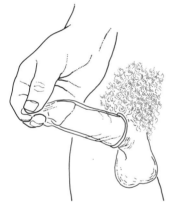

FIGURE 8.8

Condom use. *Hints:* (1) Avoid prolonged heat or pressure—condoms should not be stored in glove compartments or wallets. (2) Use only once and throw away. (3) If condom should break, use an extra dose of spermicide. (4) Put condom on an erect penis *before* it comes in contact with the vagina. (5) Hold onto the rim of the condom as the penis is withdrawn from the vagina. (6) Do not use petroleum-based lubricants with condoms. (7) Latex condoms are more impermeable to AIDS virus.

partner to take an active role in birth control. The lubrication on prelubricated condoms may help to reduce friction during lovemaking and reduce the risk of vaginal or penile irritation. Condoms should be stored in a cool, dry place. Storage in a heated unit (such as a glove compartment) can result in deterioration. They should not be lubricated with a petroleum jelly (such as Vaseline), which can weaken the latex. If extra lubrication is desired, a water-soluble lubricant (such as K-Y Jelly) or lubricated condoms can be used.

If a couple selects condoms as the method of birth control, it is essential that a condom be used for every lovemaking event. Condom use requires commitment and discipline for effective birth control. A spermicide-coated condom affords the most effective birth control protection as well as additional protection from sexually transmitted diseases. The clear fluid that collects on the end of an erect penis may contain living sperm so the condom should be placed on the penis before the penis comes near the vagina. It is important that room be left at the end of the condom to collect the semen. A condom that is stretched very tightly over the head of the penis is more likely to break or force the seminal fluid along the shaft of the penis and out the upper end of the condom. The penis should be withdrawn from the vagina before the erection subsides, and the condom should be held as the penis is withdrawn from the vagina. As the penis begins to lose its erection, the condom will collapse and there is a possibility for a spill of its contents. A quick visual inspection to ensure that the contents are inside and that there has been no spill or leakage is a good idea.

Couples should use condoms both during and after treatment for any reproductive tract infection as a precaution against reinfection. Condom use is encouraged with women who are at risk for sexually transmitted diseases, even for those who are using an effective form of birth control, such as the pill.

Female Condom

The female condom has recently been released as another form of barrier contraception. The female condom fits into the vagina, preventing the penis and semen from direct physical contact with the vagina. Two forms of the female condom are available. The first is a latex rubber G-string that contains a condom pouch located in the crotch. When the penis enters the vagina, it pushes the latex pouch into the vagina. The second type is placed in the vagina with an inner circular rim going deep into the vagina and an outer rim that is outside the vagina.

Contraceptive Sponge

The **contraceptive sponge** is a modern version of a historical form of birth control. For centuries, women have soaked small sea sponges in various solutions and placed them inside the vagina to prevent conception. The sponge acts both as a cervical barrier and a source of spermicide, and the sponge absorbs the ejaculated semen. One side of the sponge has a dimple in it that fits against the cervix, and the other side has a nylon loop for easy removal. It is available without fitting or prescription. Sponge effectiveness depends somewhat on a woman's previous pregnancy history because this product is less effective for women who have previously completed a full-term pregnancy and delivery than for women who have not done so.

An advantage of the contraceptive sponge is that it is portable and disposable. It can be inserted up to 24 hours before intercourse and need not interrupt lovemaking. It does not require a repeat application of spermicide for a second round of lovemaking, and it is less messy than other spermicidal agents. Before inserting the sponge, it is necessary to moisten the sponge with a small amount of tap water. It is held between two fingers and inserted into the vagina with the dimple side against the cervix. It is a good idea to check for proper placement by feeling the cervix through the sponge. The sponge can absorb vaginal lubrication, so some women use additional lubricant such as K-Y Jelly or spermicidal jelly after the sponge is in place. The sponge is designed for 24 hours of use and should remain in place for 6 hours after the last round of intercourse. Care should be taken to ensure that the sponge is not left in place longer than necessary. Before discarding a used sponge, it is best to check to make sure that it is intact. If the sponge is not intact, it is necessary to check the vagina for fragments.

Permanent Methods

Healthy women and men usually have many years of fertility after they have completed their childbearing. Surgical **sterilization** offers permanent birth control for those individuals who do not wish to have any more children. Surgical sterilization has become the most popular method of birth control among married couples in the United States (see Figs. 8.1 and 8.3). Advantages of sterilization include a high rate of effectiveness with relatively quick, simple procedures that have minimal complications and side effects.

Female Sterilization

Trends among contracepting older reproductive-age US women show a dramatic increase in sterilization rates (see Figs. 8.1 and 8.3 and 8.9). Sterilization of women has been made much easier in recent years by the development of new instruments and new techniques that have replaced laparotomy, surgically opening the abdomen and tying off the fallopian tubes. Because there were a significant number of unwanted subsequent pregnancies with this procedure, newer techniques have evolved that add destruction or removal of part of the fallopian tube. Laparoscopic sterilization, also known as "band-aid" surgery, is one of these techniques and uses a surgical instrument, the **laparoscope**, which is a tube equipped with light and magnification lenses. The laparoscope is inserted into the abdomen and provides a view of the uterus and tubes. The fallopian tubes are sealed with a cauterizing instrument or with rings or clips. Minilaparotomy is the latest technique for tubal ligation. It requires a small

We have three children and that is our family. The decision for sterilization was not difficult once we realized that we did not wish to become pregnant again. Our sex lives have improved—there is no need to worry about birth control anymore.

35-YEAR-OLD WOMAN

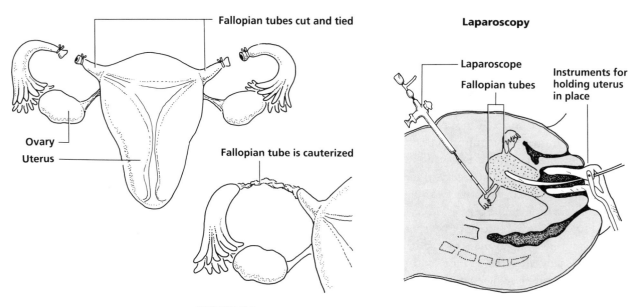

FIGURE 8.9

Female sterilization. *HInts:* (1) Resume normal activity slowly after procedure. (2) Most sutures are dissolvable. (3) Take mild analgesic for discomfort. (4) Resume sexual activity when comfortable. (5) Seek medical attention if temperature rises above 100°F, acute pain, discharge from incision, or bleeding.

abdominal incision and is performed under local or general anesthesia. The fallopian tubes are lifted out through the incision, cut, sealed, and replaced. The entire procedure takes a few minutes, and the woman requires a few hours' rest and observation and is then able to go home.

Sterilization should be undertaken with the expectation that the procedure is not reversible. Some reversal procedures, however, have been successful. The chances of repairing the tubes for future pregnancy depend on the amount of fallopian tube that was destroyed at the time of the sterilization procedure. Silicone plugs have been placed into tubal openings of recent sterilization procedures with the theoretical possibility that the procedure would be reversible, but sufficient data are not yet available on the procedure to date.

Male Sterilization

Male sterilization is accomplished with a surgical procedure known as a vasectomy. It is usually performed under local anesthesia in a physician's office. Usually one or two small incisions are made just through the skin of the scrotum. The vas deferens is lifted through the incision where it is cut. The two ends are tied or cauterized to seal them. Most men are able to return to work and normal activities the day after surgery but are advised to avoid strenuous activities, such as straining and lifting, for the first week after surgery. Vasectomy does not provide immediate contraceptive protection. Live sperm may remain in semen for some time because mature sperm are stored in the vas deferens above the surgical site. Vasectomy offers several advantages in birth control. It is extremely effective as a permanent form of birth control with very low risk of problems or complications compared with temporary forms of birth control or tubal ligation for women. Vasectomy does not cause any change in hormone levels or in the appearance or volume of semen. It also permits the male partner to take an active role in contraceptive responsibility.

Other Forms of Contraception

In addition to the temporary and permanent methods of birth control discussed, other forms of contraception have been used. Some of these methods are valid approaches to birth control but are associated with fairly high failure rates, even among motivated partners. These methods include abstinence, withdrawal, and breastfeeding.

Abstinence refers to no penis-in-vagina intercourse and depends on total willpower. Other forms of sex such as oral sex or mutual masturbation do not result in pregnancy and may be considered a form of abstinence.

Withdrawal is also known as coitus interruptus and refers to interrupting intercourse before ejaculation of the semen. Although it is logical to believe that if there is no ejaculate, there is no sperm and thus no conception, withdrawal can fail as a form of birth control when the man is unable to remove his penis in time or because some sperm are released before ejaculation. The failure rate for withdrawal as a form of birth control is fairly high because it is difficult for a man to know exactly when ejaculation will occur, and it is difficult to override mentally the physical activity of intercourse.

Breastfeeding is not considered an effective form of birth control. Although breastfeeding does delay the return to fertility after birth, it is not possible to calculate exactly when fertility returns. One study found that more than half of the breastfeeding women who did not use birth control were pregnant again within 9 months after delivery.

Intrauterine Devices

An IUD is an object placed in the uterus through the cervix. The IUD is left in place for an indefinite period and prevents pregnancy from the time it is placed in the uterus until it is removed. The IUD was a popular form of birth control in the 1970s. Since then, its popularity has declined. Medical problems and lawsuits against the manufacturers have led to decreased production and use of the IUD as a form of contraception. An IUD is inserted by a clinician into the uterus via the cervix with special instruments. There is a string attached to the IUD for identification and removal of the device.

The presence of the IUD inside the uterus alters a number of factors necessary for pregnancy. IUDs reduce the number of sperm cells that reach the oviducts and decrease the viability of those sperm cells that do reach the oviducts. It was once proposed that the primary mode of action of the IUD was to prevent implantation, and therefore it induced abortion.[7] Numerous studies of the mode of action have not found frequent evidence of fertility (as evidenced by biochemical markers of early pregnancy in blood and urine.) Thus it is proposed that IUDs interfere with fertilization and not implantation.[7,8] Most likely the IUD acts on both fertilization and implantation, with the major action on fertilization.

Pelvic inflammatory disease (PID) has been identified as a significant risk associated with the IUD. In an international study, researchers learned that the risk of PID among IUD users appears highest in the first 20 days after it is inserted. Women who received their IUDs before the age of 25 and before 1980 were more likely to contract PID than those who did not. The researchers also concluded that PID among IUD users is more strongly related to the insertion process and a background risk of sexually transmitted disease than to the type of IUD or to long-term use.[9]

Some women should not have an IUD inserted. Anyone with an active pelvic infection, including gonorrhea, or a pregnant woman should never have an IUD placed in her uterus. Insertion of an IUD is strongly contraindicated if a woman has recent or recurrent pelvic infections, inflammation of the cervix or vagina, history of ectopic pregnancies, valvular heart disease, and abnormal Pap smears.

Advantages of the IUD include no supplies or equipment for lovemaking, normal hormonal cycles are not manipulated, and it is a highly effective form of contraception. Health risks are the primary disadvantage with the IUD. Risk of infection is a major concern with IUDs because IUD-related infection can lead to illness, infertility, and, in rare cases, even death. Total amount of menstrual bleeding tends to increase with the IUD, and spotting between periods commonly occurs. The IUD remains as a birth control choice for a woman who has finished childbearing and whose risk of infection is very low.

Emergency Birth Control

A woman who engages in unprotected sexual activity runs the risk of both sexually transmitted diseases and pregnancy. Birth control measures must be used in accordance with the manufacturer's guidelines. Removing a diaphragm too early, failing to use a spermicidal agent with the diaphragm, and using too little foam are all examples of increasing the risk of an unplanned pregnancy. Occasionally accidents happen. A condom may tear or slide off, or a diaphragm may dislodge from the cervix. In these situations, one option is to use a spermicidal agent immediately. Foam or cream would be more immediately effective than a vaginal suppository, which takes time to dissolve. There are no guarantees, but the spermicide may help reduce the risk of an unplanned sperm/egg union. If spermicides are not available, a douche with warm water is another alternative, but no guarantees are offered.

Another form of emergency birth control includes medications containing synthetic estrogens or progestins (or both), which may be taken within 72 hours of unprotected intercourse to prevent implantation. These are considered emergency methods only and should not be considered as a regular form of birth control. These medications, such as Ovral (high estrogen and progesterone levels) and high-dose progesterone-only pills carry the same risks as oral contraceptives. The synthetic estrogen diethylstilbestrol (DES) is no longer approved for use in the United States as a postcoital contraceptive.

The European drug RU486 has received recent media attention as the "abortion pill." The drug antagonizes the actions of progesterone and has been used extensively throughout Europe. Some experts argue that even if available in the United States, RU486 would not be the drug of choice as a postcoital contraceptive and that Ovral is preferred immediately after unprotected intercourse.[7]

Informed Decision Making About Contraception

An array of effective birth control methods are available to women today. The decision-making challenge is to determine which method or combination of methods best meets each woman's unique needs. Safety and reliability are the

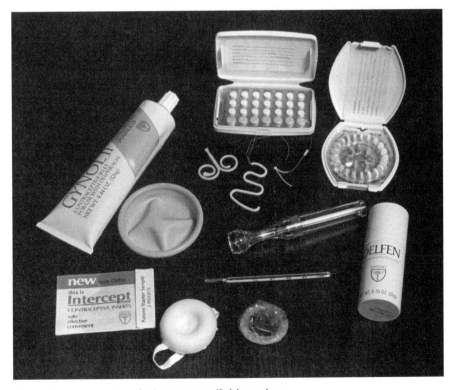

Several contraceptive choices are available today.

first concern. Other factors such as health status, lifestyle, financial considerations, and patterns in sexual activity also determine which method is best suited. Many women will decide to change to a different method as factors change. Communication is an essential component of contraceptive decision making. It is important that couples talk about feelings, needs, and fears.

Determining Personal Needs

Sexual urges and sexual activity are normal events for men and women, but for women, a very real possible consequence of heterosexual intercourse is pregnancy. For both technological and sociological reasons, there has been a traditional tendency for women to assume the major responsibility for contraception. This has been both unfair and unreasonable for women. Although most of the current contraceptives require primary use by women, there are a number of ways couples can share the responsibility for contraception. Open and honest communication, sensitivity to each other's needs and feelings, and awareness of each method's strengths and weaknesses are essential components for effective decision making.

Specific strategies to informed consumer contraceptive decision making include the following (Self-Assessment 8.1):

1. *Review needs.* It is important to consider when or if pregnancy may be desired. If never, perhaps sterilization is a more logical option. If pregnancy is desired in a few years, the more effective methods such as the pill may be preferable. If pregnancy is desired later on this year,

---

SELF-ASSESSMENT 8.1

Strategies for Contraceptive Decision Making

Contraceptive decision making is a personal and private decision between a woman and her partner. Several factors should be carefully considered when making the decision:

1. Review needs:
   When/if pregnancy will be desired
   How disruptive would an unplanned pregnancy be
   Frequency of intercourse
   Number of partners
   Risk of STDs
   Personal preferences for lovemaking
   Level of partner cooperation
   Significance of spontaneity
2. Medical history:
   Cardiovascular risk factors

   Smoking status
   Allergies
   Circulatory disorders

3. Put risks and benefits of methods in perspective:
   Weigh all the advantages and disadvantages of each method in a personal perspective

4. Reevaluate decision periodically:
   Assess level of compliance
   Assess level of satisfaction

one of the barrier methods may be a better choice. If a woman does not want to become pregnant and an abortion is out of the question, she may wish to consider a combination of two good birth control methods, such as foam and condoms, or pills and condoms, or a diaphragm and condoms. Frequency of intercourse is another major consideration to review. If intercourse occurs frequently, barrier methods may prove to be inconvenient. Number of partners should be considered. If a woman has more than one partner, or her partner has another partner, she has a greater risk for infection. In this case, a condom with spermicide in addition to birth control pills would provide the best protection against both sexually transmitted diseases and pregnancy. Emotional, behavioral, and psychological needs must also be considered. Even though a method may appear perfectly logical from a medical point of view, if it is distasteful or undesirable, the chances are that compliance with that method would be poor. The degree of partner cooperation is another important consideration. Barrier methods are more likely to be successful if there is partner cooperation and support. If spontaneity is an important consideration, barrier methods that require time-out for insertion may not be desirable and represent additional risk for pregnancy. Perhaps one of the most important considerations is an evaluation of partner feelings and support. Ideally the contraceptive choice is a joint decision made by a couple with open honest discussion of all the considerations and issues. With less than an ideal situation, the woman would be unwise to depend on her partner for contraception decision making or use.

2. *Consider medical factors.* Medical factors such as risk factors for cardiovascular disease, smoking status, and circulatory disorders must be carefully reviewed before deciding on birth control pills.

3. *Review failure rates.* It is important to compare typical failure rates with best observed failure rates for the method selected. The difference can provide insight into what the relative margin of error is in that method. For example, foam has a best reported failure rate of 3 to 5 percent with an average failure rate of 18 percent. Clearly these differences indicate that typical users are different from the study population that achieved the best reported rates. At best, however, failure rates can provide only a general idea of how successful other couples have been with a selected method in the past.

4. *Put risks and benefits of the methods in perspective.* It is important to weigh all the dimensions and issues of the relationship carefully with the advantages and disadvantages of each method. The risks and benefits of each method need to be carefully assessed for each method in terms of the individuals involved and the relationship. Some couples find that they can use a numerical rating scheme to determine the best contraceptive that meets their unique needs.

5. *Periodic reevaluation of decision.* At regular intervals, contracepting couples need to reevaluate the level of effectiveness and their individual level of satisfaction with the selected method. Reevaluation requires review of each of these steps and consideration of any new contraceptive developments, possible medical contraindications, and a current assessment of their needs, feelings, and family planning goals.

When to See a Health Care Provider

It is necessary to see a clinician for prescription of the diaphragm, cap, pill, or IUD. Other forms of birth control do not require a clinician's prescription, but conditions associated with these forms may warrant a clinic visit. In general, a clinician should be consulted any time that there is pain during intercourse or any unusual bleeding, spotting, discharge, or odor. Any burning or itching associated with spermicide use may be an indication of an allergy to the agent. A clinician should be consulted in the event of toxic shock syndrome symptoms. With a diaphragm, it is wise to check with a clinician any time that the diaphragm does not seem to be fitting properly or there is discomfort, pain, or recurring bladder infections. After having a baby, it may be necessary to be refitted for a different sized diaphragm because vaginal depth and muscle tone are usually altered by full-term pregnancy.

Abortion

Abortion may be defined as the spontaneous or induced expulsion of an embryo or fetus before it is viable or can survive on its own. Complications may occur with the development of a fetus during pregnancy. These complications may be due to various genetic, medical, or hormonal problems, and the result is termination of the pregnancy. This termination of pregnancy is called a **miscarriage** or a **spontaneous abortion.** In contrast to a spontaneous abortion, an **induced abortion** involves a decision to terminate a pregnancy by medical procedures.

I am an organized and responsible person. I was a victim of contraceptive failure. It was impossible for me to have a child at that time in my life. It would have destroyed everything that I had worked years for. So I had an abortion. I am not proud of it, but I am grateful that I was able to go to a safe facility.

32-YEAR-OLD WOMAN

Abortions are a critical facet of women's health. Each year, more than 6 million American women become pregnant, and more than half of these pregnancies are unintended. Of these unintended pregnancies, approximately 1.6 million terminate their unintended pregnancy through abortion.[10]

Historical Overview

Induced abortion has been both controversial and widely practiced for centuries. The history and politics of abortion is long and complex. Anthropological studies have revealed that abortion practice was widespread in ancient and preindustrial societies. In the Western World before Christianity, Greeks and Romans considered abortion acceptable during the early stages of pregnancy. A proscription for abortion has been found in the Hippocratic oath taken by

Greek physicians. Until the late 1800s, women healers in Western Europe and the United States provided abortions and trained other women to do so, without legal prohibitions. The movement to establish abortion as both criminal and sinful was led by male physicians as part of a crusade from 1860 to 1880 to outlaw all forms of contraception. By 1965, all 50 states had passed legislation prohibiting abortion during all stages of pregnancy. The issue of equity entered abortion public policy considerations. Women with greater personal financial resources were able to arrange for safer, more "legal" abortions by traveling to less rigid jurisdictions or by persuading physicians to make therapeutic exceptions. Women with fewer financial resources were more likely to suffer from unsafe abortions and incompetent abortionists. Legal prohibition did not have the effect of reducing the incidence of abortions. Estimates of the annual number of illegal abortions in the 1950s and 1960s ranged from 200,000 to 1.2 million.

In the early 1970s, legal challenges were increasingly mounted against any prohibition of a woman's ability to obtain an abortion. Abortion was legalized in the United States on January 22, 1973, through the landmark Supreme Court decision *Roe v. Wade.* This decision declared unconstitutional all state laws that prohibited or restricted abortion during the first trimester of pregnancy. The decision stated that the "right of privacy . . . founded on the Fourteenth Amendment's concept of personal liberty . . . is broad enough to encompass a woman's decision whether or not to terminate her pregnancy." The ruling also limited state interventions in second-trimester abortions and left the issue of third-trimester abortions up to each individual state.

The *Roe v. Wade* decision was immediately greeted with opposition. "The "right-to-life" movement was originally a creation of The Family Life division of the National Conference of Catholic Bishops (NCCB), the directive body of the Catholic Church in the United States. Immediately following the Supreme Court decision of *Roe v. Wade,* the NCCB Pro-Life Affairs Committee declared that it would not accept the Court's judgment and called for a major legal and educational battle against abortion. A religious pro-abortion group, the religious coalition for abortion rights, was formed in 1973 to support the Supreme Court decision and preserve the right of women, regardless of income, to have their choice of legal abortions.

A number of states in 1974 and 1975 instituted restrictions in the ruling by enacting laws requiring teens seeking abortion to have parental permission. This legislation, however, was declared unconstitutional by the Supreme Court in 1976. The decision stated that a minor should have free access to sex-related health care and that a third party such as a parent could not veto a decision made by the physician and the patient to terminate the patient's pregnancy.

In 1976, the Hyde Amendment was introduced and passed in Congress. This legislation was a major setback to the abortion movement because it banned Medicaid funding for abortion unless a woman's life was in danger. It has been argued that this amendment disproportionately affected low-income women. A temporary injunction stalled the Hyde Amendment for a year. Meanwhile in June 1977, the Supreme Court ruled that states did not have to fund what they considered "medically unnecessary" abortions. In December

1977, a compromise version of the amendment added exceptions for promptly reported rape and incest cases in which two physicians would testify that the woman's health would be seriously impaired by maintaining the pregnancy. Many groups fought against the Hyde Amendment, but the final ruling of the Supreme Court upheld it in the 1980 *Harris v. McRae* decision. Although the Supreme Court reaffirmed the central holding of *Roe v. Wade* in 1986, a newly constituted court agreed to hear *Webster v. Reproductive Health Services* in 1989. The Supreme Court decision on the *Webster* case returned to the states the authority to limit a woman's right to a legal abortion. The saga continues into the 1990s.

Epidemiology

Induced abortions have been legal throughout the United States since 1973. Data on pre-1973 illegal abortions are not valid or reliable indications of actual prevalence. After an initial rise in the 1970s following legalization, the number of induced abortions stabilized in the 1980s at about 1.6 million a year.[10] Fig. 8.10 shows abortion rates for selected years since 1972. The stabilization in rates during the 1980s may have been caused by changes in the use of abortion services or by the increased number of older women (due to the aging of the baby boom cohort) because older women have lower abortion rates than younger women.[11] Other possible sociocultural reasons for the reduction may include reduced access to abortion services, changing attitudes toward abortion, or continuation of unplanned pregnancies.[11]

Women having abortions in the United States in 1987 were predominantly white (65.2 percent), unmarried (82.4 percent), and young (25.1 percent were under age 20, and 33.1 percent were 20 to 24 years of age).[10] For both white and nonwhite women, the highest abortion rates are seen among women 20 to 24 years of age, and the lowest rates are among women 40 and older

FIGURE 8.10

Legal abortion rates, United States, selected years, 1972–88.

SOURCE: Adapted from Centers for Disease Control (1991). Special Focus on Reproductive Health Surveillance—Abortion Surveillance, United States, 1988. *Morbidity and Mortality Weekly Report.* 40(33-2), 15–42.

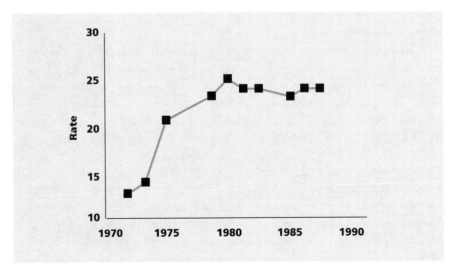

(Information Box 8.4). When the same age groups are compared in white and nonwhite women, nonwhites have significantly higher rates of abortion at all ages.

Adolescent females are a special population of concern with abortions. Factors contributing to adolescent pregnancies and decisions about keeping or terminating the pregnancy depend on several sociodemographic considerations. Data indicate that 58 percent of adolescents having an abortion are less than 17 years of age, 55 percent of them are white, and 79 percent are experiencing their first pregnancy.[12] One study found that 61 percent of the adolescents indicated that one or both parents knew about the abortion. Of those who did not tell their parents, 30 percent had experienced violence within the family, feared that violence would occur, or were afraid of being forced to leave home.[12] Previous studies have found that a teen's decision about an unintended pregnancy—whether to carry it to term and, if she does, whether to marry to legitimate the birth—are strongly affected by her age and her parents' level of education.[13]

Abortion Procedures

Vacuum curettage is the most widely used abortion technique in the United States. This procedure is performed while the woman is under local anesthesia.

INFORMATION BOX 8.4

Abortion Rate by Race, According to Age and Marital Status, 1987

Age and Marital Status	Race	
	White	Other
Age (years)		
<20	37.3	78.1
<15	5.8	26.4
15–19	36.3	73.0
20–24	41.3	103.2
25–29	23.2	66.0
30–34	13.5	38.8
35–39	7.6	21.0
≥40	2.2	6.2
Marital status		
Married	6.9	27.6
Unmarried	38.2	71.1

SOURCE: Reproduced with the permission of The Alan Guttmacher Institute from Stanley K. Henshaw, Lisa M. Koonin and Jack C. Smith, "Characteristics of U.S. Women Having Abortions, 1987," *Family Planning Perspectives,* Vol. 23, No. 2, 1991.

Approximately 96 percent of all legal abortions done in the United States use this procedure.[14] The procedure involves the dilation of the cervix, and a vacuum curette, an instrument consisting of a tube with a scoop attached for scraping away tissue, is inserted through the cervix into the uterus. The other end of the tube is attached to a suction-producing apparatus, and the contents of the uterus are aspirated into a collection vessel. Vacuum curettage is usually performed during the first trimester of pregnancy, or until 13 weeks, but can be done up to 20 weeks. The length of pregnancy is determined from the onset of the last menstrual flow or the last missed period. Through 13 weeks of pregnancy, this procedure can be performed in a clinical office setting with appropriate backup facilities for unexpected medical problems.

Dilatation and curettage (D&C) is a technique used for many gynecological procedures but rarely in abortions.[7] A sharp curette is used to scrape out the contents of the uterus. This procedure requires that the woman be under general anesthesia. The reasons that it is rarely used in abortions in the United States are that it is more painful than the vacuum curettage method, causes more blood loss, and requires larger cervical dilation.[7]

Dilatation and evacuation is a procedure that combines the D&C and vacuum curettage approaches. It is usually done between 13 and 16 weeks' gestation. At this time, the cervix needs to be dilated to a greater extent because the products of conception are larger.

Nonsurgical methods can also be used to terminate a pregnancy. The use of prostaglandins, which are potent biochemical compounds produced by the male and female, has increased in recent years to terminate pregnancies. The prostaglandin compounds may be used intraamniotically, injected into the amniotic sac that surrounds the uterus, or inserted into the vagina as suppositories. Prostaglandins are used in second-trimester pregnancies (14 to 24 weeks of gestation). Prostaglandins cause the uterus to expel the fetus. Hypertonic saline may also be used in second-trimester abortions. In such instances, the saline is infused slowly into the amniotic cavity to cause fetal death and expulsion of the fetus from the uterus. A hypertonic solution of urea is also used to induce abortions. The urea is infused into the amniotic cavity and works in the same manner as the saline.

In some abortions, laminaria, a type of seaweed, is used to dilate the cervix. In a few hours, the laminaria dilate the cervix sufficiently for the abortion procedure. Oxytocin, a product produced in the posterior pituitary and also commercially manufactured, is often used to facilitate uterine contractions. It is commonly used with the D&C method and with hypertonic saline during second-trimester abortions.

As with all medical procedures, health risks are associated with the various abortion techniques. Abortion-related health risks are greatly reduced if the pregnancy is terminated as early as possible, if the woman is healthy, if the clinician is skilled, and if the woman is confident in her decision to have an abortion.[7] The risk of death or serious complications increases dramatically as the gestation period increases. The most common postabortion problems include infection, retained products of conception in the uterus, continuing pregnancy, cervical or uterine trauma, and bleeding.

Other Abortion Techniques

Terms such as "menstrual induction," "menstrual extraction," and "aspiration without dilation" have been used in the past to refer to vacuum procedures performed very early in pregnancy before a routine urine pregnancy test could confirm pregnancy. The technique for menstrual induction or extraction is identical to that for early vacuum abortion. Because it is now possible to confirm pregnancy as early as 1 week after conception, these terms are no longer meaningful. In many ways, these terms are "word games." A woman who requests "menstrual induction" because her period is a few days late can now find out for certain whether or not she is pregnant. If her pregnancy test is positive, the vacuum procedure is an abortion. If the test is negative, there is no need for the procedure. Another major area of concern is in the preparation, training, and skill of the person performing such a procedure. A lack of training and the nonavailability of emergency medical backup in the event of a problem are potentially life-threatening conditions.

Current Perspectives

Abortion is one of our nation's most widely debated and controversial topics. There are basically two opposing perspectives on abortion and each side of the issue is filled with intense feelings and social, moral, and religious ramifications. The two opposing perspectives are known as "pro-life" and "pro-choice."

Pro-Life

Pro-life advocates argue that the human fertilized ovum is a human being that should be afforded legal protection. Pro-life efforts to overturn abortion public policy have taken three major approaches: human life amendments to the US Constitution, human life statutes and governmental action through legislation, and other means to restrict access to abortion services. Antiabortion groups have been lobbying for legislation and raising revenue for electoral campaigns targeting pro-choice electoral candidates. The National Right to Life Committee, which includes most pro-life groups, claims a membership of 11 million and has a 3-million-dollar annual budget.

Pro-Choice

Pro-choice advocates favor legalization and ready availability of abortions. From their perspective, for women in one of the most industrialized countries in the world to have a personal issue played out in a political arena is deplorable. They believe that the pregnant woman has the right to freedom of choice as to whether or not she will terminate an unwanted pregnancy because a woman has the right to exercise control over her own body. Many also believe that a fertilized ovum is not yet "human." Feminists have argued that the concerns generated from abortion politics have more to do with compulsory heterosexuality, family structure, the relationship between men and women, parents and children, and women's employment than they do with the fetus.

Middle Ground?

Unfortunately, the polarization of the issue in exclusive terms of these positions prohibits dialog and an opportunity to find common ground of interest and concern. One recent nonpolarized effort merits attention in this arena. In St. Louis, Missouri, staff from Reproductive Health Services (the plaintiff in *Webster v. Reproductive Health Services*) and local pro-life leaders have inaugurated a Common Ground Project. The groups have agreed to disagree about abortion but to work together to increase state funding for women who want to continue their pregnancies.[15] Other groups are beginning to convene discussion sessions in an attempt to understand each other and find common ground for learning and addressing important issues in reproductive health. Perhaps in future years the polarization of these two positions will be less pronounced, the need for abortion services will be diminished, and there will be a concerted effort from both groups to prevent unwanted pregnancies more effectively.

Informed Decision Making

The decisions with an unwanted pregnancy are a private, personal, and difficult process. Decisions should not be rushed, and all options should be carefully weighed. Being able to talk through the process with a trusted person is essential. Options include terminating the pregnancy, continuing the pregnancy and raising the child, or continuing the pregnancy and relinquishing the child for adoption. Many supportive services are available for each of these options.

If a woman elects to have an abortion and is confident in her decision, she can reduce her risk of medical complications from the procedure by making arrangements in a timely fashion. In selecting an abortion facility, a primary concern should be for around-the-clock emergency care services. Infection, bleeding, and other complications can almost always be treated successfully if treatment begins promptly. Other activities to minimize risks from an abortion include making sure that the surgeon who performs the procedure is well trained and experienced and making sure that the facility provides comprehensive care to include postoperative instructions, education, and supportive services. Abortion counseling services are perhaps one of the most important features of a comprehensive facility.

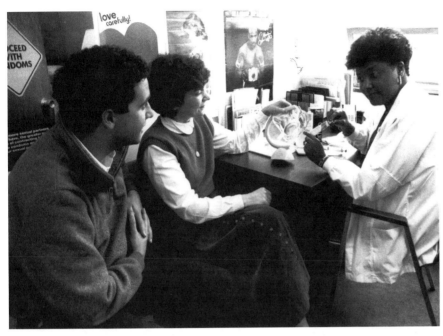

The decision as to which contraceptive to use is a shared responsibility.

Summary

Birth control is an important issue for most American women. Being able to control reproductive functioning is a necessary component of career preparation and family growth management. Many methods of contraception are available today. Information Box 8.5 provides a comparison overview of the methods

Abortion Remains an Important Legal Issue

In June 1992, the Supreme Court upheld a Pennsylvania law that places restrictions on abortions in that state. The state law specified that women seeking abortions must receive counseling on risks and alternatives and must wait at least 24 hours after counseling to have the abortion. Minors under the age of 18 must obtain one parent's informed consent or judge's approval for an abortion. No abortions are to be performed after 24 weeks of pregnancy unless needed to protect the woman's life or prevent permanent physical harm. Physicians must keep detailed records on abortions and reasons for performing late-term abortions. Married women must notify their husbands if they plan to have an abortion (few exceptions were available to this requirement).

The only restriction that the Supreme Court ruled as unconstitutional was the one requiring spousal notification. The other restrictions were upheld by the Court and are allowed to stand in all cases of abortion in the state of Pennsylvania.

While upholding the Pennsylvania law, the Supreme Court declined, by a 5–4 margin, to overturn *Roe v. Wade* at this time.

Comparison Issues: Contraceptives

	Birth Control Pills	Intrauterine Device (IUD)
Estimated Effectiveness	98% (combination) 97% (mini)	95%
Typical Effectiveness	97–98%	95–98%
How It Works	Prevents the release of eggs from the ovaries	Prevents implantation and first stage of pregnancy
Advantages	Most effective temporary form of contraception; lighter and more regular periods; protective factor for ovarian and uterine cancer; decreases risk of PID, fibrocystic breast disease, and benign ovarian cysts; does not interfere with sexual activity	Once inserted, remains in place; remains effective while in place; does not interfere with sexual activity
Disadvantages	Contraindicated for women with cardiovascular risk; some women experience minor side effects during first 3 mos of use; major complications occur in women who are over 35 and who smoke; must be taken daily	May cause bleeding and cramping; increased risk of PID; increased risk of ectopic pregnancy
Availability	By clinician examination and prescription only	Limited availability—by examination and fitting only
Comments	Combination pills contain both synthetic estrogen and progesterone. Minipill contains only progesterone and may produce irregular bleeding	Better for those women who do not desire future pregnancies

	Condom	Cervical Cap
Estimated Effectiveness	90%	95%
Typical Effectiveness	80–90%	80–90% (estimated)
How It Works	Prevents sperm from entering the vagina	Blocks sperm from reaching egg; kills sperm
Advantages	Protects against STDs, including AIDS and herpes; may help protect against cervical cancer; can be used as a backup device for other methods; no hormonal or systemic effects; easy to use; male shares responsibility	Smaller than a diaphragm; may be left in place longer than diaphragm; does not require additional spermicide for repeated intercourse like the diaphragm
Disadvantages	Must be applied in midst of lovemaking; rare cases of allergy to latex; may break and have diminished sensation	More difficult to position properly; may become dislodged during intercourse
Availability	Widely available in over-the-counter purchase	Must be fitted by clinician; not widely used in US
Comments	More effective when used with a spermicide	

	Vaginal Spermicide	Diaphragm
Estimated Effectiveness	70–80% (used alone)	90–95% (with spermicide)
Typical Effectiveness	80–90%	80–90%

	Vaginal Spermicide	**Diaphragm**
How It Works	Kills sperm	Blocks sperm from reaching egg; kills sperm
Advantages	Able to use it only as needed; few side effects and contraindications; protects against STDs; provides additional lubrication	No side effects (rare allergies to latex or spermicide); can be inserted up to 6 hours before intercourse
Disadvantages	Messy; must be applied just before intercourse; effective for only 30–60 min; may be awkward or embarrassing to use	Must be used with a spermicide; proper fit is essential; may be awkward or inconvenient to use
Availability	Available over-the-counter as foam, jelly, cream, film, or suppository	Clinician examination and fitting required
Comments	Best results when used with a barrier method such as condom or diaphragm	Requires repeat application of spermicide with repeat intercourse

	Contraceptive Sponge	**Withdrawal**
Estimated Effectiveness	76–83%	85%
Typical Effectiveness	75–90%	75–80%
How It Works	Kills sperm; absorbs ejaculate; blocks sperm from entering vaginal tract	Keeps sperm from reaching egg
Advantages	Easy to use—spermicide is contained in sponge; may be inserted up to 24 hours before intercourse; helps protect against STDs; continuous protection for 24 hours	Free; causes no health problems—no side effects or contraindications; no supplies or advance preparation; shared responsibility by male
Disadvantages	May be difficult to remove; may fragment; may cause irritation to vaginal lining; cannot be used during period	Unreliable; requires considerable control and discipline; may decrease pleasure
Availability	Available over the counter; relatively expensive	No purchase required
Comments	Must be left in place for 6 hours after intercourse; must be moistened before use	Not reliable form of contraception

	Tubal Ligation	**Vasectomy**
Estimated Effectiveness	99.9%	99.9%
Typical Effectiveness	99.8%	99.8%
How It Works	Prevents egg from traveling into uterus	Prevents sperm from being in ejaculate
Advantages	Permanent; removes fear of pregnancy; no interruption of lovemaking	Permanent; removes fear of pregnancy; no interruption of lovemaking; shared responsibility by male
Disadvantages	Surgery-related risks; irreversible	Irreversible
Availability	Surgical expense	Surgical expense

discussed in this chapter. No one contraceptive method is perfect. The risk for sexually transmitted diseases must also be assessed with contraceptive decision making. Contraception is a shared responsibility. The best method is one that a woman and her partner feel comfortable using, and one that they will use correctly and consistently. Abortion is another dimension of birth control. Preventing unwanted pregnancy is a primary responsibility of all sexually active couples. In the event of an unwanted pregnancy, understanding all options and risks are critical prerequisites for effective decision making.

Philosophical Dimensions: Preventing Unwanted Pregnancy: Contraception and Abortion Issues

1. What are some possible reasons to explain the higher contraceptive failure rate among younger women compared to older women?

2. What are some of the common reasons for birth control?

3. What are some reasons that couples fail to use contraceptives or fail to use them correctly?

4. How can couples share in the responsibilities associated with contraception?

5. When are contraceptive "risky" times likely to occur in a relationship?

6. How can a couple improve their communication about sexuality issues, including contraception?

7. How may socio-cultural beliefs and practices influence contraceptive decision making?

References

1. Mosher, W.D. (1990). Use of family planning services in the United States, 1982 and 1988. *Advance Data, 184,* 1–6.

2. Mishell, D.R. (1981). Clinical and legal implications of contraception in the 80's. *The Female Patient, 1*(Suppl.), 2.

3. Mosher, W.D., and Pratt, W.F. (1990). Contraceptive use in the United States, 1973–1988. *Advance Data, 182,* 1–7.

4. Mosher, W.D. (1990). Contraceptive practice in the United States, 1982–1988. *Family Planning Perspectives, 22,* 198–205.

5. *Contraceptive Report* (1991). Breast cancer, cervical cancer, and oral contraceptives. Vol II, 1–15.

6. *Population Reports* (1988). Lower dose pills. Series A (No. 7), 1–31.

7. Hatcher, R.A., Stewart, F., Trussell, J., Kowal, D., Guest, F., Stewart, G.K., and Cates, W. (1990). *Contraceptive technology* (15th ed.). New York: Irvington Publishers, Inc.

8. Sivin, I. (1989). IUD's are contraceptives, not abortifacients: A comment on research and belief. *Studies on Family Planning, 20,* 355–359.

9. Farley, T.M.M., et al. (1992). Intrauterine devices and pelvic inflammatory disease: An international perspective. *Lancet, 339,* 785.

10. Gold, R.B. (1990). Abortion and women's health: A turning point for America? New York: The Alan Guttmacher Institute.

11. Henshaw, S.K., Koonin, L.M., and Smith, J.C. (1987). Characteristics of U.S. women having abortions, 1987. *Family Planning Perspectives, 23,* 75–81.

12. Henshaw, S.K., and Kost, K. (1992). Parental involvement in minor's abortion decisions. *Family Planning Perspectives, 24,* 196–207.

13. Cooksey, E.C. (1990). Factors in the resolution of adolescent premarital pregnancies. *Demography, 27,* 207–210.

14. Centers for Disease Control (1988). Abortion surveillance, United States. *Morbidity and Mortality Weekly Report, 38,* 11–45.

15. Kissling, F. (1992). Books in review—"A call to embrace ambivalence." *Family Planning Perspectives, 24,* 279–280.

Resources

CENTER FOR POPULATION OPTIONS	NATIONAL ABORTION FEDERATION	PLANNED PARENTHOOD FEDERATION OF AMERICA
1025 Vermont Avenue Suite 210 Washington, DC 20005 202-347-5700	1436 U Street NW Washington, DC 20009 202-667-588 800-772-9100	810 Seventh Avenue New York, NY 10019 212-541-7800

CHAPTER 9

Pregnancy and Childbirth

CHAPTER OBJECTIVES

On completion of this chapter, the student should be able to discuss:

1. Historical dimensions of pregnancy and childbirth in the last three centuries.
2. Why the "natural childbirth" movement evolved in the 1950s.
3. How the "medicalization" of childbirth has influenced women's role in birthing.
4. How a pregnancy due date is calculated.
5. How conception occurs and the process of cell division after fertilization.
6. Hormonal changes that occur during pregnancy.
7. The two-step process of pregnancy confirmation.
8. The monthly changes in fetal development.
9. The nutritional and weight gain recommendations of pregnancy and exercise concerns with pregnancy.
10. The detrimental effects of smoking, alcohol, and drugs on pregnancy.
11. The concern with heat exposure and pregnancy.
12. The four major techniques for prenatal testing.
13. Ectopic pregnancy and laparoscopy.
14. The events associated with spontaneous abortion.
15. Four major genetic disorders and the populations most vulnerable to each.
16. The prenatal concern with cytomegalovirus.
17. The symptoms that may indicate problems with pregnancy or premature labor.
18. The significance of childbirth preparation.
19. The concerns with pain relief during childbirth.
20. How birthing position affects delivery.
21. Possible problems with the fetus and possible problems with the birth passage that may influence the decision for a cesarean delivery.

22. The recent trend with vaginal birth after cesarean delivery (VBAC).

23. The concepts of fecundity, infertility, and sterilization techniques.

24. The influence of the baby boom cohort on the proportion of reproductive-age women.

25. The trend in birth rates among unmarried women.

26. How the trend in maternal mortality has changed since the early 1900s.

27. Which groups of women are at greatest risk for ectopic pregnancy.

28. The relationship between prenatal care and pregnancy outcome, including the most frequent complications of pregnancy.

29. Which group is at greatest risk for infant mortality and neonatal deaths.

30. What conditions have led to the misconception of increased infertility.

Introduction

Pregnancy and childbirth are exciting and complex facets of women's health. In addition to the obvious biological aspects, pregnancy and childbirth are greatly influenced by social, cultural, historical, legal, and ethical dimensions. This chapter provides an overview of pregnancy, childbirth, and infertility.

Historical Dimensions

> There is a realization that women's attitudes toward and behavior during birth are shaped and conditioned by the demands and expectations of family, peers, community, and often religion. What a woman expects from her childbirth experience, what she will do, what she will fear and not fear, how she will interpret what is happening to her, and what in fact will happen when she gives birth, depend in large measure upon how her society defines what birth should be and where she fits in the various hierarchies of that society.
>
> JANET CARLISLE BOGDAN

The academic examination of childbirth as a social phenomenon did not really begin until the 1960s. Before that time, knowledge about childbirth had been derived principally from the writings of medical historians who stressed the progressive history of scientific advances in obstetrics. This medical and historical account provided little insight into how the management of pregnancy or birthing affected women's experience of birth or about women's reactions to and participation in such changes. The accounts also failed to document how the birth experience felt to the woman.

Today there is considerably more focus and investigation on the whole social, racial, economic, and ethnic spectrum of childbirth. Childbirth history is now studied in a variety of contexts, including medical, demographic, cultural, social, economic, professional, and symbolic. The term "childbirth," however, generally evokes an image of a medical environment, with physicians and nurses, surgical drapes, intravenous poles, and fetal monitors. In the early United States, childbirth did not have an association with medical personnel or equipment except when a woman's life was threatened. Childbirth was part of a woman's domestic responsibilities, both among immigrants and native populations.[1] Although there were specific cultural and ethnic variations in the management of the birthing process, all shared the tradition that only women attended other women. Women were the experts about birthing.[1]

During the mid-eighteenth century, the expertise of women in birthing began to be questioned. Women in France were beginning to deliver babies in hospitals under the watchful eyes of not only traditional midwives, but also physicians. Although physicians had previously witnessed or participated in abnormal birthings, the hospitalization practices enabled them to study and understand the normal childbirth process. Consistent with the Age of Enlightenment, birth was perceived as a natural process that proceeded by natural laws. Through close observation, measurements, and recordings, French physicians attempted to describe these natural laws and explain the mysterious process of childbirth.[2] During the same period, the English focus became more oriented to surgical techniques, specifically the development of instruments known as **forceps** to assist in the extraction of the fetus from the woman. The European obstetrical knowledge quickly crossed the Atlantic, and American physicians began appearing at the births of middle-class and upper-class urban women. At first, physicians attended along with traditional midwives but soon replaced them. Medical schools began to certify men as birth attendants and traditional midwifery began a decline. By the end of the eighteenth century, physicians had established roles in managing childbirth experiences throughout urban areas, including those for poor women.

With the medical presence during childbirth came a widening array of interventions, including medications, anesthesia, and birthing instruments. Accompanying the increasing technologies were additional problems of birth accidents, including tears and infections. Physician attitudes had changed from observing and learning to affecting and controlling. Women continued actively to participate in determining the terms of their childbirths only as long as the home was the birthing environment. When birthing moved to the hospital, women lost this power.[3] The American medical management of childbirth originated in urban northeastern areas. Childbirth retained much of its traditional aspects during the nineteenth and early twentieth centuries in the South and in some religious communities. Immigrant groups were also more likely to continue with traditional practices.

The twentieth century brought additional medicalization and hospitalization to childbirth. Midwives remained in the more inaccessible portions of the United States. Despite the increased technology and promises of greater safety, some authors point out that women were exposed to greater mystification of childbirth than they had ever known.[3] It was in some ways ironic because women were electing to control their fertility and have fewer children, thereby increasing the significance of the childbirth experience. Yet they understood less about the process and were less in control of birthing than their grandmothers had been. This trend continued until the late 1950s and 1960s when women began openly to express dissatisfaction with medicalized births. Europe again was leading in a new trend of childbirthing experiences that suggested that childbirth should be anticipated with joy and knowledge, not fear and ignorance, and could be accomplished with less pain, less medication, and less of the medical and surgical control that was typical of American births. These natural-birth relaxation techniques are the foundation of modern "prepared childbirth" efforts.

Pregnancy

Pregnancy lasts an average of 266 days from the time of fertilization or 280 days from the first day of the last menstrual period. The gestational period is divided into three phases or trimesters of approximately 3 months each. Not all women have 28-day menstrual cycles, so due dates cannot be precisely determined. Information Box 9.1 provides guidance on calculating the expected due date. Fig. 9.1 shows many of the physical changes that accompany pregnancy.

Conception

Conception, also known as **fertilization,** is the union of the male sperm cell and the female egg cell. Before conception is possible, certain changes must take place within the sperm cells. They must mature in the male reproductive tract before ejaculation and undergo still more biological changes in the female reproductive tract before they can fertilize the egg. The human egg, **ova,** is far more rare than the sperm. Each woman is born with her lifetime supply of ova, and usually 300 to 500 mature eggs eventually leave her ovaries during the monthly process of **ovulation.**

INFORMATION BOX 9.1

Calculating a "Due Date"

To calculate the expected due date of a pregnancy:

1. Determine the first day of the last menstrual period.
2. Add 1 week to the first day of the last menstrual period.
3. Subtract 3 months.
4. Add 1 year.

For example, if the first day of the last menstrual period was February 8, 1992, add 1 week (which is February 15, 1992), subtract 3 months (which makes it November 15, 1991) and then add 1 year, which is November 15, 1992.

It is important to remember that this is an estimate, although approximately 60% of births occur within 5 days of the dates predicted in this manner.

FIGURE 9.1

Physical changes in pregnancy.

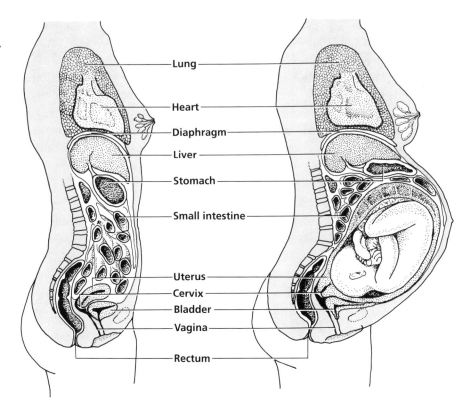

Lung

Heart

Diaphragm

Liver

Stomach

Small intestine

Uterus

Cervix

Bladder

Vagina

Rectum

The sperm cell is one of the smallest cells in the body. Mature sperm cells swim like miniature tadpoles with an undulating movement of a threadlike tail. During the process of ejaculation, the sperm cells are combined with secretions from the male reproductive tract to form semen. If ejaculation occurs into or around the entrance of the vagina, there is a possibility of fertilization. It has been estimated that up to 300 million sperm are deposited with ejaculation, but fewer than 20 actually arrive anywhere near the unfertilized egg.[4] The semen coagulates after it is deposited in the vagina and becomes gelatinous. If the woman is in the early or middle segment of her menstrual cycle, the cervical mucus is of a consistency to allow the sperm to pass into the uterus. If progesterone is the dominant hormone, as in the late segment of the menstrual cycle, the cervical mucus inhibits sperm penetration past the cervix.

The traditional explanation of conception has been one of a passive egg and aggressive sperm. **Capacitation** has been described as the process of biochemical changes in the sperm cell that permit the sperm to penetrate the egg. This traditional explanation has been challenged. Instead of a passive egg, it has been suggested that it is a "chemically active sperm catcher," that actually sperm are trying to get away but are held in place by molecules on the surface of the egg that hook together with counterparts on the sperm's surface, fastening the sperm until the egg can absorb it.[5]

Regardless of whether the sperm or the egg is the aggressor, conception usually takes place in the fallopian tube. The sperm releases an enzyme called hyaluronidase, which works to dissolve the outer layer of the egg cell and allows the sperm cell to advance toward the center of the egg to join with its nucleus. At fertilization, the 23 chromosomes from the sperm combine with the 23 chromosomes of the egg to form the **zygote.** The zygote is the fertilized egg and contains the full complement of 46 chromosomes. The genetic information from the sperm cell combines with the genetic information from the egg to form a unique set of **chromosomes.** This genetic information determines the unique characteristic of the individual, including eye and hair color, height, and all the other physical characteristics that are passed from one generation to the next. One pair of chromosomes determines the sex of the individual, with males having one X and one Y chromosome and females having two X chromosomes.

Cell division of the zygote usually occurs within 36 hours and continues as the dividing cell mass is propelled by the cilia in the oviducts toward the uterus. It generally takes 3 to 5 days to reach the uterus, and at this stage, the cell mass is known as a **blastocyst.** The blastocyst usually freely floats within the uterus for 1 to 2 days before implanting into the lining of the uterus. Implantation is often the marker for the beginning of a pregnancy. The products of conception are generally referred to as the **conceptus.** For the first 8 weeks of gestation, the material is known as an **embryo,** and from then to birth it is known as a **fetus.**

Hormonal Changes During Pregnancy

The maternal system undergoes dramatic changes in estrogen and progesterone levels during pregnancy. Secretion of the follicle-stimulating hormone (FSH) and luteinizing hormone (LH) by the anterior pituitary gland is suppressed throughout pregnancy. There are an additional two pregnancy-specific hormones that also influence the course of the pregnancy. **Human chorionic gonadotropin** (HCG) prevents the corpus luteum from degenerating. Specific cells in the outer portion of the developing embryo secrete HCG shortly after implantation. The presence of this hormone in the woman's system produces a positive pregnancy test result because HCG can be detected in the woman's blood and urine. Large amounts of HCG are produced during the first trimester and stimulate the corpus luteum to secrete estrogen and progesterone. The corpus luteum is essential for the maintenance of early pregnancy. If it regresses, a **spontaneous abortion,** or miscarriage, results. After the first 3 months, HCG levels drop off.

The second hormone unique to pregnancy is human placental lactogen (HPL). HPL is believed to stimulate breast growth during pregnancy and to prepare the breasts for lactation. HPL also has growth-promoting properties and may be responsible for the physical changes that occur in the maternal system to accommodate the growing fetus. HPL levels rise throughout the pregnancy, and as birth approaches, the levels become reduced.

After the first 3 months of pregnancy, the corpus luteum is no longer essential to maintain the pregnancy because the placenta is producing large amounts of

Early Signs of Pregnancy

Symptoms of pregnancy that often occur in the first 6 weeks:

Missed period(s)

Breast swelling and tenderness

Fatigue

Queasiness or nausea, vomiting

Slightly elevated body temperature

Mood swings

estrogen and progesterone. Progesterone suppresses uterine contractions during pregnancy and stimulates the alveoli of the breasts. Progesterone production and secretion by the placenta increase continuously during pregnancy and rapidly decline at birth.

The fetus plays a role in maintaining the pregnancy. The fetus' adrenal glands produce a precursor hormone during the first 3 months of pregnancy that is converted to estrogen in the placenta. The growing fetus and placenta contribute increasing quantities of estrogen and progesterone to the maternal blood system as the pregnancy progresses. Estrogen levels rise throughout the pregnancy and then rapidly fall off at birth.

Confirming Pregnancy

The benefits of early diagnosis of pregnancy are immeasurable. When pregnancy is desired, good prenatal care can begin immediately, and extra efforts can be made to protect the vulnerable embryo from chemical and physical agents. When pregnancy is not desired, early detection permits early decision making, and if an abortion is elected, risks of complications are reduced. As shown in Information Box 9.2, several symptoms often occur in the first 6 weeks of pregnancy. Most women begin to have symptoms 2 or 3 weeks after conception. An overdue period is usually the first definitive sign of pregnancy, although it is important to note that there are many reasons for missed periods other than pregnancy. The bottom line is that some women do not always miss periods when are pregnant, and missed periods do not always signal a pregnancy.

Confirming a pregnancy is a two-step process that includes a pregnancy test and a pelvic examination. HCG is easily detectable in blood and urine throughout the first 5 months of pregnancy. All pregnancy tests use chemical procedures to detect the presence of HCG. Home pregnancy tests can be purchased without a prescription. Home tests are fairly expensive but quite simple to use. It is important to follow directions carefully for accurate results. If an initial test is negative and the menstrual period has still not started, it is often a good idea to repeat the test in a week or so. Tests are most reliable with urine that is most concentrated; hence women are advised to use early morning urine. Home pregnancy tests are valuable sources of information, but they are only the beginning. If the findings are positive, it is important to set up an appointment for a pelvic examination, and if the findings are negative, there is a need to determine why the menstrual period is late or missed.

Fetal Development

The process of development for the fertilized egg is both fascinating and complex. When the cluster of cells reaches the uterus, it is smaller than the head of a pin. Once the cells are embedded into the uterine lining, they are collectively known as an embryo. The embryo soon takes on an elongated shape that is rounded at one end. A sac known as the **amnion** envelops it. As water and other small molecules cross the amniotic membrane, the embryo floats freely. The fluid provides protection from shocks and bumps and helps maintain a **homeostatic,** or constant, environment for the developing embryo. A primitive placenta soon forms. The **placenta** is an organ that supplies the growing embryo with food, water, and nutrients from the maternal bloodstream and serves as a conduit for the return of waste products back to the mother for disposal.

Major changes occur with the developing embryo as it evolves into a fetus (Fig. 9.2).

First month.   The embryo grows to about ¼ in. in length and ½ oz in weight. Foundations are formed for the nervous system, genital-urinary system, skin, bones, and lungs. Arm and leg buds begin to form. Rudiments of the eyes, ears, and nose appear. The head is disproportionately large because of early brain development.

Second month.   The embryo's length is about 1.2 in., and it weighs about ⅙ oz. Fingers and toes are distinct structures. The circulatory system is closed. At about 8 weeks, the embryo is termed a fetus.

Third month.   The fetus' length is about 2 in., and the weight is nearly ½ oz. The sex of the fetus is defined. The fetal kidneys excrete urine, and the heart beats. The nose and palate take shape.

Fourth month.   The fetal length is 4 in., and the weight is 2 oz. Fetal movements can be discerned by the mother. Heart sounds can be monitored with external instruments.

Fifth month.   The fetal length is 8 in., and weight is 1.4 lb. The skin is loose and wrinkled. Eyebrows and fingernails develop.

Six month.   The length is 11.5 in., and weight is 2.1 lb. The skin is red. Eyelids remain sealed. If born, the infant will cry and breathe but rarely survives.

Seventh month.   The fetal length is 14 to 15 in., and the weight is 3 lb. The fetus is generally able to survive if born at this time. Eyelids open. Fingerprints are set. The fetus is capable of vigorous movements.

Eighth month.   The fetal length is 15 to 17 in., and weight is 4 to 5 lb. The face and body have a loose and wrinkled appearance.

Ninth month.   The overall length is 16 to 19 in., and the weight is 6 to 7 lb. The skin is filled out and smooth. The skull bones have hardened, and the baby is ready for survival outside the womb.

FIGURE 9.2
Fetal development.
Photos courtesy of Landrum B.
Shettles.

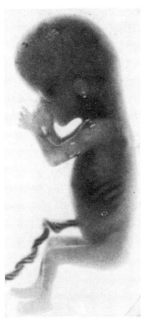

(A) 12 weeks.

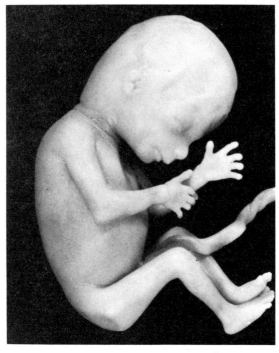

(B) 15 weeks.

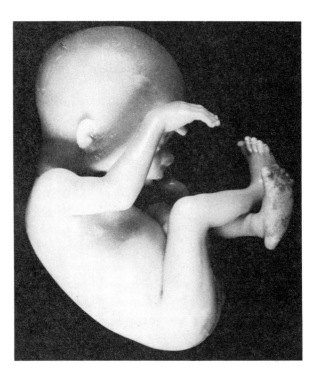

(C) 20 weeks.

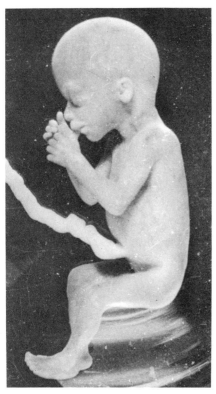

(D) 26-29 weeks.

Prenatal Care

A pregnant woman needs to take good care of herself to ensure proper development of her unborn child. Good prenatal care includes a spectrum of topics from proper nutrition to regular prenatal health care.

Nutrition

Pregnant women today receive different nutritional advice from a generation ago. It has been standard practice for health care providers to promote the use of prenatal vitamins. Now a blanket vitamin recommendation for all pregnant women is not practiced. The previous recommendations were based on data from studies that indicated that women who took a simple daily multivitamin before conception cut in half the risk that their children would suffer neural tube defects, including spina bifida.[6] It has been determined that the specific vitamin providing this protective factor appears to be folic acid (see Current Events Box, page 287.) A successful pregnancy is not solely dependent on adequate levels of folic acid. Throughout pregnancy, a well-balanced diet is critical. Pregnancy increases a woman's need for other nutrients, such as calcium and vitamin C. The National Research Council (NRC) recommends that these nutrients be taken not by supplements but through the daily consumption of wholesome nutritious foods.[7] Any supplementation should be discussed with a physician because large quantities of certain nutrients can pose hazards to a developing fetus. Vitamin A, for example, can cause abnormal fetal development. Iron is the one exception to the NRC's no-supplement guide. Pregnant women are advised to take a low-dose iron pill (30 mg in the ferrous iron form) because most female iron stores are not adequate to supply both mother and unborn child with the large demand for iron throughout the pregnancy.

Weight gain is another important prenatal nutrition issue. Only as recently as a generation ago, obstetricians were advising pregnant women not to gain more than 20 pounds during their pregnancies so they would have small, lightweight, easy-to-deliver babies. Today's medical experts advise otherwise. The NRC recommends a weight gain of 25 to 35 pounds for a pregnant woman.[7] Failure to gain adequate weight increases the risk of problems for the baby. Low infant birth weight is associated with higher infant morbidity, including physical and mental retardation and mortality. Steady weight gain is important. Erratic weight gains may be symptomatic of an underlying problem such as **toxemia,** in which fluid is retained, and toxic substances end up in the blood.

Sensible eating is important throughout a woman's life. This is particularly true during pregnancy. Sensible eating during pregnancy includes the basic concepts discussed in Chapter 1. Pregnant women should consume approximately an additional 300 calories a day after becoming pregnant. It is important *not* to diet during pregnancy but rather to eat sensibly. Salt should not be restricted unless specifically advised to do so by a clinician.

Exercise

Proper exercise during pregnancy can have many benefits. For a woman who enjoyed regular workouts before becoming pregnant, it can be important psychologically to continue with a regular exercise program. Moderate exercise during pregnancy can help prevent excessive weight gain and help expedite recovery after childbirth. The exercise program of a pregnant woman must be geared to her current level of fitness, medical history, past pregnancies, the stage of fetal development, and maternal complicating factors.

Generally women are advised not to take up a new exercise program during pregnancy. It is better to stay with usual routines. Pregnancy places a significant extra demand on the heart and lungs. Oxygen consumption and heart rate increase during pregnancy. As pregnancy advances, breathing becomes more difficult because of the displacement of the enlarging uterus downward with each inhalation. Walking and swimming are particularly good for pregnant women who have previously had rather sedentary lifestyles.

Activities that involve bouncing, jarring, or twisting and any activity that places the abdomen in jeopardy should be avoided during pregnancy. Contact sports are too risky, as is any activity that requires rapid stops and starts. The center of gravity for the body changes during pregnancy, increasing the risk of balance loss. A specific exercise position to be avoided during pregnancy is lying on the back, particularly after the fourth month. This position can block the blood supply to the uterus and depress fetal heart rate. A resting position on the side does not compromise fetal blood supply.

Avoiding an elevated body temperature is an important consideration of exercise during pregnancy. This is particularly important in hot, humid weather. To avoid dehydration, plenty of water should be consumed before and after exercising. The American College of Obstetricians and Gynecologists (ACOG) recommends that the body temperature of pregnant women not rise to more than 100°F or the heart rate climb above 140 beats per minute.

The question of exercise during pregnancy is important, and many questions regarding the safety and benefits remain unanswered. In a comprehensive review of the subject, researchers concluded that the interaction between exercise and pregnancy is complex and concern may not be warranted in healthy women with clinically normal pregnancies and that significantly more multidisciplinary study on the subject is indicated.[8]

Along with exercise, proper posture is important for women during pregnancy. Maintaining proper body alignment helps general circulation, helps fetal circulation, and reduces discomfort associated with fetal growth and displacement.

Avoiding Toxic Substances

Maternal exposure to many substances during pregnancy has been shown to have detrimental effects on the developing fetus. Many of these topics are discussed in detail elsewhere in the text. Cigarettes, alcohol, and drugs have specific detrimental effects on the fetus.

Cigarette smoking is detrimental to both mother and her developing baby. Maternal smoking has been clearly identified as the single most important determinant of low birth weight and perinatal death in the United States.[9] Low birth weight (5.5 lb or less) has been associated with many physical and mental infant problems.[10] Links have also been reported between maternal smoking and infertility; spontaneous abortions; ectopic pregnancies; placental irregularities; infant death; and long-term effects on the physical, emotional, and intellectual development of the child.[11]

Alcohol also is detrimental for both mother and her developing baby. Heavy alcohol consumption during pregnancy is known to cause alcohol-related defects among infants and **fetal alcohol syndrome** (FAS), which is characterized by growth retardation, facial malformations, and central nervous system dysfunctions, including mental retardation.[12] Although the lower limit of safe alcohol consumption during pregnancy has not been established, there appears to be a dose-response relationship; that is, the most known adverse effects in infants are associated with heavy maternal alcohol use. Alcohol appears to act in concert with other factors in the development of FAS in infants. These factors include differences in the degree of prenatal exposure to alcohol, maternal drinking patterns, possible genetic susceptibility to FAS, differences in maternal metabolism of alcohol, time of gestation during heavy alcohol consumption, interactions of alcohol use with other drugs and medications, and the maternal nutritional status. It has been suggested that the fetus may be especially vulnerable during the first trimester of pregnancy when central nervous system development occurs, and during this vulnerable period, effects on the infant may be more related to peak blood ethanol level in the mother rather than overall consumption throughout the pregnancy. Without further information, no safe level of alcohol consumption can be established or assumed for women during pregnancy.

Like alcohol and cigarettes, drugs can adversely affect a developing fetus. No medications or over-the-counter preparations should be taken during pregnancy without first consulting with a clinician. Illicit drug use, most notably the use of cocaine, is associated with fetal distress and impaired fetal growth. The consequences of drug use during pregnancy include severe damage to the baby's brain and nervous system and other birth defects. Compared with mothers who did not smoke marijuana, smokers had smaller, sicker babies and higher risk of stillbirths. Drug use may also lead to neurochemical birth defects by disrupting normal development of the brain. Cocaine use increases the risk of premature birth, stillbirths, and malformations.[13,14]

Environmental Risks

High levels of radiation of the type used for cancer therapy have been associated with birth defects. Diagnostic x-rays should be avoided if possible throughout the pregnancy or if there is the possibility of pregnancy. Although data are scarce, it is believed that the rapidly developing fetus is especially vulnerable to pollutants, toxic wastes, heavy metals, pesticides, gases, and other hazardous compounds.

Another environmental risk to be considered during pregnancy is heat exposure. Women who use hot tubs and saunas or who have high fevers early in pregnancy have been found to be at greater risk of having children with such neural tube defects as spina bifida. Although more research is indicated on this subject, it appears that the greatest risk is early in the pregnancy when the fetus' central nervous system is developing.

Prenatal Testing

All mothers worry to a certain degree whether or not their unborn baby is normal and healthy. Sophisticated testing has evolved so that some questions can be answered about specific diseases and birth defects. These procedures include ultrasound, alpha-fetoprotein screening, chorionic villus sampling (CVS), and amniocentesis (Fig. 9.3).

Ultrasound is a procedure that uses high-frequency sound waves to project an image of the fetus. The procedure is valuable for ascertaining fetal age and detecting certain birth defects. Ultrasound may be performed at any time in the pregnancy; however, first-trimester procedures may not be effective in detecting fetal abnormalities.

FIGURE 9.3

Prenatal diagnostic procedures. (A) In chorionic villus sampling, fetal cells from the chorionic villi, fingerlike projections on the developing placenta, are suctioned out through the cervix. (B) In amniocentesis, cells shed by the developing fetus are extracted from a sample of the amniotic fluid withdrawn from the mother's uterus.

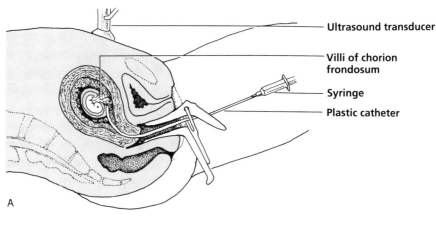
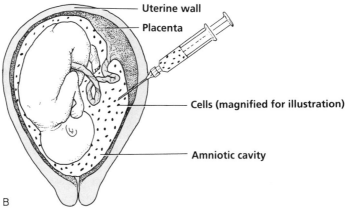

Alpha-fetoprotein screening measures a substance produced by the baby's kidneys between the 13th and 20th week of pregnancy. These levels are measured in the maternal blood. High levels could be an indication of neural tube defect, and levels that are abnormally low may be an indication of Down syndrome.

Amniocentesis is a procedure performed in the 14th to 16th week of pregnancy. It involves the removal of a small amount of the **amniotic fluid** surrounding the fetus. The fluid contains cells shed by the fetus, which are grown in tissue culture and then checked for any chromosomal, biochemical, or genetic defects. There is a slight risk of fetal loss associated with the procedure.

Chorionic villi sampling (CVS) is another prenatal screening procedure. It can be done as early as six weeks after conception. CVS is generally performed in the 10th to 12th week of pregnancy and involves suctioning a small sample of the chorionic **villi,** the tissue surrounding the fetus, for laboratory analysis. Major concerns are associated with CVS. The chromosome results may be inconclusive and require a follow-up amniocentesis procedure. Although the risk appears low, concern exists that there is a possible link with the procedure with infant limb abnormalities, premature birth, and fetal loss.[15] The advantage of the procedure is that it is performed during the first trimester, permitting a greater range of options with decision making about the pregnancy.

It is difficult to calculate risks associated with these procedures. Risks for ultrasound and AFP are considered to be very low. For both CVS and amniocentesis, there is about a 1 to 3 percent chance of miscarriage.[16,17] Therefore these tests are generally recommended only if the mother is over age 35, has already had a child with a genetic disorder, or is known to be a carrier of a detectable genetic disorder.

Complications of Pregnancy

Ten to 15 percent of all pregnancies have an increased risk of complications. Perinatology is the medical specialty concerned with the diagnosis and treatment of pregnant women with high-risk conditions and their unborn babies.

Ectopic Pregnancy

Ectopic pregnancy is a hazard for women in the early months of a pregnancy. A fertilized egg that implants and begins to grow outside the uterine cavity results in an **ectopic pregnancy**. Ectopic pregnancy occurs in about 1 percent of pregnancies and can be a life-threatening condition. Ectopic pregnancies have become of the leading causes of maternal death during the first trimester.[18] Most occur inside a fallopian tube. As the tubal pregnancy advances, the tube stretches and can tear or rupture. Symptoms of ectopic pregnancy usually begin at about the seventh or eighth week of gestation. Tubal rupture can cause sudden, massive internal bleeding and is a serious condition that is a leading cause of pregnancy-related death. An overdue menstrual period and pain are the most common symptoms of an ectopic pregnancy. The pain can be quite subtle initially and progress in severity if tearing of the fallopian tube causes internal bleeding. Abnormal vaginal bleeding or spotting also occurs in a majority of cases of ectopic pregnancy.

If symptoms are severe or internal bleeding is suspected, hospitalization is indicated for further assessment. Evaluation usually consists of a pregnancy test and ultrasound assessment. **Laparoscopy** is often indicated to assess the situation further. With laparoscopy, the physician is able to visualize the uterus, tubes, and ovaries through a lighted tube inserted near the navel. Laparoscopy is considered to be a surgical procedure and requires general anesthesia. In the event of significant internal hemorrhage, immediate surgery is necessary as a life-saving procedure. In some cases, an ectopic pregnancy may degenerate on its own and require no intervention. In most cases, however, surgery is indicated to remove the fertilized egg. When ectopic pregnancy is diagnosed early, conservative surgery to remove only the fertilized egg and spare the tube may be possible.

Several risk factors and a few protective factors have been identified for ectopic pregnancy. Pelvic inflammatory disease has been shown to be the major risk factor. Other risk factors, such as past use of an intrauterine device, infection of the lower genital tract, tubal infertility, pelvic surgery, and postabortion infection, are probably associated with ectopic pregnancy through their relationship to pelvic infection. Protective factors for ectopic pregnancy include the use of barrier methods of contraception and oral contraceptives.

Miscarriage

A miscarriage is also known as a spontaneous abortion. It is defined as a pregnancy that ends before the 20th week of gestation. It is estimated that about 1 in every 10 pregnancies ends in miscarriage. A miscarriage can occur early in the pregnancy, and many women who miscarry are not aware of their pregnancy. A miscarriage may be characterized by bleeding and cramping. Generally when a woman experiences bleeding or cramping early in the pregnancy, she is advised bed rest. In some cases, these symptoms stop, and the pregnancy proceeds normally. In other cases, the bleeding may become intense, the cervix dilates, and the embryo is released from the body. If the miscarriage is complete, the bleeding stops and the uterus returns to its normal shape and size. If the miscarriage is incomplete, any remaining fragments must be removed. This procedure is known as a **dilation and curettage** (D&C).

Genetic Disorders

Genetic disorders are responsible for a significant number of miscarriages. It is estimated that 3 percent of all newborns have a genetic abnormality. These abnormalities include a spectrum of conditions of varying seriousness. Certain genetic disorders are more prevalent among specific populations; for example, the most common genetic disorder among American whites is cystic fibrosis, an abnormality of the respiratory system and the sweat and mucous glands. Four other major genetic disorders include Down syndrome, sickle cell anemia, phenylketonuria, and Tay-Sachs disease.

Down syndrome is caused by an extra number 21 chromosome. This abnormality presents in about every 800 births. The condition is characterized by varying degrees of physical and mental retardation. A woman's risk of having a baby with Down syndrome increases as she gets older. Amniocentesis and alpha-fetoprotein screening may indicate the presence of Down syndrome.

Sickle cell anemia is a blood disorder that primarily affects African Americans. This condition occurs when **hemoglobin,** the oxygen-carrying protein of red blood cells, is abnormal and causes red blood cells to assume a crescent or sickle shape. The sickled cells are unable to provide adequate oxygen to vital organs of the body. The victim becomes tired and lethargic. Other symptoms include pain and a loss of appetite. Transfusions provide some relief but do not cure the condition. Many victims die before the age of 20.

Phenylketonuria (PKU) is a genetic disorder in which a crucial liver enzyme needed by the body for the metabolism of the amino acid phenylalanine is absent, resulting in severe mental retardation if not treated. In most states, laws require the prompt testing of all newborns for PKU. Treatment for the condition is a long-term therapeutic diet, which reduces the effect of the disorder.

Tay-Sachs disease is a genetic disorder resulting in death by age 5 or 6 years. It presents almost exclusively among Jews of Eastern European ancestry. Tay-Sachs victims appear normal at birth but experience gradual physical and mental deterioration. Carriers of the condition may be identified by a blood test.

Infections

Any infection in the mother can potentially cause harm to an unborn fetus. Sexually transmitted diseases, including human immunodeficiency virus (HIV) (see Chapter 10), are particularly dangerous during a pregnancy. The most common prenatal infection today is cytomegalovirus (CMV), a viral infection that causes mild flulike symptoms in adults but that can cause brain damage, mental retardation, liver dysfunction, cerebral palsy, hearing problems, and other malformations in unborn babies.[19] The infectious disease most clearly linked to birth defects is **rubella,** also known as German measles. All women of reproductive age should be vaccinated against rubella if they have not had this formerly common childhood illness.

Premature Labor

Pregnancy usually lasts from 38 to 42 weeks. Babies born before 37 weeks may have problems with breathing, eating, and temperature control. Approximately 10 percent of all babies are born too early. Labor that starts this early is called **premature labor.** Information Box 9.3 lists symptoms that may indicate problems with the pregnancy or premature labor.

INFORMATION BOX 9.3

Warning Signs of Premature Labor

A clinician should be consulted if any of the following symptoms develop during pregnancy:

Vaginal bleeding

Abdominal pain

Persistent nausea, vomiting

Unusual thirst

Fever or chills

Facial, feet, or finger swelling

Continuous or severe headaches

Blurring or dimness of vision, "spots"

Vaginal fluid leaks

Childbirth

The concern expressed by most women in regards to childbirth is "I hope that the baby is healthy." Many women have special concerns about the childbirth experience. It is important to discuss these concerns with the clinician early in the pregnancy. Self-Assessment 9.1 provides a checklist for childbirth considerations. This list can serve as a basis for further questions and decision making.

Preparation for Childbirth

Preparation for childbirth is a concept that has been popular in the United States for the last 40 years. "Preparation" usually means attending organized classes that provide learning and experiences to prepare a woman and her partner for labor and delivery. Some individuals anticipate or desire having a "natural childbirth," and others wish to learn more about the birthing events. Regardless of the plans for the childbirth experience, organized classes provide an opportunity to learn about local birthing options and a chance to discuss personal issues and concerns. The classes also provide an opportunity to gain knowledge about pregnancy and childbirth and develop pain management skills. Strategies such as different positions that facilitate labor and promote an uncomplicated birth are taught. Perhaps the greatest advantage of childbirth education is the opportunity to prepare for a more satisfying birth experience.

Labor and Delivery

Labor and delivery can be a rewarding and satisfying experience when a woman anticipates the sequence of events and is prepared for the process. Many factors affect the progress of labor, including the position of the baby and the shape of the mother's pelvis. Each labor is different, although each labor progresses through three distinct stages. Stage I is from the onset of labor to full dilation of the cervix. Stage II begins when the cervix is completely dilated and ends with the birth of the baby. Stage III is from the completion of delivery of the baby to completion of delivery of the **afterbirth,** or placenta.

Long before any of these stages begin, the uterus changes and prepares itself to function efficiently during labor and delivery. By the end of the pregnancy, the uterus measures about 10×14 inches. Its capacity has increased nearly 500 times during the pregnancy, and it has increased in weight from 1.5 oz. to 30 oz. The uterine muscle fibers have grown to 10 times their original thickness. The uterus is one of the strongest muscles in a woman's body, and it contracts powerfully during labor. Throughout pregnancy, the uterus contracts at slightly irregular intervals. These irregular contractions are known as **Braxton-Hicks contractions.** These contractions are not like "real" labor contractions in that they do not gradually increase in frequency, intensity, or duration. They serve to increase the blood circulation and help the uterus to accommodate the growing baby.

Childbirth Considerations

Birthing Issues	Very Important	Not Important	Don't Want
Hospital delivery room	_____	_____	_____
Hospital birthing room	_____	_____	_____
Birthing center	_____	_____	_____
Home	_____	_____	_____
Obstetrician	_____	_____	_____
Family practitioner	_____	_____	_____
Certified nurse-midwife	_____	_____	_____
Partner/coach			
Present during labor	_____	_____	_____
Present during delivery	_____	_____	_____
Present for all procedures	_____	_____	_____
Present during Cesarean	_____	_____	_____
Present during recovery	_____	_____	_____
Early labor			
Stay home as long as possible	_____	_____	_____
Arrive early and settle in	_____	_____	_____
Wear own clothes	_____	_____	_____
Perineal shave	_____	_____	_____
Enema	_____	_____	_____
IV	_____	_____	_____
First stage labor			
Labor room	_____	_____	_____
Birthing room	_____	_____	_____
External fetal monitor	_____	_____	_____
Internal fetal monitor	_____	_____	_____
Second stage labor			
Labor room	_____	_____	_____
Delivery room	_____	_____	_____
Birthing room	_____	_____	_____
Family present	_____	_____	_____
Delivery position flexibility	_____	_____	_____
Episiotomy	_____	_____	_____
After delivery			
Prolonged holding of baby	_____	_____	_____
Warm water bath for baby	_____	_____	_____
Breastfeeding in birthing area	_____	_____	_____
Postpartum			
Private room	_____	_____	_____
Baby rooming in with mother	_____	_____	_____
Breastfeeding	_____	_____	_____
Bottle-feeding	_____	_____	_____
Length of stay in facility	_____	_____	_____
Sibling/family visitation	_____	_____	_____

Three distinctive signs indicate that labor is beginning (Fig. 9.4). These include regular, progressive uterine contractions that occur every 5 minutes or so and last from 45 seconds to a minute. They are uncomfortable but not necessarily painful. In contrast to Braxton-Hicks contractions, they gradually become longer, stronger, and closer together. They are accompanied by a definite hardening of the uterus. The second distinctive sign is the rupture of the membranes, or "bag of waters." This rupture may be a "slow leak" or a gush. The fluid is usually clear. If the membranes break at home, the clinician should be alerted and arrangements made for the impending labor and delivery. The third distinctive sign is the "bloody show." This is the passage of small amount of bloodstained mucus that served as a mucous plug of the cervix during pregnancy. As the cervix begins to dilate, this plug is released. Other less distinctive signs of approaching labor include diarrhea, backache, and an increase in Braxton-Hicks contractions. The only confirmation that labor has begun is an internal examination that reveals a softening, thinned out, and dilating cervix.

In the *first stage of labor,* the tightening or contractions of the uterus open or dilate the neck or **cervix.** Stage I labor has three parts: early labor, active labor, and transition. Early labor occurs as the cervix opens to 4 cm (Fig. 9.5). Before labor begins, the wall of the uterus is thin, the cervix is long and thick, the **birth canal** is narrow, and the membranes may still be intact. The bands of longitudinal muscle fiber in the upper part of the uterus contract and thus gradually draw up, thin, and open the mouth of the cervix. The cervical canal shortens until the cervix is of the same thickness as the uterine wall. This process, in which the cervix is "taken up" into the uterus, is known as **effacement.** Once the cervix is effaced, the force of uterine contractions begins to dilate the cervix, although effacement and dilation may occur simultaneously. **Dilation** refers to the size of the round opening of the cervix. It is measured in centimeters or finger widths. Full dilation is 10 cm or five finger widths. Dilation is slow during early labor. It usually takes much longer to go from one to three fingers' dilation than from three fingers to full dilation. Early labor is often the easiest

FIGURE 9.4

Labor begins.

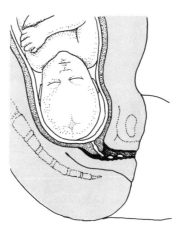

Mucous plug and bloody show

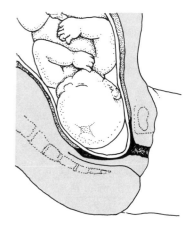

Effacement and dilation

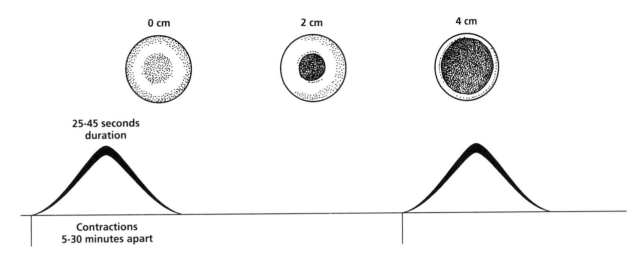

FIGURE 9.5

Early labor.

part of labor to handle and the most comfortable. Because this phase may last up to 6 hours or more, most women stay at home until this phase is over.

Active labor is the part of first-stage labor during which the cervix dilates from 4 to 7 cm (Fig. 9.6). The contractions in this part are very strong and gradually increase in frequency until they occur every 2 to 3 minutes and last about 60 seconds. Transition is the last part of the first stage and is characterized by cervical dilation from 8 to 10 cm (Fig. 9.7). This is considered to be the most difficult part of labor. Fortunately it is also the shortest, usually lasting 20 to 90 minutes. Transition may be characterized by generalized symptoms,

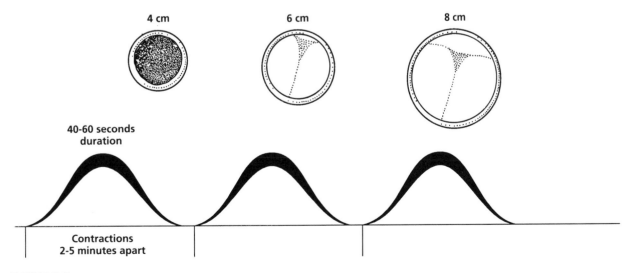

FIGURE 9.6

Active labor.

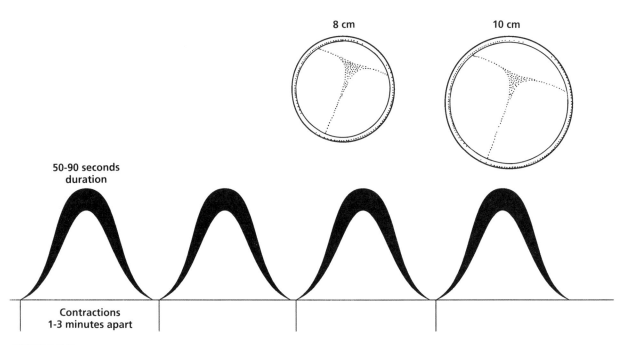

8 cm   10 cm

50-90 seconds
duration

Contractions
1-3 minutes apart

FIGURE 9.7

which include irritability, shaking, chills, nausea, vomiting, leg cramps, and perspiration. Through the combined force of maternal pushing and the uterine contractions, the baby's head descends and stretches the pelvic floor so that it comes into contact with the muscular outlet of the pelvis, known as the **perineum.**

The presentation of the baby—the part of the body positioned to emerge first—is usually by the top of the head, **vertex** presentation. When the feet or buttocks present first, it is known as a **breech** presentation. The breech position occurs in about 3 percent of deliveries. A breech presentation usually results in a longer labor. Because a breech delivery presents greater risks to the mother and baby, a cesarean delivery is often performed.

During the *second stage of labor,* the baby is pushed from the mother's body. This stage begins when the cervix is completely dilated at 10 cm (Fig. 9.8). The baby moves down the birth canal and out the mother's body with strong uterine contractions. This stage may last up to an hour. Contractions may last 60 to 90 seconds each and occur every 2 to 3 minutes. As the baby's head descends into the birth canal, the mother feels an overwhelming urge to bear down or push. As the baby's head appears, or crowns, an **episiotomy** may be performed. The episiotomy is an incision in the perineum that enlarges the vaginal opening for birth. The traditional argument for an episiotomy is that a surgical incision heals better and faster than a jagged tear. Data do not generally support this position, but factors affecting the need for such a procedure include the mother's skin elasticity and the size of the baby's presenting part. Some

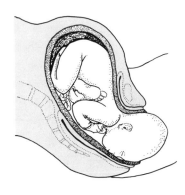

FIGURE 9.8
Birth.

mothers find that a sitting or squatting position facilitates the second stage. Such positions permit gravity to help with the birth. Squatting specifically enlarges the pelvic opening. Under usual circumstances, the birth of the baby is a gradual process with head first, then shoulders, and then the body.

In the *third stage of labor,* the uterus contracts firmly after the delivery of the baby. The placenta separates from the uterine wall and is expelled. The third stage generally last about 5 minutes. If an episiotomy has been performed, it is sutured at this time. The top of the uterus, the **fundus,** is usually massaged to stimulate **involution,** or the downsizing of the uterus to its pre-pregnant size and position. Breastfeeding also stimulates these uterine contractions.

Pain Relief in Childbirth

A few years ago in the early phases of the childbirth education movement, "natural childbirth" advocates promoted measures that implied a "painless" childbirth. Different women experience different levels of pain during childbirth. The reality of childbirth is that it usually involves some physical hurt. The physical and psychological techniques promoted in childbirth preparation classes can dramatically influence the perception of pain and the confidence to deal with labor difficulties. These pain relief measures have the inherent advantage of not producing any chemical disruption in the mother's body, which could then affect the baby or the birthing process. Medication choices should also be understood before labor. Most decisions about medications are actually personal choices, not medical decisions. Therefore it is important for the pregnant woman to learn about possible medications before going into labor. Medications may have no apparent ill effect on mother or baby, but medication always carries some potential drawbacks. It is best to use painkillers only if the possible benefits outweigh the potential risks or side effects.

A variety of pain-relieving medications are available for childbirth. Tranquilizers and analgesics are often used together for general relaxation and for taking the edge off contractions. Demerol (meperidine hydrochloride) is the drug most widely used for analgesia. Other narcoticlike drugs are also available for use in labor. Gas anesthetics such as nitrous oxide are sometimes used for the actual delivery. Although the mother experiences relief from her pain, she often misses the birth event. Babies also are affected by these products. Local or regional anesthetics include paracervical blocks, spinal anesthesia, pudendal blocks, and epidurals. These anesthetics can also cross the placenta, but they are least likely to affect the baby if they are injected into the area around the vagina and the perineum. When local anesthetics are used to bathe nerves that cover a large area of the body, they are called regional anesthetics.

Birthing Positions

Labor contractions are the signal that the body is pushing the baby out from the uterus. Traditional positions during this process have included standing, sitting, squatting, or kneeling. For many recent generations, however, women

I had some rather severe abdominal pain and some bleeding. I knew my period was late, but I was shocked to learn from my doctor that I had had a miscarriage. I didn't even know that I was pregnant.

24-YEAR-OLD WOMAN

have been giving birth on their backs in a supine position. Until recently, this has been the preferred position by physicians, who were not compromised in observing and facilitating the birthing process. Each of the traditional childbirth positions has certain mechanical advantages for delivery. An upright or standing position can help both mother and baby because when her spine is vertical, her uterus falls forward away from the diaphragm and the major blood vessels supplying the uterus and baby. Standing also maximizes the beneficial effects of gravity, and this position makes it easier for the mother to breathe and helps protect the baby's blood supply.

When a pregnant mother bends forward, her baby is aligned in the direction of the birth canal. This helps the baby enter her pelvis and facilitates the progression backward into the wider, rear part of the birth canal. Sitting can also make the birth easier by increasing the size of the birth canal. Any upright position helps delivery by using gravity and the full force of arm, chest, and abdominal muscles to help bear down and push the baby out.

No single position is ideal for all stages of labor. Walking during the first stage of labor often helps to make contractions stronger, longer, and more effective. Labor can be managed by trying various positions. Different positions are also effective for pushing in the second stage of labor. By working with their bodies and responding to body signals, women are able to facilitate their birthing process more effectively.

Cesarean Delivery

Considerable controversy exists today over whether cesarean births are being performed too often. There are undoubtedly times, however, when a cesarean birth is necessary for the safety of the mother or the baby. A **cesarean delivery** is the birth of a baby through surgical incisions in both the wall of the mother's abdomen and her uterus (Fig. 9.9). Anesthesia is required for the procedure. Cesarean births may be indicated for problems with the baby, problems with the passage area, and problems with the delivery process.

Problems with the fetus include fetal distress. A number of factors can produce this distress, in which some aspect of labor or the baby's environment places the baby at risk. For example, the baby's oxygen supply might be cut off owing to **abruptio placentae**, in which the placenta separates prematurely from the wall of the uterus. This not only threatens the baby, but also the mother with a risk of hemorrhage. A **prolapsed cord** is another risky situation in which the umbilical cord comes through the pelvis before the baby and can result in a disrupted flow of oxygen to the baby owing to a compressed cord.

Problems with the birth passage also influence the decision for a cesarean delivery. **Cephalopelvic disproportion** is a term meaning the baby is too large for the pelvis. Cephalopelvic disproportion is a common reason for cesarean delivery. Often a fetus indicates that the pelvis may not be a comfortable "fit" by assuming a position other than the normal head-first position for birth. A woman in labor whose baby is in a **transverse lie**, crosswise position in the

Uterine incisions

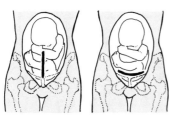

Vertical   Low transverse

FIGURE 9.9

Cesarean birth.

uterus, will need a cesarean delivery because neither the head nor the buttocks are in the pelvis. Multiple births are also more likely to require cesarean delivery. When a baby is in a breech position, the buttocks emerge before the head. The head has a larger diameter than the buttocks and the risk is that it will not fit well through the passage because it has not had the opportunity to mold and nestle into the pelvis throughout the labor process. A relatively rare complication of the passageway is the obstruction by a **fibroid,** benign tumor, or even by the placenta, **placenta previa.** Usually these obstruction or problems with fetal passage can be diagnosed in late pregnancy, which permits time to discuss various options with the health care provider.

Other conditions may also be an indication for cesarean delivery. One of the most common reasons for cesarean deliveries is failure to progress. This term refers to cervical failure to dilate adequately despite regular uterine contractions. To avoid prolonged distress to mother and baby in this situation, a cesarean delivery may be performed. Herpes is another reason for a cesarean delivery. If a woman has active lesions in the birth canal, a cesarean delivery is indicated to avoid infecting the fetus.

Vaginal Birth After Cesarean Delivery

For many years, a widely held philosophy about childbirth was "once a cesarean, always a cesarean." This philosophy may be partially responsible for the overall increase in cesarean birth rates.[20] There has been a movement to encourage vaginal birth after cesarean delivery (VBAC), both to control the morbidity associated with a major abdominal surgical procedure and to help reduce the spiraling cost of health care. The ACOG revised its standards of practice in 1985 and recommends a trial of labor in selected women.[21] There has been a steady increase in VBAC in the 1980s. ACOG has found that the mother usually experiences fewer complications with VBAC than with cesarean birth in such areas as infection, bleeding, and anesthesia. Other advantages of VBAC include a shorter hospital stay and recovery period as well as significant cost savings.

Infertility

Fecundity refers to the physical ability of a woman to have a child. Women with impaired fecundity include those who find it physically difficult or medically inadvisable to conceive or deliver a child. The term, impaired fecundity, is also used to described women, who, although having sexual intercourse on a regular basis without contraception for 36 months or more, fail to become pregnant.[22] This definition of reduced ability to bear children differs from the medical definition of **infertility,** which is the inability of couples who are not surgically sterile to conceive after 12 months of regular intercourse without contraception.[22]

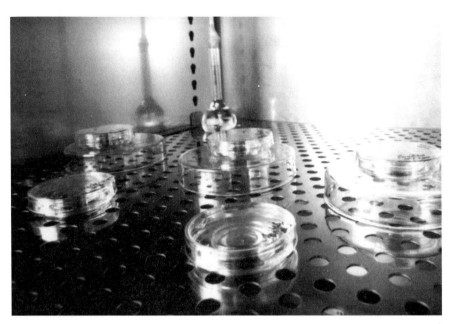

In vitro fertilization involves the fertilization of an ova in the laboratory and transfer of the conceptus to the uterus for continued embryonic and fetal development.

We had been trying to have a baby for several years. It was so frustrating because all of our friends were having babies, and our parents really wanted to be grandparents. We felt so many things—guilt, embarrassment, fear, and anger. Finally, after a lot of testing, we tried IVF and it worked! We have a little girl . . . it was a long and difficult journey to have her, but we are so pleased.

35-YEAR-OLD WOMAN

New approaches to infertility include microsurgery, sometimes with lasers to open destroyed or blocked egg or sperm ducts, new hormone preparations to induce ovulation, and the use of ultrasound to monitor ovulation. Other techniques that have shown success to date include **in vitro fertilization** (IVF), **gamete intrafallopian transfer** (GIFT), **embryo transfer, host uterus,** and **surrogacy.** Each procedure, while offering hope to infertile couples, raises significant ethical and legal questions.

IVF involves removing the ova, often with a long needle, from a woman's ovary just before normal ovulation would occur. The woman's egg and her partner's sperm are placed in a special fertilization medium for a specific period of time and are then transferred to another medium for continued developing. If the fertilized egg cell shows signs of development, within several days it is returned to the woman's uterus by means of a hollow tube placed through the vagina and cervix. The egg cell implants itself in the lining of the uterus, and the pregnancy continues as normal. Data indicate that 15 to 20 percent of these procedures are successful.[23]

GIFT is a procedure that involves placing sperm and eggs into the fallopian tubes. This procedure is less time-consuming and less expensive than IVF. GIFT mimics nature by permitting fertilized eggs to divide in the fallopian tubes. It has similar success rates to IVF.

Embryo transfer is a procedure in which the sperm of the infertile woman's partner are placed in another woman's uterus during ovulation. Approximately

5 days later, the fertilized egg is transferred to the uterus of the infertile woman, who then carries the developing embryo.

Host uterus is a procedure in which the sperm from a man and the egg from a woman are combined in a laboratory. The fertilized egg is then implanted into the uterus of a second woman who agrees to bear the child, which is not genetically related to her.

Surrogacy occurs when a woman is artificially inseminated with the sperm of an infertile woman's partner. She carries the baby to term, usually for an established fee and the provision of her health care. After delivery, the baby is turned over to the couple. This procedure received considerable publicity with the recent "Baby M" case.

Epidemiology—Pregnancy, Childbirth, and Infertility

Traditional epidemiological data on pregnancy and childbirth have focused on issues of maternal and child morbidity and mortality. In recent years, an expanded focus has provided insight into other important epidemiological considerations of pregnancy, childbirth, and infertility.

Reproductive-Age Women

The large number of births that occurred after World War II is known as the "Baby Boom." As a result of this postwar birth explosion, the number of women aged 30 to 44 is currently larger than at any time in American history.[24] This large cohort has been followed by a much smaller cohort, which reflects a period of lower birth rates. As seen in Figure 9.10, the combination of these two cohorts means that older women now make up a larger proportion of women of childbearing age in the United States.

Birth Rates

Patterns of childbearing among women of various ages differ. Birth rates in almost all age groups of women between 15 and 44 years have increased between 1980 and 1989. Fig. 9.11 provides a comparison of 1980 and 1988 birth rates (live births per 1,000 population) for African-American and white women. In both 1980 and 1989, African-American women had significantly higher birth rates among younger women. Birth rates for Hispanic-American women have followed trends similar to those for African-American and white women, but they have been consistently higher.[25] Another group of interest for birth rates is unmarried women. There has been a dramatic increase in the number of births to unmarried women 20 years of age and older.[25] This trend corresponds to the national pattern of increasing numbers of formerly married and never married women.[24]

FIGURE 9.10

Percent distribution of US women by reproductive age, 1982 and 1988.

SOURCE: Adapted from Forrest, J.D., and Singh, S. (1990). The sexual and reproductive behavior of American women, 1982–1988. *Family Planning Perspectives; 22,* 207.

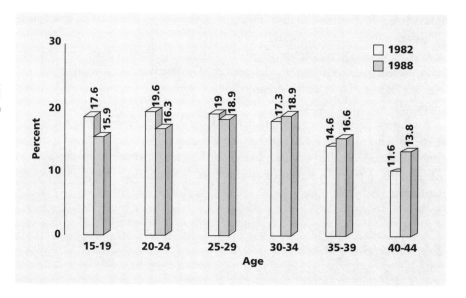

FIGURE 9.11

Birth rates by age of mother and race of child, United States, 1980 and 1988.

SOURCE: Adapted from USDHHS (1991). *Health United States, 1990.* (DHHS Pub. No. 91-1232.) Washington, DC: US Government Printing Office. p. 52.

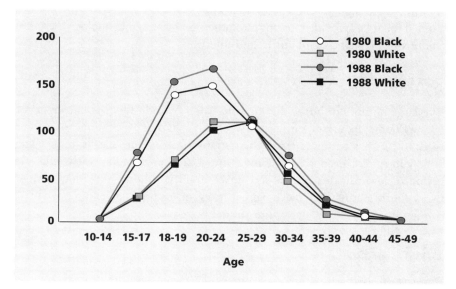

Maternal Mortality

The leading causes of maternal death are **toxemia**, hemorrhage, embolism, and ectopic pregnancy.[27] In the early 1900s, 1 in 150 women died from causes related to pregnancy with the death rate among nonwhite women nearly double that of white women.[27] These deaths were caused by infection, toxemia, abortion, and hemorrhage. Today most of these deaths would be considered preventable. In 1989, 320 maternal deaths were reported among the 3.8 million live births in the United States.[25] Although this reduction in maternal mortality is impressive, data (Fig. 9.12) indicate that nonwhite women are still more than three times as likely as white women to die of pregnancy-related causes, and the risk for African-American women is the highest of all racial groups. The data indicate that older women are also at increased risk for maternal mortality.

Ectopic Pregnancy

Ectopic pregnancy is a major factor contributing to maternal mortality. In 1987, ectopic pregnancy accounted for more than 12 percent of maternal deaths and was the leading cause of maternal mortality in the first trimester.[26,28] Ectopic pregnancy rates have steadily increased in recent years. The risk of ectopic pregnancy is greater for nonwhite women and increases with age among women of all races, with the highest ectopic pregnancy rate among women aged 35 to 44 years.[26]

Prenatal Care

Early prenatal care is important for women because it permits timely, appropriate intervention to improve maternal health and pregnancy outcome. Studies have shown prenatal care to be associated with a reduction in infant death and illness.[29–31] The risk of low birth weight is reduced among women who initiate prenatal care early in the pregnancy.[7] Approximately 75 percent of mothers initiate care in the first trimester, and about 6 percent of mothers do not receive prenatal care or wait until their third trimester.[25] Studies have shown that prenatal care has the greatest impact in those women who are at highest risk for poor pregnancy outcome, such as adolescents, unmarried women, and

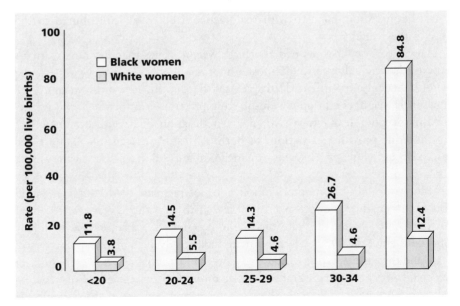

FIGURE 9.12

Maternal mortality rates for complications of pregnancy, childbirth, and the puerperium, according to race and age, United States, 1988.

SOURCE: Adapted from USDHHS (1991). *Health United States, 1990.* (DHHS Pub. No. 91-1232.) Washington, DC: US Government Printing Office. p. 94.

minority women.[34,35] In 1989, African-American women were more than twice as likely as white women to receive little or no care, and Hispanic-American women were almost as likely as white women to receive care.[25]

Place of Delivery

Nearly 99 percent of births in the United States occurred in hospitals in 1989.[25] The remaining 1.2 percent of births took place in free-standing birthing centers or at home. Although the proportions were small, white mothers were more likely than African-American mothers to deliver outside a hospital. Nearly 96 percent of all deliveries were attended by physicians.[25]

Complications of Pregnancy and Childbirth

Pregnancy and childbirth are safe experiences for most women, with 40 percent of women experiencing no medical or obstetrical complications during the prenatal or intrapartum period.[36] The remaining 60 percent of women experience some type of complication. About half of these complications are considered to be major medical problems. Adolescents, poor women, and older women are most likely to experience these problems. The most common problems are those that occur during labor or delivery, with approximately 30 percent of women experiencing umbilical cord complications, obstructed labor, breech presentation, severe lacerations and tears during delivery, and severe postpartum hemorrhage.[36]

Cesarean delivery can be considered a complication of pregnancy. In the United States, approximately 25 percent of babies are born by cesarean delivery.[20,37,38] In 1970, the national rate for cesarean delivery was 5 percent, and by 1988 the rate had risen to over 24 percent. There is a general consensus that the increasing concern with malpractice liability has contributed to the rise in these rates.[21]

Low birth weight is defined as a birth weight of less than 2,500 gm. Infant low birth weight is the single most important predictor of survival.[39] In the United States, most infant deaths are associated with low birth weight. The low-birth-weight condition may result from preterm birth (before 37 weeks' gestation) or poor fetal growth for a given duration of pregnancy, known as **intrauterine growth retardation,** or both. African-American infants are twice as likely as white or Hispanic-American infants to have low birth weight (Fig. 9.13).

Infant mortality is another complication of pregnancy. Although in 1991, the infant death rate of 9.8 per 1,000 live births was the lowest ever recorded in the United States, the rate of decline has slowed.[40] The decline in infant mortality since the 1970s is largely attributable to advances in neonatal intensive care and the dissemination of these advances.[41] Data analyses, however, indicate that still African-American infants die at more than twice the rate of white or Hispanic-American infants.[25] The neonatal period consists of the first month of life, and about two-thirds of infant deaths occur in this time frame. The

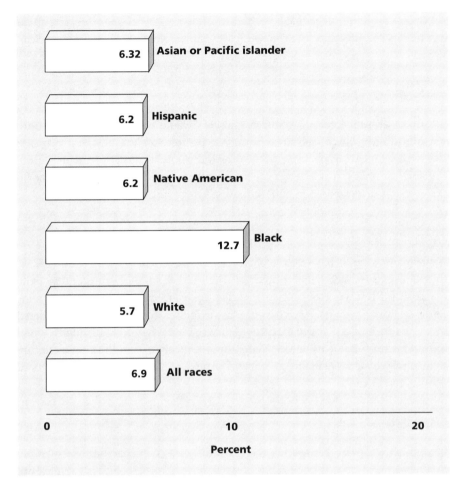

FIGURE 9.13

Percent low birth weight, by specified race of the child, 1987.

SOURCE: Adapted from Tauber, C. (1991). *Statistical Handbook on Women in America.* Phoenix: Orynx Press, p. 33; and National Center for Health Statistics (1991). Advance report of final natality statistics, 1989. *Monthly Vital Statistics Report, 40*(8) (Suppl).

leading causes of neonatal death are birth defects and respiratory distress syndrome.[25]

Infertility

Nearly 1 in 12 reproductive-age women in the United States have reported difficulty in becoming pregnant.[22] About half of these women were childless, and the other half had given birth one or more times before experiencing difficulty in conceiving further pregnancies. Data from a 1988 national survey reveal that there has been no change in the proportion of infertile couples since 1982.[22] Despite these data, a common perception is that infertility is on the increase. This perception may be due in part to changes in the composition of the population. Although the proportion of couples who are considered infertile has remained stable, the number of childless women aged 25 to 44 years is increasing as a result of the aging of the baby boom cohort and to the tendency of this group to delay marriage and childbearing.[42] Another factor contributing to the perception is the availability of new drugs and treatment technology for infertility and the willingness of couples to request these services.

Informed Decision Making

Informed decision making about pregnancy should begin before conception, not after. The newly conceived offspring is dependent on its mother for nutrition and well-being weeks before the mother knows that she is pregnant. If the potential mother is a smoker or is abusing alcohol or drugs during this critical early period of development, the offspring is at a decided disadvantage.

Pregnancy

A pregnant woman has to take good care of herself to provide the best care for the unborn child. Regular prenatal care that begins early in the pregnancy is essential. Most women see their clinician once a month during the pregnancy until the 28th week. As they enter the last trimester, this frequency is increased to every other week until the 36th week, when weekly visits until delivery are indicated. Proper nutrition; adequate and appropriate exercise; and avoidance of alcohol, tobacco, caffeine, and illegal drugs are all essential components of good prenatal care.

Childbirth

Childbirth is a personal, special, one-time-only event. Preparation for birthing ensures the best possible childbirth experience. Childbirth education classes provide many valuable opportunities for learning, practical preparation, and skills building for a rewarding and facilitated childbirth experience. The classes provide an opportunity to share concerns and discuss plans. Local resources for childbirth options, such as birthing centers or home deliveries, can be evaluated. Classes provide motivation to learn relaxation and pain management techniques.

Resources in childbirth preparation vary. Some communities have many resources, and in other communities, resources other are rather few and far between. To maximize the benefits from a childbirth education class, qualifications of the instructor, class size, and class focus should be carefully evaluated. Instructors in childbirth education should be certified. The most prestigious certification program for childbirth educators is conducted by the American Society for Psychoprophylaxis in Obstetrics, Inc. (APSO/Lamaze). Educators with this certification use the credential ACCE (member, American College of Childbirth Education). Those who have made significant contributions to the field may use FACCE, indicating that they are Fellows of the College. The most appropriate class size is 8 to 12 couples. This allows for individual attention, time for discussion, and adequate floor space for practice. In addition to providing the basic information on pregnancy and childbirth, classes should discuss birthing options and developing personal plans for birth based on personal medical requirements and resources.

Infertility

Nearly 1 in 12 women reports difficulty in becoming pregnant.[24] Infertility should be recognized as a problem of a couple, not the woman or her partner. Because the factors that reduce fertility are shared, both partners must be evaluated when initiating an infertility workup. Infertility services are more widespread today, and evolving technologies have assisted many couples in having a child. Infertility clinics can offer couples information, support, and procedures to address their specific needs. Identification of infertility services is often facilitated through referral from a gynecologist.

Summary

Pregnancy and childbirth are exciting yet complex dimensions of women's health. In addition to the biological aspects, pregnancy and childbirth are greatly influenced by social, cultural, historical, legal, and ethical dimensions. Informed decision making is a critical determinant throughout pregnancy and childbirth.

CURRENT EVENTS

Folic Acid Supplements Backed

Washington Post
September 14, 1992

To reduce the risk of serious birth defects, all women of childbearing age should take folic acid supplements or include more foods containing folic acid in their diets. These recommendations are released by the US Public Health Service (PHS) and represent the first time that the government has advocated vitamin supplements for the general population. The evidence has been accumulating for several years that folic acid, a B vitamin, can reduce the risk of neural tube defects, such as spina bifida and anencephaly. The body uses folic acid to manufacture DNA.

The PHS believes that it is possible to reduce by half the number of infants born with neural tube defects through diet or supplements. Almost 2,500 infants are born annually in the United States. These defects occur within the first month after conception, so intake of folic acid must begin at least 1 month before pregnancy. Because this is before a woman knows she is pregnant—and because close to half of all pregnancies are unplanned—the PHS recommends that all women from puberty through menopause consume 0.4 mg of folic acid daily, twice the current recommended intake.

Daily intake of folic acid should not exceed 1 mg because high intake might mask or exacerbate anemia. Good sources of folic acid include citrus juices and fruits, dark green leafy vegetables, breads, beans, and fortified cereals. Women who eat at least five fruits and vegetables daily should meet the recommendation.

Philosophical Dimensions: Pregnancy and Childbirth

1. Should childbirth retain its "medicalized" focus? Why? Why not?

2. Should pregnant women be restricted in their access to tobacco, alcohol or drugs?

3. Should prenatal testing be routine for all pregnant women?

4. Should preparation for childbirth be routine (required?) for all women?

5. Should a laboring mother be permitted all the pain medication she wants?

6. What are possible ethical and legal dilemmas associated with IVT? with GIFT? with embryo transfer? with host uterus? with surrogacy?

References

1. Bogdan, J.C. (1990). Childbirth in America, 1650 to 1990. In R. D. Apple (Ed.), *Women, Health and Medicine in America.* New York: Garland Publishers.

2. Wertz, R.W., and Wertz, D.C. (1977). *Lying-In: A History of Childbirth in America.* New York: Free Press.

3. Leavitt, J.W. (1986). *Brought to Bed: Childbirthing in America, 1750–1950.* New York: Oxford University Press.

4. Ansley, D. (1992). Spermtales. *Discover, 13*(6), 66–69.

5. Freedman, D.H. (1992). The aggressive egg. *Discover, 13*(6), 61–65.

6. Lemire, R.J. (1988). Neural tube defects. *Journal of the American Medical Association, 259*(4), 558–562.

7. Institute of Medicine (1985). *Preventing low birthweight.* Division of Health Promotion and Disease Prevention, Committee to Study the Prevention of Low Birth Weight. Washington, DC: National Academy Press.

8. Clapp, J.F., Rokey, E., Treadway, J.I., Carpenter, M.W., Artal, R.M., and Warrnes, C. (1992). Exercise in pregnancy. *Medicine and Science in Sports and Exercise, 24*(6), Suppl., S294–S300.

9. Longo, L. (1982). Some health consequences of maternal smoking: Issues without answers. *Birth Defects: Original Article Series, March of Dimes Foundation, 18,* 13–31.

10. Cunningham, F.G., Mac Donald, P.C., Grant, N.F., Leveno, K.J., and Gilstrap, L.C. (1993). *Williams Obstetrics* (19th ed.); Norwalk, CT: Appleton and Lange.

11. Cefalo, R., and Moos, M. (1988). *Preconceptual Health Promotion: A Practical Guide.* Rockville, MD: Aspen Publishing.

12. Rossett, H.L., and Weiner, L. (1984). *Alcohol and the Fetus: A Clinical Perspective.* New York: Oxford University Press.

13. MacGregor, S.N., Keith, L.G., Chasnoff, I.J., Rosner, M.A., Chisum, G.M., Shaw, P., and Minogue, J.P. (1987). Cocaine use during pregnancy: Adverse perinatal outcome. *American Journal of Obstetrics and Gynecology, 157,* 686–690.

14. Zuckerman, B., Frank, D.A., Hingson, R., Amaro, H., Levenson, S.M., Kaye, H., Parker, S., Vinci, R., Aboagye, K., Fried, L.E., Cabral, H., Timperi, R., and Bauchner, H. (1989). Effects of maternal marijuana and cocaine use on fetal growth. *New England Journal of Medicine, 320,* 762–768.

15. Firth, H.V., Boyd, P.A., Chamberlain, P., MacKenzie, I.Z., Lindenbaum, R.H. and Huson, S.M. (1991). Severe limb abnormalities after chorion villus sampling at 56–66 days gestation. *Lancet, 337,* 762–763.

16. Rhoads, G.G., Jackson, L.G., Schlesselman, S.E., de la Cruz, F.F., Desnick, R.J., Golbus, M.S., Ledbetter, D.H., Lubs, H.A., Mahoney, M.J. and Pergament, E. (1989). The safety and efficacy of chorionic villus sampling for the early prenatal diagnosis of cytogenic abnormalities. *New England Journal of Medicine, 320,* 609–617.

17. Simpson, J.L. (1990). Incidence and timing of pregnancy losses: Relevance to evaluating safety of early prenatal diagnosis. *American Journal of Medical Genetics, 35,* 165–173.

18. Centers for Disease Control (1986). Ectopic pregnancy surveillance, United States, 1970–83. In: Surveillance summaries, August 1986. *Morbidity and Mortality Weekly Report, 35*(2SS), 29SS–37SS.

19. Panjvani, Z.F.K., and Hanshaw, J.B. (1981). Cytomegalovirus in the perinatal period. *American Journal of Diseases in Children, 135,* 56–60.

20. Taffel, S.M., Placek, P.J., and Moien, M. (1989). Cesarean section rate levels off in 1987. *Family Planning Perspectives, 21,* 227–228.

21. Martin, J.N., Morrison, J.C., and Wiser, W.L. (1988). Vaginal birth after cesarean section: The demise of the routine repeat abdominal delivery. *Obstetrics and Gynecology Clinics of North America, 15,* 719–736.

22. Mosher, W.D., and Pratt, W.F. (1990). Fecundity and infertility in the United States, 1965–1988. *Advance Data, 192,* 1–6.

23. In vitro fertilization-embryo transfer (IVT-ET) in the United States: 1989 results from the IVT-ET Registry. (1991). *Fertility and Sterility, 55,* 14–23.

24. Forrest, J.D., and Singh, S. (1990). The sexual and reproductive behavior of American women, 1982–1988. *Family Planning Perspectives, 222,* 206–214.

25. National Center for Health Statistics. (1991). Advance report of final natality statistics, 1989. *Monthly Vital Statistics Report, 40*(8), Suppl., 39–40.

26. Lawson, H.W., Atrash, H.K., Saftlas, A.F., and Finch, E.L. (1989). Ectopic pregnancy in the United States, 1970–1986. *Morbidity and Mortality Weekly Report, 38,* Suppl. 2, 1–10.

27. Rochat, R.W., Koonin, L.M., Atrash, H.K., and Jewett, J.F. (1988). Maternal mortality in the United States: Report from the Maternal Mortality Collaborative. *Obstetrics and Gynecology, 72,* 91–97.

28. Nederlof, K.P., Lawson, H.W., Saftlas, A.F., Atrash, H.K., and Finch, E.L. (1989). Ectopic pregnancy surveillance, United States, 1970–1987. *Morbidity and Mortality Weekly Report, 39,* Suppl. 4, 9–17.

29. Shapiro, S., Schlesinger, E., and Nesbitt, R. (1968). *Infant, Perinatal, Maternal, and Childhood Mortality in the United States.* Cambridge: Harvard University Press.

30. Moore, T.R., Origel, W., Key, T.C., and Resnik, R. (1986). The perinatal and economic impact of prenatal care in a low socioeconomic population. *American Journal of Obstetrics and Gynecology, 154,* 29–33.

31. Kotelchuck, M., Schwartz, J.B., Anderka, M.T., and Finison, K.S. (1984). WIC participation and pregnancy outcomes: Massachusetts Statewide Evaluation Project. *American Journal of Public Health, 74,* 1086–1092.

32. Heins, H.C., Miller, J.M., Sear, A., Goodyar, N., and Garder, S. (1983). Benefits of a statewide high-risk perinatal program. *Obstetrics and Gynecology, 62,* 294–296.

33. Leveno, K.J., Cunningham, F.G., Roark, M.L., Nelson, S.D., and Williams, M.L. (1985). Prenatal care and the low birth weight infant. *Obstetrics and Gynecology, 66,* 599–605.

34. Greenberg, R.S. (1983). The impact of prenatal care in different social groups. *American Journal of Obstetrics and Gynecology, 145,* 797–801.

35. Peoples, M.D., and Siegel, E. (1983). Measuring the impact of programs for mothers and infants on prenatal care and low birthweight: The value of refined analyses. *Medical Care, 21,* 586–608.

36. Gold, R.B., Kenney, A.M., and Singh, S. (1987). *Blessed Events and the Bottom Line: Financing Maternity Care in the United States.* New York: Alan Guttmacher Institute.

37. Taffel, S.M., Placek, P.J., and Moien, M. (1990). U.S. Cesarean section rate at 24.7 per 100 births: A plateau? *New England Journal of Medicine, 323,* 199–200.

38. Myers, A.A., and Gleicher, N. (1988). U.S. Cesarean rate: Good news or bad? *New England Journal of Medicine, 323,* 200.

39. Hogue, C.J.R., Strauss, L.T., Beuhler, J.W., and Smith, J.C. (1989). Overview of the National Infant Mortality Surveillance (NIMS) Project. *Morbidity and Mortality Weekly Report, 38,* Suppl. 3, 1–46.

40. USDHHS (1991). *Healthy People 2000: National Health Promotion and Disease Prevention Objectives.* (DHHS Pub. No. (PHS) 91-50212.) Washington, DC: US Government Printing Office.

41. Beuhler, J.W., Kleinman, J.C., Hogue, C.J.R., Strauss, L.T., and Smith, J.C. (1987). Birthweight-specific infant mortality, United States, 1960 and 1980. *Public Health Reports, 102*(2), 151–161.

42. American College of Obstetricians and Gynecologists. (1989). *Infertility.* ACOG Technical Bulletin 125. Washington, DC: American College of Obstetricians and Gynecologists.

Resources

AMERICAN COLLEGE OF NURSE MIDWIVES

1522 K Street NW, Suite 1120
Washington, DC 20006
202-347-5445

AMERICAN COLLEGE OF OBSTETRICIANS AND GYNECOLOGISTS

409 12th Street SW
Washington, DC 20024
202-638-5577

ASPO/LAMAZE CERTIFIED CHILDBIRTH EDUCATORS

1101 Connecticut Avenue NW
Washington, DC 20036
800-368-4404

C/SEC, INC. (FOR VBAC INFORMATION)

22 Forest Road
Framingham, MA 01701
508-877-8266

CESAREAN PREVENTION MOVEMENT, INC.

PO Box 152 University Station
Syracuse, NY 13210
315-424-1942

INTERNATIONAL CHILDBIRTH EDUCATION ASSOCIATION

PO Box 20048
Minneapolis, MN 55420
612-854-8660

MARCH OF DIMES BIRTH DEFECTS FOUNDATION

1275 Mamaroneck Avenue
White Plains, NY 10605
914-428-7100

NATIONAL ASSOCIATION OF PARENTS AND PROFESSIONALS FOR SAFE ALTERNATIVES IN CHILDBIRTH

Route 1, Box 646
Marble Hill, MD 63764

314-238-2010

RESOLVE (information, counseling information on infertility)

5 Water Street
Arlington, MA 02174
617-643-2424

CHAPTER 10

Reproductive Tract Infections

CHAPTER OBJECTIVES

On completion of this chapter, the student should be able to discuss:

1. Why the emotional impact of reproductive tract infections for women is often worse than the physical impact.

2. The bacterial infection process.

3. The viral infection process.

4. STDs from a historical perspective.

5. The difference between STD prevalence and incidence data.

6. Which populations are disproportionately afflicted with STDs.

7. How women experience disproportionate STD burdens.

8. How stigma is a dimension of STDs.

9. The diagnostic strategy, symptoms (in women), special concerns, and treatment for gonorrhea, chlamydia, HPV, HSV, syphilis, hepatitis, trichomonas, yeast infections, and bacterial vaginosis.

10. The significance of PID as a major health problem for women.

11. How PID may be characterized by localized infections.

12. Diagnostic and treatment dimensions of PID.

13. The relationship between HPV and cervical cancer.

14. Special precautions to be observed when someone has HSV or HPV.

15. Why good communication is essential with STDs.

16. How contraceptive choice influences STD risk.

17. When a woman should see a clinician about STDs.

18. How AIDS compromises the body's immune system.

19. AIDS from a historical perspective.

20. Why women have not been recognized as an at-risk and HIV-susceptible population.

21. **The epidemiological data and trends with women and HIV/AIDS.**

22. **How minority women are disproportionately affected by the HIV epidemic.**

23. **Special diagnostic and treatment dimensions for women and HIV.**

24. **How pregnancy and HIV is a special issue.**

Introduction

Reproductive tract infections are infections caused by a variety of organisms that affect either the upper or the lower reproductive tract. Most women encounter at least one, probably several, reproductive tract infections in their lifetime. Most infections are transmitted by sexual intimacy. Some infections are not serious health threats: Yeast infections, for example, may be a major annoyance, but they do not have serious life-threatening sequelae. Other infections, however, are far less kind. Chlamydia, gonorrhea, syphilis, herpes, genital warts, hepatitis, and acquired immunodeficiency syndrome (AIDS) are serious threats to future reproductive capability and life itself. Although some infections attack one structure alone, such as the labia or cervix, others ascend upward from the vagina, through the cervical canal, into the uterus, where further invasion into the fallopian tubes, ovaries, and entire pelvis can occur. Bacteria and virus may also enter the bloodstream and result in systemic effects.

The emotional impact for women of reproductive tract infections is often as serious or worse than the physical impact. Sexually transmitted disease (STD) organisms know no class, racial, ethnic, or social barriers—all individuals are vulnerable if exposed to the organism. Society, however, has a tendency to look on STDs as "punishment" for immoral activity, so when a woman learns that she has an STD, her reaction may include disbelief, hurt, victimization, guilt, embarrassment, anger, fear, shame, and a feeling of loss of control over sexuality and health. In addition, with viral diseases, there is often the added pressure of worry over how the lingering virus will impact present and future relationships. Clearly knowledge and prevention are the best defenses against STDs.

Infection Process

Reproductive tract infections are caused by a variety of organisms, including bacteria, viruses, and parasites. Each organism requires a unique diagnostic strategy and treatment. Bacteria behave in different ways; some attach to the surface of normal body cells, and some live within host cells. Some are oxygen dependent (**aerobic**), and others are intolerant of oxygen environments (**anaerobic**). Antibiotics are drugs capable of killing harmful bacteria. Many kinds of bacteria normally live in the intestine and vaginal area. The normal ecosystem of these areas is a delicate balance of organisms. Taking antibiotics to kill one organism often results in the "killing off" of the normal bacteria. For women, this often results in a domino effect. When bacteria levels are reduced, yeast colonies may proliferate, and additional treatment may be necessary.

Bacteria receive nourishment from the fluid or tissue in which they reside. Waste products from the bacteria are released into these invaded tissues. The body's **immune system** senses the presence of the foreign bacteria, and white blood cells are mobilized to attack them. The infected area becomes warm, red, and swollen owing to the increased circulation and the accumulation of **pus.** The local host cells may be destroyed directly from the bacteria or indirectly from the excessive swelling and waste products. Bacterial waste products are often toxic beyond the localized area and may result in systemic conditions of aches, fever, chills, and malaise. An example of a systemic illness produced by bacterial waste products is toxic shock syndrome, which is caused by certain strains of *Staphylococcus aureus* bacteria. Although normal infection defenses routinely fight off invading organisms throughout the body, reproductive tract infections are particularly challenging. During menstruation and after a miscarriage or abortion, the pelvis contains ideal media for bacterial growth and proliferation. Bleeding seems to facilitate bacterial invasion, and blood enhances bacterial growth. Chlamydia, gonorrhea, and bacterial vaginosis are reproductive tract infections caused by bacterial organisms.

Viruses present unique invasion patterns. They are tiny organisms made of DNA or RNA. Viruses are considerably smaller in size than bacteria. Their attack mechanism is also different from bacteria. Viruses invade normal cells and take over the metabolic functions, fueling themselves on the cells' resources. Antibiotics are ineffective against viral organisms. The body's immune system is able to recognize invading viruses and mobilize responses, but a compromised immune system is ineffective against viral invaders. Viruses, such as **human immunodeficiency virus** (HIV), present incredible challenges to medical researchers because they effectively compromise the immune system of the host, allowing opportunistic infections to invade and proliferate. Research is underway to develop more effective antiviral drugs that are not too toxic to use. Herpes, genital warts, hepatitis, and AIDS are reproductive infections caused by viruses.

Sexually Transmitted Diseases

STDs were previously called "venereal diseases." STDs are a major health problem and have been identified as a national health priority.[1] Despite the availability of effective antibiotics against several of the pathogens, STD rates have continued to climb. More than 50 diseases and syndromes are currently recognized as being transmitted sexually. STDs are at epidemic proportions among reproductive-age Americans and present especially serious threats to young women. About 85 percent of all STDs occur in persons between the ages of 15 and 30.[1] STDs are biologically sexist—presenting greater risk and complications among women than among men.

Although STDs are a modern epidemic, they are not modern diseases. STDs have been referenced in medical literature for hundreds, and sometimes

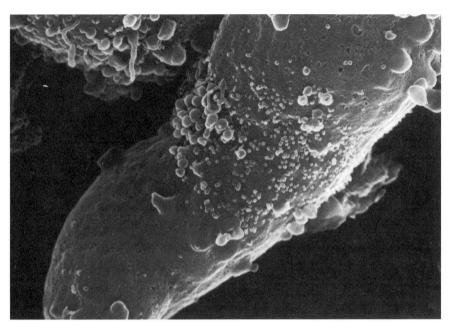

Viral infections like herpes simplex or human papillomavirus are lifelong conditions.

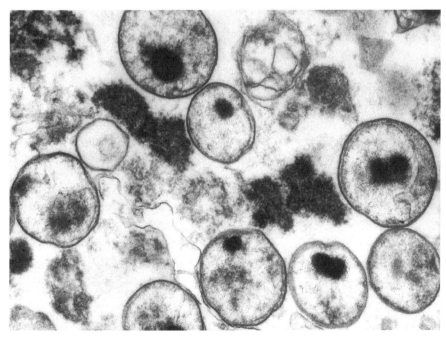

Bacterial sexually transmitted diseases can be treated with antibiotics.

thousands, of years. The oldest books in the Bible describe diseases that probably were gonorrhea and syphilis. Early Biblical descriptions of leprosy more accurately fit the conditions of diseases now called syphilis or scabies. Ancient Greek and Roman physicians identified genital warts and syphilis chancres in their writings. Hippocrates described the mechanism for gonorrhea transmission as "accesses of the pleasures of the Venus." The term "**condyloma**," now solely used for genital warts, means fig and is of Greek origin. Egyptian writings describe an herbal remedy for painful urination, and Susruta, an ancient Hindu, also described gonorrhea. In ancient Rome, Tiberius issued a decree outlawing public kissing to curb a herpes epidemic. Syphilis is reported to be one of the "gifts" of the New World brought back by early Spanish explorers. Between 1495 and 1500, the disease ravaged Europe killing hundreds of thousands. The AIDS epidemic today has been likened to these historical STD ravages.

Epidemiological Data and Trends

Epidemiological data indicate that STD rates are increasing nationally. Many STDs are reportable conditions, and national data are available. Others are not reportable diseases, and actual prevalence rates can only be estimated. The Centers for Disease Control (CDC) report that more than 12 million STDs occur among Americans each year, and more than 3 million of these STDs are among teenagers.[2] Incidence and prevalence are two important and often misused epidemiological terms. Prevalence refers to a "snapshot" picture—that is, at one point in time, how many cases of a specific STD are present in a population. Incidence refers to the number of new cases of a disease. Both incidence and prevalence rates depend on a number of factors that can greatly affect the accuracy of measurement.

The US STD epidemiological picture is dramatic. Incidence rates of several STDs are presented in Fig. 10.1. Chlamydia infections are not officially reportable diseases, but it is estimated that between 3 and 10 million cases occur each year in the United States.[3] Prevalence rates provide an even more startling picture; for example, it is estimated that 20 to 30 million Americans harbor the herpes virus,[4] and **human papillomavirus** (HPV) has been estimated to afflict 10 to 20 million people in the United States.[5] Racial and ethnic differences are also dramatic dimensions of the STD epidemiological picture. Native Americans experience higher reported gonorrhea and syphilis morbidity than non-Native Americans.[6] Racial and ethnic differences in syphilis incidence rates grew throughout the 1980s (Fig. 10.2). The African American–to–white incidence ratio almost tripled, and the Hispanic American–to–white ratio almost doubled. Gender differences have decreased in all racial and ethnic groups, indicating that women's risk of contracting syphilis is increasing more rapidly than men's risk.[8]

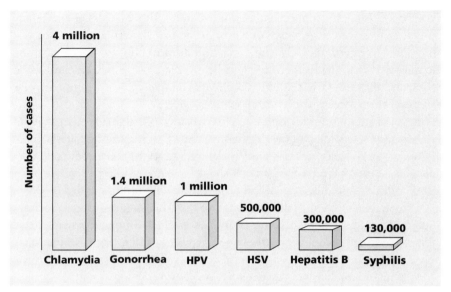

FIGURE 10.1

Annual US number of new STD cases.

SOURCE: Centers for Disease Control (1991). *Sexually Transmitted Disease Surveillance, 1989.* (DHHS Pub. No. 91-736-854R.) Washington, DC: US Government Printing Office.

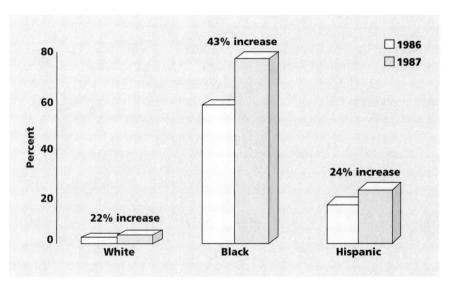

FIGURE 10.2

Race/ethnicity differences in syphilis incidence rates among women, 1986–87.

SOURCE: Centers for Disease Control (1988). Syphilis and congenital syphilis, 1985–88. *Morbidity and Mortality Weekly Report, 37,* 486–489.

Social Issues and Dimensions of Sexually Transmitted Diseases

Women experience a disproportionate amount of the STD burden and STD complications, including sterility, perinatal infections, genital tract neoplasia, and death. STDs in women are often silent, presenting as asymptomatic but damaging and infectious. Their children and unborn babies are frequently placed at risk of illness, congenital anomalies, mental retardation, and death.

Because STDs are most prevalent among women 15 to 24 years of age,[1] these women experience the greatest burden of pelvic pain, infertility, increased risk of ectopic pregnancy, and pelvic inflammatory disease (PID). Women constitute the majority of individuals living at or below the poverty line in the United States, and the poor have the added burden of limited access to comprehensive STD diagnostic, treatment, and follow-up services.

Stigma is another dimension of STDs. Considerable stigma accompanies an STD diagnosis, regardless of the culprit organism. This stigma originates because the underlying sexual behavior is often labeled as deviant. Reproductive tract infection is often perceived as dirty or shameful, and an infected woman may fear that health care providers will not care for her or will be offended by doing so. Women are more vulnerable than men to the STD stigma owing to society's double standard of women being "pure" or virginal, women's general social subordination, and women's relatively poor power position. Some women may view an STD as punishment for previous behavior. Many people still equate STDs with immorality, promiscuous behavior, and low social status.

Cultural and emotional dimensions complicate public health and education efforts. Although STD educational and behavioral issues are a common denominator across all racial and ethnic groups, the situation is far worse in poor African-American communities. Other social problems impact and complicate the STD epidemic. Anonymous sex in crack houses compounds STD transmission.[9] Many Hispanic-American communities have a traditional outlook that winks at male philandering but regards condom use as immoral and contrary to principles of machismo. Emotional dimensions often dominate logical behavior and rational thinking—for example, prostitutes who wear condoms with clients but not with boyfriends and teenage girls who believe that condoms are unnecessary when a boyfriend declares his love.

Clinical Dimensions and Treatment Issues of Sexually Transmitted Diseases

Because STDs are caused by a spectrum of organisms, there is considerable variation in the manifestation of symptoms and in treatment options. Each major STD is discussed in terms of its clinical and treatment perspectives.

Gonorrhea

Gonorrhea is a major STD in the United States. Women commonly do not experience any symptoms with gonorrhea, especially in the early stages. Gonorrhea in women is often detected at routine gynecological screening or when their male partners develop symptoms that lead to clinical treatment. When symptoms do present in women, they may include unusual vaginal discharge or bleeding, painful urination, painful intercourse or bleeding after intercourse, pelvic pain or tenderness, or fever. The gonococcus bacterium thrives in moist warm cavities, such as the mouth, throat, rectum, cervix, and urinary tract. Therefore gonococcal infections may present in the reproductive tract, the throat, eyes, and rectum. Accurate diagnosis of gonorrhea requires a culture, although a clinician may examine a sample of vaginal discharge under a microscope.

Treatment for gonorrhea is with antibiotics (ampicillin, amoxicillin, or penicillin) and probenecid, a drug that helps to maintain and sustain a high blood level of antibiotic. Gonorrhea treatment is complicated by the frequent coexistence of unrecognized chlamydial infection and the increasing incidence of infection owing to gonorrheal antibiotic-resistant strains. Because neither of these conditions may be apparent on physical examination, gonorrhea treatment usually includes additional antibiotics to treat chlamydia effectively and screening for resistant strains. The sequelae of gonorrhea are so severe and threatening to general health and reproductive capability that any woman exposed to a partner with gonorrhea, even in the absence of symptoms, should be treated. If a woman has symptoms that would indicate gonorrhea spread, longer, more intensive antibiotic treatment is indicated. This often means hospital admission for intravenous antibiotic therapy. In about a week after antibiotic treatment for gonorrhea, reculture is necessary for a woman and her partner(s). This follow-up is especially important because some strains of gonorrhea are resistant to penicillin, and further treatment may be necessary to eliminate the disease. Reinfection with gonorrhea is common, so sexual intercourse should be avoided until confirmatory cultures indicate that treatment was successful. Untreated or unsuccessful treatment of gonorrhea may result in PID or a syndrome caused by disseminated gonococcal infection, which can include septicemia (blood poisoning), arthritis, skin problems, and heart and brain infections.

Chlamydia

Chlamydia is not a reportable disease, but it is ranked as the most common STD in the United States (see Fig. 10.1). Chlamydia infections are caused by a bacterium that is transmitted sexually. Symptoms may not present with chlamydia for weeks or months after transmission. The most common symptom for women is a yellowish vaginal discharge or general pain in the lower abdomen. Chlamydia can invade the uterus and fallopian tubes, and even then symptoms may not be present. It has been hypothesized that swimming sperm cells may be the transportation mechanism for carrying chlamydial organisms into the **cervix** and uterus. Chlamydia usually attack the reproductive tract in women but may also attack the urinary tract. Chlamydia urinary tract infections are characterized by frequent burning urination. An association between oral contraceptive use and chlamydia has been suggested. It is not known if oral contraceptives actually promote the growth of chlamydial infections of the cervix or perhaps enhance the detection of chlamydia from the cervix.

Definitive diagnosis of chlamydia requires fairly expensive sophisticated testing, although new diagnostic strategies are being tested that will be less expensive and provide definitive information in a more timely manner. Clinician suspicion of chlamydia is heightened in a woman with a reddened, swollen cervix and a yellowish cervical discharge. Because gonorrhea and chlamydia often coexist, culture for gonorrhea is usually a standard procedure with a suspicion of chlamydia. A woman may be treated for chlamydia, even without a confirmed diagnosis, based on symptoms and physical examination. A 7-day regimen of doxycycline or tetracycline is the preferred treatment for chlamydia. Partner(s) should be treated at the same time, and a follow-up examination is usually indicated about a week after treatment to ensure that it was successful. Sexual intercourse should be avoided until after treatment is successful.

Aggressive treatment is necessary with chlamydia because uterine invasion occurs fairly rapidly, and the invasion process may be asymptomatic. Full PID treatment is indicated if there is any evidence that the organism has invaded the uterus. Treatment delay may result in the organism reaching the fallopian tubes with resultant scarring, tubal obstruction, infertility, and ectopic pregnancy. Pregnant women infected with chlamydia may be at increased risk for spontaneous abortions, stillbirth, and postpartum complications. Transmission of the organism to the baby may result in eye infections and pneumonia.

Pelvic Inflammatory Disease

PID is a serious and the most frequent complication of bacterial infections, particularly chlamydia and gonorrhea. Each year more than 1 million women experience an episode of PID, with an estimated total cost of $4.2 billion annually.[10] PID may result in an annual involuntary sterilization of 100,000 women. It is also a leading cause of ectopic pregnancies. More than 300,000 women are hospitalized annually for PID. PID has been estimated by the Centers for Disease Control (CDC) to afflict 11 percent of reproductive-age women in the United States: 1 in 10 white women and 1 in 6 African-American women.[11] Chlamydia or gonorrhea are responsible for more than half the cases of PID. Pelvic infection and PID disease are general terms for an infectious process that occurs anywhere in a woman's pelvic organs (Fig. 10.3). The infection process may be diffuse, spread out throughout the pelvic cavity, or it may be localized in specific areas. Terms that indicate localized infections include:

- Endometritis—infection of the lining of the uterus.
- Myometritis—infection of the muscular layers of the uterus.
- Salpingitis—infection of the fallopian tubes.
- Oophoritis—infection of the ovaries.
- Peritonitis—infection of the lining of the abdominal cavity.

There is considerable variability with PID symptoms. Some women experience very insidious symptoms. These may include a vaginal discharge, mild but persistent abdominal or back pain, or pain during intercourse. Other women experience sudden and severe pelvic pain, elevated temperature, shaking chills, or heavy vaginal discharge or bleeding. Gonorrhea PID is more likely to present with the latter set of symptoms, and chlamydial PID is more likely to present with the former, more subtle symptoms.

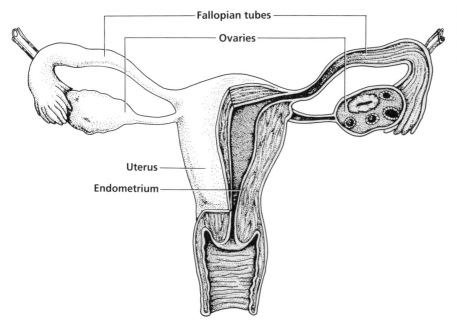

FIGURE 10.3
Pelvic inflammatory disease can affect any or all of a woman's reproductive organs.

Clinical evaluation is necessary for PID diagnosis. Although uterine tenderness is an indication of possible infection, bacterial culture is necessary to identify the causative bacteria and to determine the most appropriate treatment course. A sonogram may be performed if there is suspicion of an abscess and helps to determine whether or not surgery is indicated to drain the abscess. Permanent damage from PID is more likely if the infection has invaded the fallopian tubes. The tubes are fragile and easily damaged by an infectious process. Infection causes swelling and scarring of the tubes, which can lead to blockage and distortion, impairing future fertility. Pelvic abscess is another serious PID complication. Pus and live bacteria may leak from the open end of a fallopian tube and result in peritonitis and an abdominal abscess. Surgery may be indicated to drain the abscess. If PID is limited to the uterus, antibiotic treatment usually is sufficient to resolve the problem with little likelihood of permanent damage or future complications. Infection in the fallopian tubes, ovaries, or abdominal cavity is a cause for significant concern. Possible sequelae include infertility, ectopic pregnancy, repeated episodes of infection, and continuing pelvic pain. Women who have had PID must take elaborate precautions to avoid reinfection. Present and previous partner(s) must be treated whether or not they have symptoms.

Human Papillomavirus

HPV is also known as genital warts, venereal warts, condylomata, or condylomata acuminata. Although genital warts were long considered as trivial annoyances, they are now considered to be major STDs. The warts are very contagious and are the most common viral STD in the United States.[12] An accurate determination of HPV prevalence is difficult because genital HPV infections are not reportable conditions, and many infections are subclinical in nature, but it has been estimated that up to 10 percent of the sexually active population may harbor these viruses.[13] HPV is spread by direct contact, sexual and otherwise. It affects both males and females of all ages. Because HPV transmission may occur with nonsexual contact, a HPV-infected woman should advise her clinician to ensure that adequate precautions may be taken to avoid transmission. Likewise, clinicians should avoid risk of iatrogenic transmission from patient to patient via a contaminated speculum or by not changing gloves.

HPV infection is usually characterized by **lesions** or warts, which may first appear as small wens (round elevations in the skin) but which can generally grow in size and number and blend together in a cauliflower-like growth. Genital warts vary in size, may exist in single or multiple units, and may be raised or flat. In women, these lesions may occur on the buttocks, **anus,** inner thighs, vulva, vagina, and cervix. The lesions may be accompanied by heavy vaginal discharge, odor, and occasionally bleeding. The lesions may increase in size during pregnancy and regress, that is, spontaneously disappear, after delivery. When warts regress, the HPV is still present, just not readily apparent. Once contracted, HPV has a variable incubation period during which there are no symptoms and the person is not yet infectious. Warts usually appear 1 to 8 months after exposure. A **prodrome** period follows the **incubation** period, during which there are still no symptoms but the disease is contagious. This is the most dangerous period because the infected person does not know that she or he is capable of transmitting the virus to others. HPV lesions develop in more than 50 percent of the sexual partners of infected individuals.

Diagnosis is usually based on visual detection during clinical examination. Because warts are dry and painless and usually present on the vulva, cervix, inside the vagina, or around the rectum, women often are unaware that they are infected. Diagnosis may be difficult because many HPV infections are not macroscopically visible. Often the first indication of an abnormal condition is a routine Pap smear that identifies cervical cellular changes consistent with HPV infection. The virus cannot be cultured, but its presence can be firmly established by electron microscopy and strain identified by specific DNA hybridization techniques.

Because warts are highly contagious and likely to grow and spread, prompt treatment is essential. HPV infections can be quite persistent and have a tendency to recur regardless of treatment method. Treatment is easier and less painful in earlier stages, and if lesions are left untreated, serious complications, such as infection, may occur. There is no completely safe and effective HPV treatment modality. The particular treatment modality depends on the extent of HPV infection and its location. Treatment options include topical caustic agents, **electrocautery** (burning of warts), **cryotherapy** (freezing of warts), **chemotherapy,** laser surgery (vaporization of warts), and surgical **excision.** Local or general anesthesia is usually used with each of these treatments depending on the location and severity of the warts. The Food and Drug Administration (FDA) has approved the use of alpha interferon for the treatment of genital warts. Initial studies indicate that alpha interferon was effective against the most disfiguring type of genital warts, condylomata acuminata. Sexual partners should also be treated, and use of a condom is recommended during treatment and follow-up.

HPV presents special concerns with women. An increased risk of HPV infection is associated with the start of sexual activity at an early age, the number of sexual partners encountered, the use of nonbarrier methods of contraception, and the status of the host immune system. Certain conditions appear to enhance wart growth as well as interfere with treatment regimens. These conditions include other vaginal infections, poor personal hygiene, birth control pills, and any condition that alters the immune system. HPV can also present special problems in pregnancy. Occasionally the warts may become large enough to interfere with labor. Although it is relatively rare, a pregnant woman with HPV may pass the virus to her child during vaginal delivery.

Relationship with Cervical Cancer

One of the most important concerns with respect to HPV infection is its relationship to cervical and other lower genital tract cancers. Data suggest that cervical HPV infection is associated with about 90 percent of all cervical dysplasia and that there is a relationship between HPV-induced cellular changes and cervical cancer.[14] There are more than 50 identified strains of HPV. Some of the strains are believed to be responsible for genital cancers, including cervical cancer, vaginal cancer, vulvar cancer, and penile cancer. The cancer-causing strains may be rather inapparent to visual inspection or smooth and flat in appearance. Research suggests that these warts may be precursors or possibly co-carcinogens that work with other factors that lead to the development of cervical cancer. Strains 16, 18, 31, 33, 35, and 39 have been specifically implicated in cervical cancer development.[15] Although all women with HPV should exercise care and seek regular medical evaluation, women with these specific HPV strains are considered to be at high risk for the development of cervical cancer and should seek aggressive treatment and lifelong close medical monitoring. As shown in Information Box 10.1, the risk factors for cervical cancer coincide with STD risk factors. Cervical cancer itself has long been considered to be an STD. HPV does not appear to pose a direct threat for PID and future reproductive capability. Cervical cryosurgery or laser treatment to extensive wart growth, however, may result in tissue damage. Damage to cervical mucous glands is possible, and this may impair fertility. Cervical cancer resulting from HPV may require hysterectomy.

Special Precautions

Women with genital warts, especially in the cervical area, should seek aggressive treatment. Colposcopic examination and biopsy of suspicious areas are indicated. It is also important to be diligent about personal care, medical follow-up care, and annual Pap smears and pelvic examinations. Because it is possible for an infected person to **autoinoculate,** spread the disease from one part of the body to another part, women should take extra care when wiping the genital area or drying after bathing. Clinicians should be advised of previous genital wart

Risk Factors for Cervical Cancer

Intercourse before age 20

Multiple sex partners

Partner with multiple sex partners

Previous STD infection(s)

Cigarette smoking

Long-term use of oral contraceptives

history. Anyone with HPV should be extremely cautious because any form of direct contact can spread the virus. Condoms afford some protection against HPV. They may protect a woman against penile warts that are entirely covered by a condom. Also, condoms may afford a male partner protection from cervical lesions. Because genital warts may be present throughout the genital regions, however, there are no guarantees with condom usage.

Herpes Simplex Virus

Herpes simplex virus (HSV) has two types, HSV-1 and HSV-2. It used to be thought that HSV-1 was geographically localized above the waist, and HSV-2 was localized below the waist. It is now known that HSV-1 and HSV-2 are capable of invading each other's territory. HSV-1 causes infections of the mouth area and is commonly known as cold sores or fever blisters. HSV-2 has been traditionally known as genital herpes. Herpes genital infections are recurrent and incurable STDs. It is estimated that perhaps 30 million Americans have HSV.[4]

The first infection of HSV is usually the most severe. It may appear as soon as 1 day or as late as 3 to 4 weeks after exposure. Lasting about 12 days, it generally manifests as blisters in the genital area, fever, enlarged lymph nodes, and malaise. Recurrent attacks are usually milder in severity and shorter in duration, usually lasting about 5 days. Herpes presents as single or multiple small, painful blisters that generally appear in the vulva or buttocks of women. If they are present on the cervix, they usually are unnoticed. The blisters evolve into painful ulcers in a couple of days. These symptoms may be accompanied by vulvar swelling, fever, and enlarged and tender lymph nodes. These symptoms are more acute during the initial outbreak. A prodrome or warning phase often precedes a herpes outbreak. The warnings may consists of tingling or itching sensations in the area where sores later appear. Sores generally heal in 1 to 4 weeks with little or no scarring. It is not known what causes repeat outbreaks of herpes. Some individuals note that triggers such as sunlight exposure, menstrual changes, stress, poor nutrition, lack of rest or sleep, illness, and exposure to extreme heat or cold seem to prompt an outbreak, whereas others are unable to notice any triggering events.

Herpes outbreaks show considerable variability. Some herpes outbreaks last as long as 3 weeks, and others are as short as a few days. Some outbreaks are characterized by multiple blisters, others by a single blister. Some individuals experience outbreaks every few months, and others have one or more a month. A very few more fortunate individuals never experience recurrent outbreak symptoms after the initial event. Although some individuals may not be aware of herpes symptoms, infectiousness remains an important concern.

Active herpes sores are contagious during both the initial attack and recurrences. Both HSV-1 and HSV-2 can be spread from sores to the eye, where serious infection is possible. Herpes may be spread to infants and children via kissing or casual contact. Viral shedding is a term used when a culture of genital secretions shows definite evidence of the herpes virus, even though the individual may have not have apparent herpes sores at the time. Viral shedding has been shown to occur 2 to 20 days during an initial outbreak and 2 to 5 days during recurrent outbreaks. Viral shedding has been also demonstrated during latent periods. Researchers have not been able to determine exactly how infectious an individual is when viral shedding occurs in the absence of symptoms. Herpes transmission has been known to occur in the absence of symptoms. The risk of transmission is considerably higher when active sores are present because active sores demonstrate hundreds of times more virus than viral sheddings from genital secretions.

Herpes may be suspect for diagnosis based on history or recurrent pattern of illness. Diagnosis of herpes is made by culture or immunological test smear of cells taken with a cotton swab from an active herpes blister or sore. Presently there is no effective biomedical cure for herpes. Medications may be prescribed to relieve pain, and antibiotic ointment may be applied to help prevent a secondary bacterial infection of the sore. Acyclovir is the present treatment of choice for herpes, not curing the condition but helping to relieve symptoms and shorten healing time. Acyclovir works by inhibiting the virus' ability to use proteins and thereby reducing its ability to replicate. Three different acyclovir treatment regimens have received FDA approval. They are for (1) initial outbreak, (2) short-term recurrence therapy, and (3) long-term recurrence therapy. The drug should be avoided if a woman is pregnant or breastfeeding. Most clinicians advise that acyclovir be taken at the earliest signs of a herpes outbreak, including any prodromal symptoms such as itching or tingling. Although various other forms of herpes treatment have been advocated, such as photoinactivation, ether, nitrous oxide, lysine, and smallpox vaccination, none of these strategies have demonstrated clinical effectiveness in reducing symptoms or recurrences.

Special Precautions

Good personal hygiene is essential during a herpes outbreak. The infected individual must exercise great caution with handwashing if the herpes sores are touched. Care should be taken to avoid spreading the virus to others, including infants and children. If active herpes are present in or near the mouth, kissing should be avoided, and personal objects such as washcloths, toothbrushes, drinking cups, and towels should not be shared. These are precautionary measures, for although clinical studies have not demonstrated effective indirect transmission, the virus can remain alive outside the body for several hours in a moist environment.

Herpes sexual transmission is an important issue. Viral shedding can occur even in the absence of symptoms, so there are no guarantees of a "safe sex" time with herpes. At a minimum, sexual intercourse, including oral sex, must be avoided when active herpes sores are present. Because viral populations are so high in sores, individuals should wait until the sores are completely healed before resuming sexual activity. Because it is difficult to tell when a herpes outbreak is beginning, open communication about risks and feelings is essential. Condoms may help to provide a degree of protection, but because herpes sores can be present in areas not covered by the condom, again there are no guarantees against transmission. Condoms are especially important in a situation in which the male partner has herpes, and the female partner does not and she is pregnant. An initial attack of herpes during pregnancy presents serious risks to the developing fetus.

Women with herpes should be especially diligent about annual Pap smears and routine gynecological examinations. Women with herpes are at increased risk for cervical cancer and HPV. Pregnant women with herpes need to begin prenatal care early. If active lesions are present in the vaginal canal at the time of birth, a cesarean delivery will probably be done to avoid exposing the infant to the virus. Infant exposure to the virus may cause severe systemic illness and death.

Communication

Communicating about sex is often difficult, but it is especially so when the topic is incurable STDs. Risk of transmission is real. Timing of the communication is obviously important—after sex is an inappropriate time to tell or find out about herpes. Many communities have herpes support groups, which are good sources of practical information and solace. Studies have found that psychosocial adjustment to recurrent genital HSV infections is facilitated by sharing and communicating the diagnosis with a supportive spouse or lover and by avoiding denial as a coping mechanism.

Comfort Measures

Keeping the genital area clean and dry minimizes discomfort during a herpes flareup. A hair dryer on a cool setting may be used to dry the area thoroughly without irritation or discomfort. Genital cleansing must be gentle because rubbing can cause lesions to break and bleed. Many women find **sitz baths** comforting during outbreaks of herpes. Domeboro solution or baking soda may be added to the sitz bath. Cold wet compresses or individually wrapped cleansing pads containing glycerol and witch hazel applied to the sores may also provide temporary relief of discomfort, especially during oozing. Some women also find icepacks helpful in reducing discomfort during outbreaks.

I don't sleep around a lot. I have been with only three guys. But I have herpes. I can't tell where I got it . . . I mean, it's like I have slept with not only those guys, but everyone else they have had sex with. How can a person really trust someone not to have an STD these days?

21-YEAR-OLD WOMAN

Syphilis

In comparison to other STDs, cases of syphilis are relatively rare (see Fig. 10.1), but long-term effects when untreated are devastating. Reported syphilis rates have doubled in the United States since 1984.[1] Syphilis is caused by the bacterial organism, *Treponema pallidum.* It has also been known in history as the "Great Pox." Although syphilis rates are not nearly as high as gonorrhea, recent increases have caused public health officials to become quite concerned. Syphilis is highly infectious and has a long, varied clinical course but is treatable and curable in its early stages. If untreated, syphilis may result in serious consequences, including cardiac and neurological damage and ultimately death. Diagnosis of syphilis is confirmed by identification of antibodies in a blood test, although the antibodies do not appear until 6 to 7 weeks after exposure. The syphilis organism may sometimes be visualized with darkfield microscopy from sore secretions. High doses of antibiotics are prescribed for early-stage syphilis. More prolonged, intensive treatment is indicated if the individual has been infected for a year or more. Antibiotics can stop the course of syphilis progression but cannot undo its damage. For all stages of syphilis, sexual partners(s) must be concurrently treated.

There are three major stages of syphilis, which present with unique symptoms. Primary syphilis is the first disease stage. It usually occurs about 3 weeks but can occur up to 12 weeks after sexual contact with an infected individual. Usually the first symptom is an open sore, called a chancre, at the site of sexual contact. Only a small portion of women who develop a chancre know it because it is often located deep inside the vagina. The chancre is usually painless, regardless of its location, although from its appearance, it would not appear to be so. The chancre heals and disappears without scarring within 2 to 6 weeks, whether or not the individual receives treatment. The secondary stage of syphilis is variable as well and occurs within 1 week to 6 months after the primary stage. The secondary stage symptoms include a range of conditions, such as a fever; flulike symptoms; rash, most notably on the palms of the hands and soles of the feet; sore mouth and throat; joint pain; loss of appetite; nausea; headache; and inflamed sensitive eyes. Some individuals experience a patchy loss of scalp hair. Condylomata, broad-based moist sores, may appear around the genital and anal areas. Individuals are highly infectious in the secondary stage of syphilis. Symptoms usually last 3 to 6 months but may appear and then disappear again for several years. Tertiary syphilis symptoms appear 10 to 20 years after initial exposure if the individual has not received treatment. These symptoms may include heart disease, brain damage, spinal cord damage, and blindness. A special concern to women is that syphilis can also pass from an infected woman to her developing fetus. Syphilis infection during pregnancy often results in miscarriage, stillbirth, or severe birth defects.

Special Precautions

Syphilis is a highly infectious, destructive disease. Prevention measures are the same as for other STDs (see under Informed Decision Making—Reproductive Tract Infections). A person infected with syphilis and sexual partner(s) should be treated at the same time and avoid intercourse and all sexual intimacy for at least a month until repeat blood tests indicate that treatments have been effective. Effective treatment in the primary and secondary stages can prevent further serious, permanent damage.

Hepatitis

Hepatitis is an inflammation of the liver. It is caused by three distinctive viruses, type A, B, and non-A, non-B. Each may be transmitted via sexual intimacy. Non-A, non-B hepatitis presents as illness similar to hepatitis B, but clinicians are unable to show direct evidence of the virus for hepatitis A or B. Hepatitis A was formerly known as infectious hepatitis. It is usually a mild illness that resolves within a few weeks. It has primarily infected young adults and children and is spread through close contact and exposure to oral secretions or fecal matter of an infected person. It may also be spread through contaminated water or food, or rarely through blood products. A common source of hepatitis A is uncooked shellfish from contaminated waters. Sexual contact is another mode of transmission.

Hepatitis B is also spread by sexual contact, and this is the most important route of transmission for the virus. It may also be transmitted via shared needles among drug users and accidental needle-sticks or contaminated surgical instruments among health care workers. Active virus has been isolated from body secretions, such as tears, sweat, saliva, vaginal secretions, and semen of infected individuals. Hepatitis B was formerly called serum hepatitis and was often transmitted via contaminated blood. Today sensitive laboratory tests are available, and transmission via contaminated blood is rare. Symptoms of hepatitis B range from asymptomatic states to severe incapacitation. Liver failure is a severe complication of hepatitis B. Another serious complication is persistent infection, which can occur with no apparent symptoms, called a carrier state, or can lead to chronic liver disease. This persistent infection can result in permanent liver scarring and liver failure. Hepatitis B infects about 300,000 individuals annually in the United States (see Fig. 10.1). It is a common problem in some parts of the world, such as Africa and Southeast Asia.

Diagnosis of hepatitis is based on clinical symptoms and laboratory tests, which confirm the type of virus. Although some individuals are asymptomatic, most do have symptoms of hepatitis, which include low-grade fever, fatigue, headache, generalized aches, loss of appetite, nausea and vomiting, abdominal pain, and jaundice, a yellowish hue to the skin and eyes. There is no biomedical cure for hepatitis. Symptoms are treated along with rest and supportive care. A healthy diet is important, and alcohol should be avoided until liver function tests indicate that the liver is functioning normally again. Women on estrogen therapy, either birth control pills or replacement therapy, should discontinue these medications until normal liver function returns. Most individuals with hepatitis recover within a few weeks. Ten to 30 percent of infected individuals develop a persistent hepatitis infection, some with and without symptoms. Chronic hepatitis may lead to severe liver impairment and is associated with later liver cancer.

Special Precautions

Hepatitis should be considered an STD, and individuals need to take the same precautions against hepatitis as other viral STDs. A unique feature of hepatitis is that both hepatitis A and B may be prevented by treatment with immune globulin within 2 weeks of exposure. Immune globulin is made from pooled antibodies from blood donations, and it provides a temporary passive immune effect. Another unique feature of hepatitis B is that a vaccination is available that provides long-term immunity. The vaccination is a series of three injections that must be given in a 6-month period. The vaccination is expensive but is recommended for certain groups that are at higher risk for exposure to the virus. These groups are identified in Information Box 10.2.

Although a vaccination is not yet available for hepatitis A, it is recommended that exposed individuals receive immune globulin within 2 weeks of exposure for a temporary level of protection. Individuals who should receive immune globulin include sexual partners and household contacts of an individual with hepatitis A. If the infected person is a member of an institutional facility, such as a day care center, prison, or nursing home, staff and fellow clients should also receive immune globulin.

Vaginitis

Several kinds of vaginal infections can be transmitted through sexual interaction. Because they are also frequently transmitted through nonsexual means, they are not generally referred to as venereal diseases. *Trichomonas* infection, yeast infections, and bacterial vaginosis are fairly common reproductive tract infections. Although they are responsible for physical and emotional discomfort, they do not pose serious long-term health problems among basically healthy women.

Trichomonas Infection

Trichomonas infection is caused by a one-celled protozoan and is usually transmitted between individuals via sexual contact. The organism is capable of surviving outside a human host in a wet environment, such as a swimsuit or wet towel, and transmission between individuals can occur via these objects. Although some women do not experience symptoms with *Trichomonas* infection, when they occur they are particularly annoying. These symptoms include a frothy, thin, grayish or greenish vaginal discharge; intense itching; redness; an objectionable odor; pain; and urinary frequency. Diagnosis of *Trichomonas* infection is confirmed with a wet smear of vaginal secretions. Metronidazole (Flagyl, Metryl, Protostat, Satric) is the most effective antibiotic treatment for *Trichomonas* infection and is available in either a single-dose or multiple-dose format. Sexual partner(s) should be treated at the same time, and condoms should be used for the first 4 to 6 weeks after treatment to avoid reinfection. Because Flagyl may compromise the body's ability to produce white blood cells, a blood test may be warranted after treatment. Flagyl should be avoided during pregnancy. Also, alcohol should not be ingested while taking Flagyl.

Yeast Infections

Yeast (also known as *Candida albicans,* fungus infection, monilia, and candidiasis) organisms normally exist in the microscopic ecosystem of the body. Yeast

---

INFORMATION BOX 10.2

Individuals Considered to Be at High Risk of Exposure to Hepatitis B

Health care workers

Household contacts of a person infected with hepatitis B

Sexual partner(s) of a person infected with hepatitis B

Individuals with multiple partners

Staff and clients of residential institutions, including prisons

Individuals receiving hemodialysis or blood products

Intravenous drug users

is usually not sexually transmitted. When yeast overgrows, the symptoms are quite annoying. A thick, white, cottage cheese–type vaginal discharge; redness; swelling; and itching are common symptoms. Diagnosis is generally made by microscopic examination of a sample of the vaginal discharge. Yeast infections are usually treated with antibiotic vaginal cream (Monistat, Gyne-Lotrimin, Myceles, Femstat) with dosage regimens of 1, 3, or 7 days, depending on the medication. Treatment of partners is usually not necessary. FDA approval has made these medications available in over-the-counter forms. For women with chronic and recurrent infections, this has facilitated treatment by reducing the waiting time for a prescription and the expense of a clinical visit. For women who are not sure what type or kind of vaginal infection they may have, self-treatment is not a good idea. Although various groups have advocated treatment modalities such as yogurt douches, commercial douches, *Lactobacillus* capsules, and cranberry juice, these regimens have not been subjected to clinical trials, and their efficacy is unknown.

Although yeast infections do not usually invade the pelvis and affect fertility, reinfection is common and annoying. Recurrent attacks may occur shortly after treatment or be delayed for a considerable period of time. What causes yeast to grow out of control is unknown. Yeast is a ubiquitous inhabitant of intestinal and vaginal tracts. Persistent yeast problems often present during pregnancy and with women who take oral contraceptives. Women with diabetes and women who are overweight report higher frequencies of yeast infections. For women with recurrent infections, prolonged or intermittent treatment is often recommended to keep yeast growth under control. Concurrent treatment for yeast whenever antibiotics are prescribed may also be indicated for women with chronic yeast infections.

Bacterial Vaginosis

Bacterial vaginosis is known by many terms, including nonspecific vaginitis, *gardnerella vaginalis,* bacterial vaginitis, *Haemophilis vaginalis, Corynebacterium vaginalis,* and anaerobic vaginosis. The condition is caused by an overgrowth of normal vaginal organisms, which may be transmitted by sexual activity. Bacterial vaginosis has been found to be more prevalent among women with more than one sexual partner, intrauterine device (IUD) users, and women who have cervicitis. Symptoms include a gray or white adherent discharge that may be thick or watery, and it may have an objectionable odor. Painful urination, vaginal pain or burning during intercourse, redness, and itching may also be present. Diagnosis is made with microscopic examination of a discharge sample and ruling out the possibility of *Trichomonas* or yeast infections. Culture tests may be done to rule out the possibility of chlamydia or gonorrhea. Bacterial vaginosis may coexist with other STDs, so definitive diagnosis is important to ensure adequate treatment. Treatment of vaginosis is usually with oral antibiotics. Routine partner treatment is not standard procedure, although it may be indicated if reinfection occurs after treatment or if sexual transmission is suspected as the mode of acquisition. Antibacterial douches may also be effective in concert with oral antibiotics to relieve symptoms. Bacterial vaginosis is suspect for uterine and fallopian tube infections, so prompt, adequate treatment is indicated.

Informed Decision Making— Reproductive Tract Infections

When a woman elects to become sexually active, she must assume responsibility for the decision. This responsibility extends beyond the pregnancy protection arena to include STD protection. A strong knowledge base is the first step in STD protection. Every woman should have a thorough understanding of STD risk, symptoms to watch for, and prevention strategies. Many STDs last forever— an ounce of prevention is worth far more than a pound of cure for there are not always cures.

Apart from abstinence, the most reliable preventive for a reproductive tract infection is long-term monogamy with a partner who is also monogamous. The most significant risk factor for an STD is the woman's partner(s). The risk increases when a woman has more than one sex partner and when her partner has more than one sex partner. STDs should be considered anytime a woman is not in an exclusively (strictly) monogamous long-term relationship. STDs are transmitted by sexual intimacy. Intimacy includes "traditional" sex (penis in vagina) and other forms of intimate skin-to-skin and mucous membrane–to–mucous membrane contact. STDs can thus be transmitted with oral or anal sex. STDs can be transmitted in both homosexual and heterosexual encounters, although they are less common among lesbian women. Although the notion of "safe sex" is misleading, there are "safer sex" practices, which reduce the overall risk of acquiring STD. A comparison of safer, risky, and dangerous sex practices is provided in Information Box 10.3.

Birth control choice influences STD risk. The use of condoms or a diaphragm with spermicide helps to reduce the risk of STD transmission by about 50 percent. This is still far from 100 percent protection. Even women who are on the pill or who have been surgically sterilized may benefit from these methods. Studies have shown that women who use oral contraceptives have lower rates for PID than women who use other forms of birth control. The mechanism for this protection is not well understood. It may be that the reduction in menstrual flow caused by the pill provides a less than optimal environment for bacterial growth. Or it may be related to the thick cervical mucous plug present during most of the pill-taker's cycle, which acts as a more formidable barrier to bacteria attempting to invade the pelvis. This is somewhat contradictory because women on oral contraceptives have demonstrated a tendency for increased cervical infections. The delicate cervical canal lining extending from the cervical opening may be less resistant to infection than the hardy tissue that normally covers the cervical surface. While providing decreased risk for PID, the pill does seem to increase risk for cervical infection. Women on the pill, therefore, may want to protect themselves from STDs by using a diaphragm,

Joe had a long-term relationship with this girl and they broke up last year. I used to worry about that relationship, but now I am more worried about the insignificant encounters he had after they broke up. He doesn't know anything about them, and neither do I. How do I evaluate my risk?

23-YEAR-OLD WOMAN

INFORMATION BOX 10.3

Safer, Risky, and Dangerous Sex Practices

Safer	Risky	Dangerous
Fantasy	French (wet) kissing	Oral sex—no condom
Masturbation—single or mutual; healthy/intact skin	Masturbation on open/broken skin	Vaginal intercourse—no condom
External water sports: (urination)	Oral sex on a woman	Anal intercourse—no condom
Touching	Sexual practices involving:	Internal water sports (urination)
	Speed (amphetamines)	Sharing needles with partners
	Amyl nitrite (poppers)	
	Alcohol	Fisting (anal penetration with hand)
	Marijuana	Rimming (oral-anal sex)
	Intravenous drugs	

vaginal sponge, or condom with sexual activity. There is evidence that condoms and spermicides are effective in inactivating the viruses that cause herpes, genital warts, and AIDS. Again there are no guarantees of total protection, for viruses located at sites other than the penis, such as the scrotum, anal region, or vulva, are not affected by condoms and spermicides, and transmission from these sites can still occur.

Frank, honest communication before sexual intimacy is essential (Information Box 10.4). Although it may be hard to have an honest discussion about infections and previous risk behaviors, the price is too high not to. Honest communication is a mark of personal maturity. If a potential partner is unable or unwilling to discuss infections and intimacy concerns, it may be an indication of other issues that merit evaluation before proceeding with sexual closeness. Sexual closeness should be avoided if either partner has any symptoms of infection or if there are any suspicions of infection. It is wiser to delay activity for a few days and have symptoms evaluated than to deal with possible lifelong consequences. To be on the "safe side," many couples now see a clinician together for examination and HIV testing before initiating a sexual relationship.

When to See a Clinician

STDs present special clinical challenges for women. Symptoms may be present, absent, or mistaken for other conditions. As shown in Information Box 10.5, there are several critical times when a woman should seek assistance in evaluating

I felt weird when Karen insisted that we go to the doctor together before we had sex. I guess I was afraid that one of us would have something. But we didn't and you know, I think that our relationship is stronger because she insisted. I respect her for having the courage it took to do that. I wish that it had been my idea.

22-YEAR-OLD MAN

Questions for Women to Ask Potential Male Sex Partners*

Have you ever suspected that you had an STD?

Have you been tested or examined for STDs or HIV?

How many sex partners have you had?

Have you ever had sex with a prostitute?

Have you ever had sex with another man?

Have you ever injected drugs?

Have your sex partners ever injected drugs?

Did you have a blood transfusion or receive blood products before 1985? (when blood was not screened for HIV)

*While recognizing that there are no guarantees with answers or honesty, it is still important for women to inquire about their potential sex partner's past before becoming intimate.

Symptoms That May Suggest a Sexually Transmitted Disease and Warrant Clinical Evaluation

Unusual vaginal discharge or bleeding

Pain or burning with urination or bowel movements

Genital itching

Sores, warts, blisters, or growths in the genital area

Pain or bleeding associated with intercourse

Abdominal or back pain or tenderness

Severe menstrual cramping

Chills, fever, aches, malaise

a possible reproductive tract infection. If a woman just suspects that she may have an infection, it is important that she be evaluated. STDs have a spectrum of symptoms, including no symptoms. Waiting for symptoms to go away is an exercise in futility, because although some symptoms may in fact temporarily disappear, the disease may still be present, transmissible, and damaging. If a partner has an infection or is suspicious of an infection, it is important to curtail sexual activity, and both individuals should seek clinical evaluation. Treating one partner and not the other often results in a ping-pong reinfection process. Sharing one antibiotic prescription between two people usually means that both individuals go untreated. Using leftover antibiotics from previous infections is equally foolhardy because supplies are usually inappropriate and inadequate and may serve only to mask the symptoms, complicating an accurate diagnosis at a later time. Sexual activity should be curtailed or condoms diligently used until both partners are certain of an STD cure.

Women are often embarrassed to mention their fears of STD to a clinician. If there is a risk of infection, it is important to mention this to the clinician. Clinicians may not routinely test for STDs or look for them in a routine gynecological examination. If a woman knows she has an infectious condition such as HSV or HPV, she should advise her clinician to reduce the likelihood of accidental transmission. If oral or anal sex have been part of the sexual experience, the clinician should be advised so a comprehensive examination may be conducted for an accurate diagnosis. Antibiotic treatments vary depending on the site of the infection. A clean bill of health from a gynecologist is not of much value if an undiagnosed gonococcal throat infection is present.

The physical examination for STDs is much like a routine gynecological examination, but it is not be limited to the genital area. An examination of the mouth, throat, and lymph nodes usually precedes the genital examination. The genital examination is conducted in a lithotomy position. It begins with a careful visual inspection by the clinician. A speculum is inserted into the vagina for an internal examination. The clinician examines the vagina for discharge, odor, ulcerations, or inflammation. If a woman has douched before the visit, the clinician may not be able to diagnose the condition accurately. A bimanual examination follows the internal examination (see Chapter 7 on the pelvic examination). Any suspicious lesion in the perianal area is cultured, and a rectal culture is obtained if the woman has had rectal intercourse.

Treatment Concerns

Treatment regimens for STDs vary according to the specific pathogen, the severity of infection, location of infection, previous infections, and personal medical history. The clinician should be advised if there are any other prescriptions or over-the-counter medications that are also being used. Previous drug reactions are important information. Any previous reaction to a drug ending in "cillin" is a contraindication to any other "cillin" drug. If a woman suspects that she may be pregnant, it is important to advise the clinician. Tetracycline should not be taken by pregnant women because it produces severe staining of the permanent teeth of the developing fetus. Sulfa drugs, acyclovir, lindane, and Flagyl (metronidazole) should also be avoided by pregnant women. When medications are prescribed by a clinician, it is of paramount importance that they be taken as prescribed. If antibiotics are prescribed for 10 days, they need to be taken for 10 days even though symptoms may dissipate earlier.

Several STDs require follow-up examinations to make sure that treatment was successful. Failure to comply with follow-up guidelines may result in unsuccessful treatment and continued disease transmission and damage. Reproductive tract infections may cause abnormal Pap test findings. After an infection is cleared up, it is a good idea to have a Pap test repeated in 6 to 12 weeks. A reading at that time is a more accurate report of the cervical status than one conducted during a period of inflammation.

AIDS

AIDS is a progressive disease characterized by the destruction of the immune system. There is no effective cure or vaccine available. Prevention is the only modality currently available to interrupt the progression of this fatal disease. When the AIDS virus (HIV) enters the bloodstream, it begins to attack specific white blood cells, T lymphocytes. The virus attacks these T cells and replicates. The T cells are no longer able to stimulate a cellular defense response, and the body's systemic immune system is compromised.

Opportunistic infections present a potentially fatal risk to individuals with AIDS. **AIDS-related complex** (ARC) is a general term for an intermediate phase of HIV infection between no symptoms and full-blown AIDS. The term is not as common now as it was in the early years of the epidemic. Asymptomatic HIV-infected individuals are capable of transmitting the virus to others, even in the absence of symptoms. The AIDS incubation period ranges from a few months to several years or more. As evidenced by recent revelations from Hollywood and the national sports scene, no individual or groups of individuals are immune to AIDS. HIV is transmitted from one person to another through sexual intercourse, shared intravenous needle use, or shared blood or blood products. An individual with HIV may have no physical symptoms, so it is impossible to tell whether or not a person is infected. HIV is not spread by casual, social, or family contact. One cannot acquire the virus by touching or being near a person with AIDS.

HIV blood testing is a mechanism to detect HIV antibodies. The **enzyme-linked immunosorbent assay** (ELISA) is an HIV screening test that is repeated if positive results are found. If a repeat ELISA is also positive, a confirmatory **western blot** test should be performed. Because it may take as long as 1 year for a person to develop HIV antibodies after exposure, a negative HIV blood test is not a guarantee against exposure. HIV tests are available at local blood banks, AIDS research programs, and alternative test sites that have mechanisms in place to provide confidential results and pretesting and posttesting counseling services.

Historical Overview

Although the history of AIDS is relatively short, the human destruction of the disease cannot be calculated. It is not known for sure when or where AIDS started. Some experts have speculated that the disease originated in Africa in the 1970s. AIDS was first diagnosed in the United States in 1981. Homosexual and bisexual men currently constitute about 74 percent of US AIDS cases.[17] Their large percentage is attributed to high-risk behavior patterns, not being homosexual or bisexual. A historical myth of this disease is that AIDS is a homosexual disease; anyone, whether homosexual, bisexual, or heterosexual, who engages in risky sexual behavior or intravenous drug use behaviors is susceptible to the AIDS virus (Information Box 10.6). AIDS has now killed more Americans than the Korean and Vietnam wars combined—more than 120,000 have died from AIDS, and the numbers are accelerating to an unknown

Dispelling AIDS Myths

AIDS is not a disease of homosexual men.

AIDS may not be spread by casual contact.

Women are susceptible to AIDS.

There is no risk of acquiring AIDS by donating blood.

Information and education are the only weapons against AIDS.

Confidential, anonymous testing for AIDS is available.

level.[17] It is estimated that there are currently 1 to 2 million HIV-infected individuals in the United States, but only a fraction have developed AIDS. More than 50 percent of those with AIDS have died. No one has completely recovered from AIDS. Internationally it is estimated that 8 to 10 million people may be HIV infected.

Special Concerns for Women

Women have not been equally recognized as an at-risk, HIV-susceptible population. The initial focus on male homosexuality as a risk factor is one reason. In North America and in Western Europe, where the primary modes of HIV transmission have been homosexual and bisexual contact and intravenous drug use, the threat posed by heterosexual contact has been largely denied until recently. The World Health Organization estimates that three-quarters of the 8 to 10 million people infected with HIV worldwide have been infected through heterosexual contact.[16] The rise in heterosexually acquired infections has serious implications for women. Women are currently the fastest growing group in the United States infected with HIV. Women make up more than 12 percent of the total numbers of adult/adolescent AIDS cases.[17] Heterosexual transmission accounts for at least 34 percent of AIDS cases in women in the United States.[17]

In many ways, including a research perspective, women have been the "missing persons" in the US HIV/AIDS epidemic. Emphasis has focused on gay and bisexual men and babies.[20] In many studies, women have been seen as "vehicles" or "vectors" of transmission to men via the commercial sex industry[21] and intravenous drug abuse[22] and to their children.[23] Failure to focus on women as a unique group creates significant obstacles in epidemiological assessment.

Epidemiological Data and Trends

AIDS in women presents a different epidemiological pattern from that found among men. Presently in the United States, more than 12 percent of AIDS cases are women, but this proportion is expected to grow rapidly within the next several years.[17] Women have been identified as the fastest growing category of the AIDS

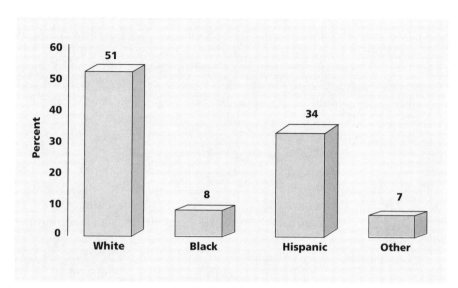

FIGURE 10.4

Race/ethnicity differences in AIDS incidence rates among women, 1991.

SOURCE: Centers for Disease Control (1991). *HIV/AIDS Surveillance Report.*

epidemic, and AIDS is now the leading cause of death of reproductive-age women in New York and New Jersey.[19] AIDS is expected to be one of the top five causes of death nationally for the group soon. Eighty-five percent of women with AIDS are of reproductive age,[18] and ethnic minority women represent the highest proportion of HIV-infected women in the United States. Although African-American and Hispanic-American women compose 19 percent of the American female population, they represent 73 percent of the AIDS cases in women[17] (Fig. 10.4). African-American women experience higher mortality from AIDS than white women: They are nine times more likely to die of AIDS than white women.[19] Nearly 50 percent of HIV-infected women are believed to have acquired the virus from intravenous drug abuse (Fig. 10.5). Others became infected from heterosexual contact with an infected partner (32 percent) or via blood transfusions.

Despite these alarming data, it is unlikely that the current prevalence rates of HIV among women accurately represent the true magnitude of the disease. The CDC have identified criteria for AIDS diagnosis. Their list of opportunistic infections has been based on symptoms of male populations who contracted AIDS via homosexual contact or intravenous drug use. HIV-infected women often develop serious gynecological problems that are HIV related, but because these problems did not meet CDC criteria, they have not been diagnosed with AIDS. Only recently have the diagnostic criteria been modified to address the gynecological symptoms consistent with the clinical picture of AIDS in women.

Clinical Dimensions and Treatment Issues

In the United States, women are actually at a greater risk for HIV than men from heterosexual intercourse.[24] It has been hypothesized that this may be due

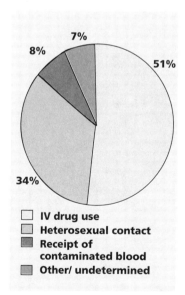

FIGURE 10.5

AIDS cases by exposure category, women, United States, 1990.

SOURCE: Centers for Disease Control, (1991). *HIV/AIDS Surveillance Report.*

to a larger pool of infected men than women or to the probability that, in heterosexual intercourse, transmission of the virus is more efficient from male to female than from female to male. Once diagnosed with AIDS, women become sicker and do not survive as long as men. It is not clear if this increased morbidity is due to social issues or clinical issues, such as delayed recognition of symptoms and diagnosis.

Perinatal transmission of AIDS is a special concern of women because the majority of HIV-infected women are of reproductive age. If a woman is infected with HIV and becomes pregnant, she is more likely to develop ARC or classic AIDS, and she can transmit the virus to her unborn child.[33] Approximately one-third of the babies born to HIV-infected mothers are also infected.[25] Most of the infected babies eventually develop AIDS and die. Pediatric AIDS is the ninth leading cause of death in children 1 to 4 years old in the United States.[26]

Although studies suggest that gynecological symptoms are often the first signs of HIV infection in women, they have only recently been included in CDC criteria for diagnosis. When women seek treatment for these gynecological conditions, HIV testing may be delayed or avoided because it is not suspected. Potential indicators of HIV infection in women include gynecological infections such as candidiasis or PID, HPV, genital ulcers, HSV, opportunistic infections, pneumonias, and sepsis.[27]

Social Issues

AIDS disproportionately affects African-American women. Many women with AIDS are socially and economically deprived. African-American women often have limited access to health care facilities. Many do not have health insurance or information on how to access and use scarce public health care services. Because of limitations with the male-based CDC diagnostic criteria for AIDS, many women are not diagnosed with AIDS and are therefore ineligible for many benefits and services available to others diagnosed with AIDS and are excluded from clinical trials.

Epidemiological efforts have viewed women as vectors of AIDS transmission to their offspring and male sexual partners. Earlier studies were limited to perinatal assessment efforts and surveys of prostitutes. Women were not considered as victims of transmission from their male partners. The identification of "high-risk groups" (homosexual and bisexual men, intravenous drug users, hemophiliacs, prostitutes, inmates, and people from specific geographical areas) served both to stigmatize the members of these groups and to promote denial of risk among nongroup members. Women are often unaware of the risks to themselves or others because they may not belong to high-risk groups, but they may practice high-risk behaviors. Or women may not be aware of the high-risk behaviors or behavioral histories of their partners. Women must understand that high-risk behaviors are of concern, not group membership.

Research on AIDS knowledge, attitudes, and beliefs among various groups

I knew that there was no way I could be positive for HIV. I am not a virgin, but I don't sleep around a lot, and I don't use drugs. I wasn't worried. I guess I should have been because here I am, 27 years old, and I have HIV. I keep thinking, why me? I don't deserve this.

27-YEAR-OLD WOMAN

of women pales in comparison with male studies. The impact of ethnicity and culture on women's attitudes and knowledge has received limited study. Findings indicate that basic information on prevention is not reaching women at highest risk for infection. A recent National Survey of Family Growth found that low-income women and non-Hispanic, African-American women were more likely to have misinformation concerning the means of HIV transmission and to say that they had a greater chance of contracting the disease.[28]

Pregnancy and HIV has been a heavily debated topic. In 1985, the CDC advised HIV-infected women to delay childbearing until more is known about perinatal transmission of the virus. Early retrospective studies of women with AIDS found a wide range of estimates for the rate of perinatal transmission.[23] Many state health departments have advised HIV-infected women unequivocally not to become pregnant. Concern has been expressed that these are quasi-coercive measures insensitive to the life experiences, feelings, and needs of women. These measures and attitudes fail to recognize that pregnancy and babies have a special symbolism for many poor African-American women. For women with few options, reproductive freedom is crucial. For many, having children is integral to their biological and social being, often tied to hopes and dreams that cannot be realized in other ways.[29] The positive cultural value attached to childbearing among African-American and Hispanic-American women may partially explain the decisions to conceive even in the threat of spreading HIV.[30] Moreover, public health efforts to prevent pregnancy are viewed by some minorities as part of a plan for genocide.[31,32]

Informed Decision Making

With the prevalence of AIDS and STDs at epidemic proportions, the most important consideration is prevention. AIDS presents special challenges because no biomedical cures or vaccinations are available. Although it is not always a reasonable solution, abstinence is the only guaranteed prevention mechanism. In the absence of abstinence, sex with a mutually monogamous HIV-negative partner is the next level of prevention (Information Box 10.7). If there is any doubt about the "mutually monogamous status" or HIV status, "safer sex" practices are necessary for prevention. Safer sex is any form of sex in which semen or vaginal secretions are not passed from one person to another. It is not as safe as not having sex, but the risk of HIV transmission is reduced. Condoms with spermicidal agents are the key ingredients of safer sex practices. They must be correctly used—if they break or fall off, their protective effect is lost. Latex condoms provide a better barrier than natural membrane condoms. Although condoms certainly provide considerably more protection than noncondom sex, it must be remembered that condom use is no guarantee against HIV infection. The risk of HIV infection also increases with the number of sexual partners: The more partners a woman has and the more her partner has, the greater her risk of exposure to the virus.

INFORMATION BOX 10.7

Strategies for Avoiding the AIDS Virus

Sexual abstinence*

Sexual fidelity with a negative partner

Avoid exchange of body fluids with condom use

Avoid sexual partners at increased risk

*Only guaranteed strategy.

I don't know if I should be upset or not. Over spring break my boyfriend went skiing and he said he "slept around a little." So what should I do about protecting myself? I'm on the pill, but should we get tested or use a condom? I really am confused.

22-YEAR-OLD WOMAN

Summary

All reproductive tract infections, including STDs and HIV, pose serious health threats to women. By understanding these conditions (Information Box 10.8) and making informed decisions about personal behavior and health-seeking behavior, women can significantly reduce their risk of exposure and the effects of disease sequelae. Personal responsibility and informed decision making are essential to the prevention and management of reproductive tract infections.

Philosophical Dimensions: Reproductive Tract Infections

1. It has been said that STDs are biologically "sexist." What does this mean?

2. Why have STD programs failed to bring the epidemic under control in recent years?

FDA Panel Recommends Approval of Female Condom

Washington Post
January 31, 1992

An advisory panel to the Food and Drug Administration (FDA) has recommended approval of the first female condom—the only contraceptive ever developed for women that is designed to protect against STDs. The panel cited an urgent social need to give women a device of their own to protect against the spread of HIV and other diseases. The product, known as Reality, is expected to appear in drug stores by early 1993.

The condom is a 7-inch polyurethane sheath. The panel members acknowledged that it is not a perfect device and that there are concerns about its effectiveness as a contraceptive and the difficulty that women have had using it in clinical trials. The condom is also known as a "vaginal pouch" and has a ring on each end. The ring on the closed end is placed over the cervix like a diaphragm anchoring it behind the pubic bone. The material that extends from it lines the vaginal wall, with the open ring on the opposite end extending outside the body to prevent any skin contact between partners that would allow transmission of STDs. The sheath is lubricated on the inside.

Several problems have been noted with the product. Slippage and premature removal occurred in trials between 6.6 and 24 percent of the time. The device was not always used properly during the trials by the participants. Pregnancy rates for those using the device were also slightly higher than those recorded for diaphragm, cervical cap, or contraceptive sponge users.

The decision for approval was based in part on the need that women have to exercise control for protection against STDs.

Summary Facts of the Major Sexually Transmitted Diseases

	AIDS	Syphilis	Gonorrhea
Also known as:	Acquired immunodeficiency syndrome	Pox, bad blood, syph	GC, clap, drip
Organism:	HIV (human immunodeficiency virus)	*Treponema pallidum*	*Neisseria gonorrhoeae*
Transmission:	Shared body fluids, intravenous drug–using equipment, perinatal (mother to baby)	Direct contact—skin-to-skin or mucous-to-mucous contact with infectious sores or rashes	Direct contact between infectious mucous membranes
Symptoms:	Fever, weight loss, fatigue, enlarged lymph nodes, diarrhea; opportunistic infections	Primary stage: painless ulceration (chancre) Secondary stage: rash, enlarged lymph nodes, hair loss Tertiary syphilis: systemic damage	Most women are asymptomatic but may have vaginal discharge, urinary frequency; pelvic pain, fever, nausea, vomiting with advanced disease
Diagnosis:	Confirmed laboratory findings, T cell counts, symptoms	Blood tests, microscopic verification of organism, physical examination	Microscopic examination of discharge; culture of organism
Treatment:	No cure or vaccine yet available; several drugs being studied in clinical trials	Antibiotics	Antibiotics
Special concerns for women:	Disease criteria based on males; women are not considered or do consider themselves to be at risk; risk to unborn babies	Long-term effects, perinatal transmission	Pelvic inflammatory disease, sterility, systemic damage, transmission

	Chlamydia	HPV	HSV
Also known as:	*Chlamydia trachomatis*	Human papillomavirus, venereal warts, condyloma acuminata	Herpes simplex virus
Organism:	*Chlamydia trachomatis*—able to coexist with *Neisseria gonorrhoeae*	Human papillomavirusvirus—>50 strains	*Herpesvirus hominis*
Transmission:	Sexual contact—highly contagious	Direct contact with warts	Direct contact with infectious blisters or sores
Symptoms:	Women often asymptomatic: slight vaginal discharge, itching, vaginal burning, painful intercourse; abdominal pain and fever in advanced stages	Some women are asymptomatic; warts may be in internal cervical areas—unknown to woman; warty growths may be in external genital area	Painful sores on genitals, rectum, or mouth that heal and crust over; females may be asymptomatic with cervical lesions; outbreaks recur in somewhat sporadic manner
Diagnosis:	Difficult to culture; often diagnosed by ruling out gonorrhea	Diagnosed by observation or biopsy	Physical examination, microscopic examination, tissue culture

(continued)

Summary Facts of the Major Sexually Transmitted Diseases

	Chlamydia	HPV	HSV
Treatment:	Antibiotics (not penicillin)	Topical caustic agents, electrocautery, cryotherapy, chemotherapy, laser surgery, surgical excision	Acyclovir to reduce duration of symptoms; no cure or vaccine available
Special concerns for women:	Pelvic inflammatory disease; sterility; systemic damage; perinatal transmission	Warts may enlarge and obstruct vagina; association with cervical cancer; perinatal transmission	Increased risk of cervical cancer; perinatal transmission

	Hepatitis	Trichomoniasis	PID
Also known as:	Hepatitis A, hepatitis B, hepatitis non-A, non-B	Trich	Pelvic inflammatory disease
Organism:	Hepatitis virus	*Trichomonas vaginalis* (protozoan)	*Chlamydia trachomatis* or *Neisseria gonorrhoeae* (usually)
Transmission:	Sexual contact, shared body fluids, fecal-oral, nonsexual transmission	Direct sexual contact—contact with contaminated wet objects (swimsuits, towels)	Not transmitted per se but is a complication of untreated gonorrhea or chlamydial infections
Symptoms:	Some asymptomatic cases; nausea, fever, anorexia, dark urine, abdominal discomfort, jaundice, enlarged liver	Many women are asymptomatic; white or greenish yellow odorous vaginal discharge, vaginal itching, soreness, painful urination	Symptoms may initially be subtle; may be severe and sudden pelvic pain, fever, vaginal discharge, bleeding
Diagnosis:	Blood tests—liver function tests and clinical symptoms	Physical examination, microscopic examination of discharge, culture	Clinical evaluation; bacterial culture
Treatment:	No medical cure; immune globulin vaccine available for hepatitis B	Oral antibiotics	Antibiotics, possible surgery
Special concerns for women:	Premature birth or spontaneous abortion; perinatal transmission	Asymptomatic states, perinatal transmission	Impaired fertility or sterility, ectopic pregnancy, recurrent infection, continued pelvic pain

3. How do cultural and emotional dimensions complicate STD public health and educational efforts?

4. Why is reinfection so common with some bacterial STDs?

5. When during the course of a relationship should a woman mention that she has HSV or HPV?

6. How far should one inquire about a person's personal past?

7. In spite of the knowledge about AIDS, people still report a strong fear of AIDS. Why? What are some of the myths associated with AIDS?

8. What should a woman do upon learning of a positive AIDS antibody test?

References

1. USDHHS (1991). *Healthy People 2000: National Health Promotion and Disease Prevention Objectives.* (DHHS Pub. No. (PHS) 91-50212.) Washington, DC: US Government Printing Office.

2. Centers for Disease Control (1990). *Division of STD/HIV Prevention Annual Report, 1989.* Atlanta: USDHHS.

3. Centers for Disease Control (1985). *Chlamydia Trachomatis Infections: Policy Guidelines for Prevention and Control.* Atlanta: USDHHS.

4. Johnson, R.E., Nahmias, A.J., Magder, L.S., Lee, F.K., Brooks, C.A., and Snowden, C.B. (1989). Distribution of genital herpes (HSV-2) in the United States. A seroepidemiological national survey using a new type-specific antibody assay. *New England Journal of Medicine, 321,* 7–12.

5. Jenson, A.B. (1989). Historical perspectives and current perception of human papillomavirus infections: Part I. *Focus in Human Papillomavirus, 1*(Winter), 1–2.

6. Rice, R.J., Roberts, P.L., Handsfield, H.H., and Holmes, K.K. (1991). Sociodemographic distribution of gonorrhea incidence: Implications for prevention and behavioral research. *American Journal of Public Health, 81*(10), 1252–1258.

7. Centers for Disease Control (1988). Syphilis and congenital syphilis, 1985–88. *Morbidity and Mortality Weekly Report, 37,* 486–489.

8. As incidence of syphilis rises sharply in the U.S., racial differences grow. *Family Planning Perspectives, 23*(1), 43.

9. Zweig Greenberg, M.S., Singh, T., Htoo, M., and Schultz, S. (1991). The association between congenital syphilis and cocaine/crack use in New York City: A case control study. *American Journal of Public Health, 81*(10), 1316–1318.

10. Washington, A.E., and Katz, P. (1991). Cost of and payment source for pelvic inflammatory disease. *Journal of the American Medical Association, 266*(18), 2565–2569.

11. Aral, S.O., Mosher, W.D., and Cates, W. (1991). Self-reported pelvic inflammatory disease in the United States, 1988. *Journal of the American Medical Association, 266*(18), 2570–2573.

12. Davis, A.J., and Emans, S.J. (1989). Human papilloma virus infection in the pediatric and adolescent patient. *The Journal of Pediatrics, 115*(1), 1–9.

13. Bartholoma, N.Y. (1989). Genital warts. *Clinical Microbiology Newsletter, 11*(3), 17.

14. Kaufman, R.H., and Adam, E. (1986). Herpes simplex virus and human papilloma virus in the development of cervical carcinoma. *Clinics in Obstetrics and Gynecology, 29*(3), 678–692.

15. American College of Obstetricians and Gynecologists (1987). Genital human papillomavirus infections. *ACOG Technical Bulletin, 105,* 1–3.

16. World Health Organization (1991, November 11). World Health Organization says three-quarters of HIV infections transmitted heterosexually. *WHO Press,* Press Release WHO/54.

17. Centers for Disease Control. (1991). *HIV/AIDS Surveillance Report,* pp. 1–18. Atlanta, GA: CDC.

18. Ellerbrock, T., Bush, T., Chamberland, M., and Oxtoby, M. (1991). Epidemiology of women with AIDS in the United States, 1981 through 1990. *Journal of the American Medical Association, 265,* 2971–2975.

19. Chu, S.Y., Buehler, J.W., and Berkleman, R.L. (1990). Impact of the human immunodeficiency virus on mortality in women of reproductive ages, United States. *Journal of the American Medical Association, 264,* 225–229.

20. Rosser, S.V. (1991). Perspectives: AIDS and women. *AIDS Education and Prevention, 3,* 230–240.

21. Campbell, C.A. (1990). Prostitution and AIDS. In D.G. Ostrow (Ed.), *Behavioral Aspects of AIDS,* pp 101–119. New York: Plenum Publishing Corporation.

22. DesJarlais, D.C., Friedman, S.R., and Woods, J.S. (1990). Intravenous drug use and AIDS. In D.G. Ostrow (Ed.), *Behavioral Aspects of AIDS,* pp. 139–155. New York: Plenum Publishing Corporation.

23. Andiman, W.A., and Modlin, J.F. (1991). Vertical transmission. In P.A. Pizzo and C.M. Wilfert (Eds.), *Pediatrics AIDS,* pp. 14–15. Baltimore: Williams & Wilkins.

24. Guinan, M.E., and Hardy, A. (1987). Epidemiology of AIDS in women in the United States: 1981 through 1986. *Journal of the American Medical Association, 257,* 2039–2042.

25. Oxtoby, M.J. (1991). Perinatally acquired HIV infection. In P.A. Pizzo and C.M. Wilfert (Eds.), *Pediatric AIDS,* pp. 3–21. Baltimore: Williams & Wilkins.

26. Novello, A.C., Wise, P.H., Willoughby, A., and Pizzo, P.A. (1989). Final report of the United States Department of Health and Human Services Secretary's Work Group on pediatric human immunodeficiency virus infection and disease: Content and implications. *Pediatrics, 84,* 547–555.

27. American Public Health Association (January 1991). *Women and HIV Disease: A Report of the Special Initiative on AIDS of the American Public Health Association.* Washington, DC: American Public Health Association.

28. McNally, J.W., and Mosher, W.D. (1991). AIDS-related knowledge and behavior among women 15–44 years of age: United States, 1988. *Advance Data, 220,* 1–7.

29. Pivnick, A., Jacobson, A., Eric, K., Mulvihill, M., Hsu, M.A., and Drucker, E. (1991). Reproductive decisions among HIV-infected, drug-using women: The importance of mother-child coresidence. *Medical Anthropology Quarterly, 5,* 153–169.

30. Mitchell, J.L., and Heagarty, M. (1991). Special considerations of minorities. In P.A. Pizzo and C.M. Wilfert (Eds.), *Pediatric AIDS,* pp. 704–713. Baltimore: Williams & Wilkins.

31. Levine, C., and Dubler, N.N. (1990). Uncertain risks and bitter realities: The reproductive choices of HIV-infected women. *The Milbank Quarterly, 68,* 321–351.

32. Thomas, S.B., and Quinn, S.C. (1991). The Tuskegee Syphilis Study, 1932 to 1972: Implications for HIV education and AIDS risk education programs in the black community. *American Journal of Public Health, 81,* 1498–1504.

33. Fox, H.E. (1991). Obstetric issues and counseling women and parents. In P.A. Pizzo and C.M. Wilfert (Eds.), *Pediatric AIDS,* pp. 669–683. Baltimore: Williams & Wilkins.

Resources

AIDS TASK FORCE FOR THE AMERICAN COLLEGE HEALTH ASSOCIATION
804-924-2670

AMERICAN FOUNDATION FOR AIDS RESEARCH
1515 Broadway, Suite 3601
New York, NY 10109-0732
212-719-0033

AMERICAN RED CROSS NATIONAL HEADQUARTERS
AIDS Education Program
17th and D Streets NW
Washington, DC 20006
202-639-3223

AMERICAN HEPATITIS ASSOCIATION (AHA)
212-599-5070
 information
212-340-8986
 hotline and referral service

AMERICAN SOCIAL HEALTH ASSOCIATION
PO Box 13827
Research Triangle Park, NC 27709
919-361-8400

AMERICAN SOCIAL HEALTH ASSOCIATION—HERPES RESOURCE CENTER
919-361-2742

NATIONAL AIDS HOTLINE
US Public Health Service
800-342-AIDS

NATIONAL AIDS INFORMATION CLEARINGHOUSE
US Public Health Service and Centers for Disease Control
800-458-5231

NATIONAL AIDS NETWORK
202-429-2856

NATIONAL ASSOCIATION OF PEOPLE WITH AIDS (NAWPA)
202-429-2856

NATIONAL HEALTH INFORMATION CLEARINGHOUSE
Health and Human Services
800-336-4797
301-565-4167 (MD residents)

NATIONAL HERPES HOTLINE
1-919-361-8488

NATIONAL STD HOTLINE
1-800-227-8922

OFFICE OF MINORITY HEALTH RESOURCE CENTER
PO Box 37337
Washington, DC 20013-7337
800-444-6472

PROJECT INFORM
800-822-7422
800-334-7422 (CA residents)
Information clearinghouse and hotline. Provides current information on AIDS/HIV experimental drug treatments. Provides information on organizations where drugs may be obtained.

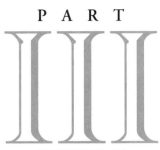

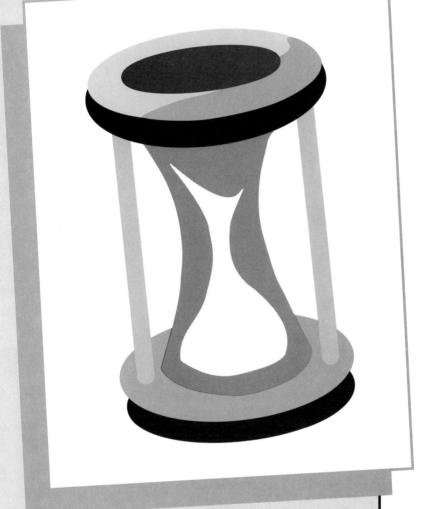

*Chronic
Conditions
and Aging
Dimensions
in Women's
Health*

Cardiovascular Disease

CHAPTER OBJECTIVES

On completion of this chapter, the student should be able to discuss:

1. How life expectancy has changed for women since 1900 and the reasons for increased life expectancy.

2. The main parts and functions of the circulatory system.

3. The primary components of blood.

4. The types of diseases that are included in the category of cardiovascular disease.

5. How atherosclerosis occurs.

6. The cause of rheumatic heart disease.

7. What happens when a heart attack occurs.

8. What types of blockages can occur in the circulatory system.

9. The major causes of cerebrovascular accidents.

10. How blood pressure is measured.

11. The significance of hypertension to cardiovascular disease.

12. The conditions that contribute to congestive heart failure.

13. The significance of angina.

14. Conditions that lead to peripheral artery disease.

15. The differences between men and women and cardiovascular disease patterns.

16. Age and race factors that place a woman at risk for cardiovascular disease.

17. The reasons why cardiovascular disease in women has not received the appropriate levels of attention.

18. What is a "silent heart attack" and its special significance to women.

19. What risk factors for cardiovascular disease are more prevalent in African-American women than with white women.

20. The major modifiable risk factors for cardiovascular disease.

21. The significance of cholesterol and cardiovascular disease.

22. **The elements that make up lipoproteins.**

23. **The differences between HDL, LDL, VLDL, and triglycerides.**

24. **How cholesterol levels can be controlled by diet.**

25. **Factors that can help control high blood pressure.**

26. **How cigarette smoking contributes to cardiovascular disease.**

27. **The relationship between diabetes and cardiovascular disease.**

28. **The contradictory findings concerning oral contraceptives and cardiovascular disease.**

29. **How menopause influences a woman's risk of cardiovascular disease.**

30. **The steps that a woman can take to reduce her overall risks of cardiovascular disease.**

Introduction

Genetics and lifestyle are major contributors to chronic diseases, including cardiovascular diseases. Genetics clearly play a role in determining those who are at highest risk for certain conditions. Lifestyle alone cannot totally counter a heavy genetic loading for certain conditions; however, among those who are genetically predisposed, changes in lifestyle can make a significant difference. This chapter provides an overview of cardiovascular disease, which today is the major killer of women. Cardiovascular disease is discussed in terms of normal heart structure and function, disease conditions, unique dimensions of cardiovascular disease and women, risk factors, and personal decision making to reduce the risk of cardiovascular disease.

Life expectancy is often a marker of a nation's health. Advances in medicine and public health over the last 100 years have had a significant impact on life expectancy and death rates in the United States. In 1900, the average life expectancy for women was 48 years. In 1990, life expectancy for women was 78 years (Fig. 11.1). Many factors have served to contribute to this expansion of life expectancy for women in the United States (Information Box 11.1). In the 1930s, life expectancy for women began to improve significantly such that a woman might reasonably expect to live into her sixties and by the 1980s into her seventies. Having survived the rigors of childbirth and infectious and parasitic diseases, women are now, however, in a position to succumb to the effects of chronic disease, particularly heart disease.

Cardiovascular Disease

Cardiovascular disease is the major killer of women today. More than 400,000 women die annually in the United States of cardiovascular diseases. Heart disease accounts for more than one-third of all deaths in women.[1] These deaths usually

---

INFORMATION BOX 11.1

Contributions to Improved Life Expectancy for Women

Identification, treatment, eradication, and/or control of some infectious and parasitic diseases

Better prenatal and antenatal care

More efficient, effective methods of assisting childbirth

Greater awareness, identification, and control of threats to health and ways to promote and maximize health

Improved protection from environmental and workplace toxins and hazards

FIGURE 11.1

Life expectancy for African-American and white women, 1900–88.

SOURCE: USDHHS (1991). *Health United States, 1990.* (DHHS Pub. No. (PHS) 91-1232.) Washington, DC: US Government Printing Office.

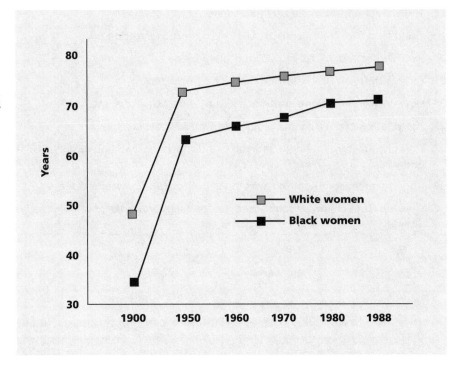

occur in later years when women are beset with a variety of morbid conditions, such as high blood pressure, high blood cholesterol, osteoporosis, and diabetes. Figures 11.2 and 11.3 dramatically show the rising death rates from heart disease among African-American and white women as they age. Cardiovascular disease is also among the leading causes of disability for women. Although it was once believed that these conditions were an inevitable consequence of aging,

FIGURE 11.2

Death rates for stroke victims among women, 15 to 84 years.

SOURCE: USDHHS (1991). *Health United States, 1990.* (DHHS Pub. No. (PHS) 91-1232.) Washington, DC: US Government Printing Office.

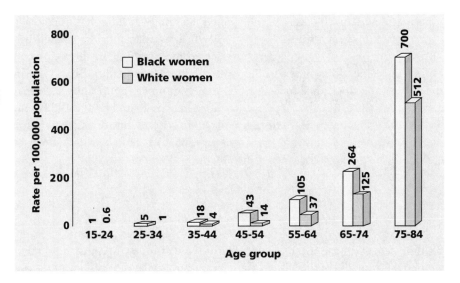

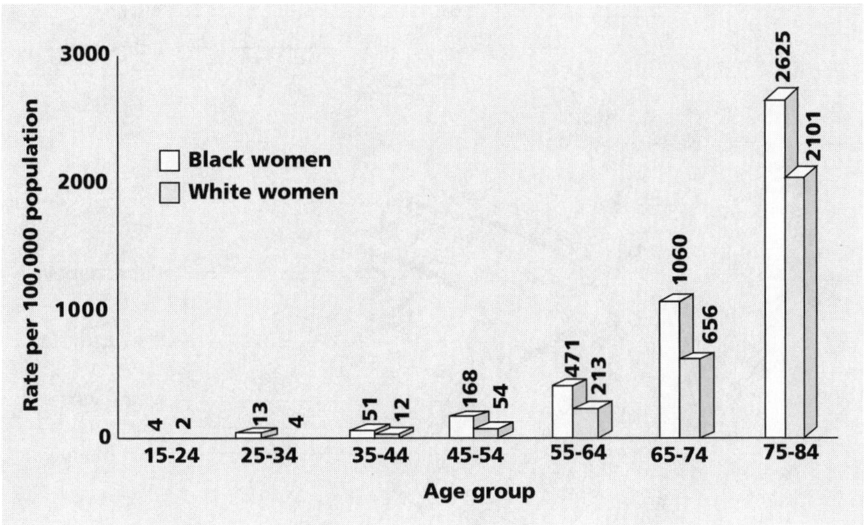

FIGURE 11.3

Death rates for corony heart disease (CHD) victims among women, 15 to 84 years of age, 1988.

SOURCE: USDHHS (1991). *Health United States, 1990.* (DHHS Pub. No. (PHS) 91-1232.) Washington, DC: US Government Printing Office.

it is now realized that these diseases are greatly influenced by negative lifestyle behaviors, such as cigarette smoking, poor nutrition, and lack of exercise.

The Heart

Cardiovascular disease cannot be understood without an appreciation of the heart as a vital organ. Not only does the heart relentlessly pump blood throughout the body, but also it has served poets, writers, composers, lovers, and countless others as an object that has been assigned traits such as love, strength, courage, pain, warmth, fullness, and emptiness. The heart is located in the chest behind the **sternum,** the breast bone. It beats an average of 72 times a minute beginning before birth and continuing on for several decades. It accelerates to meet physical demands such as physical activity and slows down during sleep or meditation. The cardiovascular system is a relatively simple circulatory delivery system of open tubing of arteries and veins through which blood is pumped throughout the body. Blood flows through the arteries and veins, delivering nutrients to cells, and returning with waste materials back to the heart.

The **cardiovascular system** consists of the heart, arteries, veins, and capillaries (Fig. 11.4). The heart has four major chambers: the **right atrium** and **ventricle** and the **left atrium** and **ventricle.** The right atrium and ventricle and the left atrium and ventricle are each separated by a valve. The right atrium and ventricle are separated by the **tricuspid valve;** the left atrium and ventricle are separated by the **bicuspid** or mitral **valve.** The right and left side of the heart are separated by a thick muscular wall known as a **septum.** On contraction of each, the blood is forced from that chamber and into circulation. Both the right and left ventricle are the pumping sections of the heart, but the major pump, the portion that

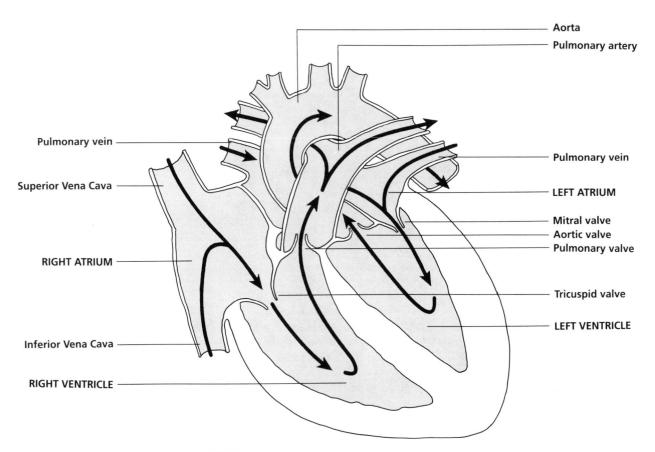

FIGURE 11.4

Cross section of the heart.

pumps blood to the body, is the left ventricle. Thus the left ventricle is a critically important part of the heart and is at particular risk in the event of a heart attack.

Contraction from the left ventricle forces oxygen-rich blood through the **aortic valve** into the **aorta** (the main artery) and from there throughout the major arteries flowing gradually into smaller and smaller arteries, arterioles, and finally capillaries. The **capillaries**, microscopic vessels with thin walls, are the sites where the nutrients and oxygen are exchanged for waste and carbon dioxide at the cellular level. From the capillaries, the oxygen-poor but carbon dioxide–rich blood flows into the venules and veins as it makes its way back to the heart. The blood then enters the right atrium of the heart from the **inferior** and **superior vena cava** (major veins) through the tricuspid valve. From the right atrium, blood flows into the right ventricle, where it is pumped to the lungs via the **pulmonary arteries** for oxygenation and then back to the heart via the **pulmonary veins,** where it enters into the left atrium passing through the mitral valve. The cycle begins again in the left ventricle. For this system to function properly, the pump must remain strong and forceful. The heart must contract forcefully and quickly when a woman runs a marathon, yet it must slow for rest during sleep. The arteries must remain supple and open. Similar to the heart, the arteries have muscles and must also expand and contract vigorously to meet demands placed on the body. Veins, although they must remain supple and open, do not themselves have muscles and must therefore rely on surrounding muscles to move the blood along through the venous system to its destination.

The heart is activated to perform its pump function through electrical stimuli pulsed from the specialized tissues called **nodes** buried in the cardiac muscle. This electrical stimulation can be detected by a special recording known as an **electrocardiogram** (ECG). An ECG can detect a normal heart rhythm or abnormalities such as a heart attack or a congenitally damaged tricuspid valve.

Blood is the vehicle for transporting the food and waste throughout the body. It is a liquid medium consisting of many critical components. The primary components are the **red blood cells,** which carry oxygen and carbon dioxide; the **white blood cells,** which act as scavengers to rid the blood and body of bacteria and waste; and the **platelets,** which cause the blood to clot. An average woman circulates about 6 quarts of blood per day.

Pathophysiology of the Heart

Cardiovascular disease is a category of diseases that includes coronary heart disease (CHD), hypertension, cerebrovascular disease (stroke), congestive heart failure (CHF), angina pectoris, congenital heart disease, rheumatic heart disease, peripheral artery disease (PAD). Each of these diseases is discussed in terms of pathology and unique dimensions in women.

Coronary Heart Disease

Atherosclerosis is the major culprit in CHD, causing the heart or the vessels to become clogged or in poor muscular condition, thereby impairing a woman's ability to function. This can happen in a variety of ways. The arteries can become clogged with waste, usually fat deposits (**plaques**). These waste deposits build up over years on the inner portion (**intima**) of the arteries, thereby impeding the flow of blood. The arteries can become stiff with age or disease, thus making the arteries less able to respond to demands placed on them. If the blood flow is compromised, the area being fed by that particular artery or arteries does not receive proper nutrients and can become damaged or die. Because the arteries surrounding the heart are so twisted and tortuous, they are particularly prone to develop atherosclerosis. When that occurs, a woman is at increased risk of suffering a heart attack.

The heart can also become damaged from other diseases or conditions, such as **rheumatic heart disease,** or from injury, such as a **heart attack,** which can lead to **congestive heart failure.** CHF is a condition in which the heart loses its ability to contract properly or sufficiently to meet the demands placed on it. Even if the arteries remain open (patent), without a strong pumping action from the heart, the ability of the nutrient-rich and oxygen-rich blood to reach

Warning Signs of a Heart Attack

Uncomfortable pressure, fullness, squeezing, or pain in the center of the chest lasting 2 minutes or longer

Pain spreading to the shoulder, neck, or arm

Severe pain, dizziness, fainting, sweating, nausea, shortness of breath

In the event of a heart attack:

Immediate action is required to prevent death or severe heart damage.

Call 911 or the local emergency system and get medical help immediately.

cells is hampered, and the cells may suffer damage or die. In addition, the heart muscle itself depends on a rich blood supply from the coronary arteries, which must remain open and supple if the heart is to function with vigor.

A heart attack, or death of a portion of the heart, occurs when one or more of the coronary arteries to the heart become damaged or clogged with waste and close off. Such blockages can occur from a clot circulating in the bloodstream (**emboli**) or a clot blocking an artery (**thrombus**). When that happens, the portion of the heart fed by the artery dies, and a heart attack (coronary event, **myocardial infarction**) occurs. If this happens to a portion of the left ventricle, the major pump of the heart, the whole ventricle can cease to pump, which stops blood flow to the rest of the body. If this situation is not reversed immediately, the person can die or suffer irreversible brain damage within a matter of minutes from lack of oxygen to the brain (Information Box 11.2).

Cerebrovascular Disease (Stroke)

Cerebrovascular accident or **stroke** is a condition in which blood vessel damage occurs in the brain. Although strokes have a variety of causes, the major causes in the brain are generally either from blood vessel blockage (embolism or thrombus) or from a ruptured artery as a result of atherosclerotic vessels (Fig. 11.5). **Cerebral aneurysm** is an abnormal outpouring of an artery in the brain that weakens and ruptures due to the stress of blood rushing through it. Although this condition has been associated with hypertension, it may also result from a congenital defect. Whatever the cause of the stroke, the damage to the artery prevents oxygen and nutrients from reaching a particular area of the brain, and as a result that portion dies. Depending on where the stroke occurs in the brain, speech, memory, thought, and movement can be affected or lost. Sometimes warning signs (Information Box 11.3) precede a stroke in the form of **transient ischemic attacks** (TIAs). A TIA is an event in which the artery may close momentarily in a spasm, and the woman may have a brief memory lapse or garbled speech. Such an event can often occur very quickly, and the woman may have little memory of it. Although a stroke can happen at any time to anyone, it is generally a condition that occurs in older individuals. The chances of having a stroke increase sharply after age 45 in white women and after age 35 in African-American women.[1]

Hypertension

Blood pressure is the pressure exerted against the walls of the arteries when the heart pumps, specifically when the left ventricle contracts. This pressure is crucial in maintaining equilibrium throughout the vascular system as different forces affect this system. For example, when an athlete runs a race, the heart must pump faster and harder to meet the demands of the cells for oxygen. As such, the arteries must constrict to keep the pressure constant to accomplish the task of running.

Blood pressure is measured with called a **sphygmomanometer.** The sphygmomanometer is a cuff device connected to a hose, which is connected to a measuring device. The cuff is wrapped around the woman's upper arm, or in rare instances the leg, and inflated, thereby constricting the underlying artery and stopping the blood flow and with it the sound of the heart beat. Gradually the pressure in the cuff is released, and the blood begins to flow back through the artery and with it the returning sound of the heart beat. The first sound heard as the blood begins to flow back into the artery is called the systolic pressure, and the last sound heard before it disappears again is called the diastolic. The measurement is shown as millimeters of mercury (mm Hg) and is expressed as 115/75 mm Hg, or a measurement of 115 mm Hg systolic and 75 mm Hg diastolic. The first number expresses the **systolic** pressure and represents the amount of force the blood exerts against the wall of the artery when the heart contracts. The second number expresses the **diastolic** pressure and represents the amount of pressure the blood exerts against the wall of the artery when the heart rests between beats. For years, a blood pressure of 120/80 was considered "normal." In fact, blood pressure varies greatly from individual to individual and throughout the day depending on the time and the activity. Many young women, especially those who are fit and slender can have blood pressure measurements of 90/70 mm Hg. In a fit person with no disease, this is a "normal" blood pressure.

   Hypertension or high blood pressure (the names are interchangeable) is a blood pressure that remains elevated above what is considered a safe level. Although there is no "normal" number at which blood pressure is considered safe, the numbers used by the National Heart, Lung, and Blood Institute's National High Blood Pressure Education Program and by the American Heart Association to indicate high blood pressure are 140 mm Hg systolic and 90 mm Hg diastolic. Hypertension is not excessive stress or tension as some individuals mistakenly imagine. Although blood pressure can reach heights such

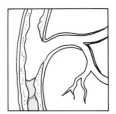

Thrombus

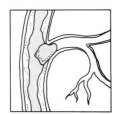

Embolism

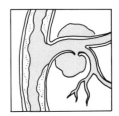

Hemorrhage

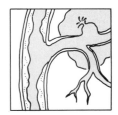

Aneurysm (ruptured)

FIGURE 11.5

Types of cerebrovascular accidents.

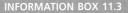

INFORMATION BOX 11.3

Warning Signs of Stroke

Temporary weakness or numbness of the face, arm, or leg, especially on one
   side of the body

Temporary loss of speech, trouble speaking, or trouble understanding speech

Temporary loss of vision or dimness in one or both eyes

Unexplained dizziness, unsteadiness, or sudden falls

In the event of a stroke:

Immediate attention is required at the first signs or symptoms.

Call 911 or the local emergency system and get medical help immediately.

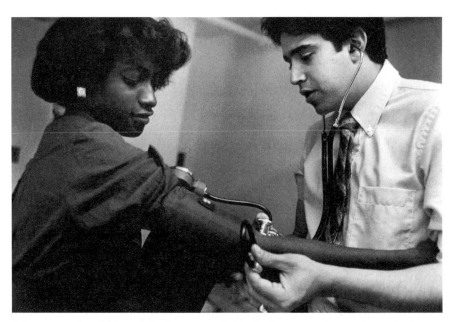

All women should know their personal risk for hypertension and regularly monitor their blood pressure.

as 140/90 mm Hg or greater in a healthy adult during exercise, these levels return to a lower level after exercise. Continuing levels of blood pressure at 140/90 mm Hg or above, however, are considered high blood pressure and as such increase an individual's risk for heart disease and stroke.

Over time, high blood pressure exerts a damaging effect on small arteries, known as **arterioles.** Arterioles become thicker and less elastic, resulting in a condition known as **arteriosclerosis.** The condition coupled with the effects from **atherosclerosis,** the narrowing of the arteries from fatty plaque deposits, creates an explosive situation. When faced with the demands of heavy exertion (such as running or shoveling snow), arterioles, particularly in the brain, heart, or kidneys, can close off, rupture, or leak, causing a stroke (in brain), a heart attack, or renal accident (in kidneys). Women are particularly at risk for stroke. Compared to men, women experience 60 percent of all stroke deaths.[1]

Congestive Heart Failure

CHF represents a heart whose muscles are weak and flabby and cannot perform the pump function with proper vigor. As a result, circulation suffers, and fluids begin to accumulate in veins causing breathing problems, kidney problems, and swelling in the extremities, particularly the legs. CHF may have many causes, but it is often a disease of older women who have suffered heart damage from high blood pressure, atherosclerosis, arteriosclerosis, or heart attack. In some cases, CHF occurs because of a congenital defect or damage to the heart from a bacterial disease, such as rheumatic heart disease.

Congenital Heart Disease and Rheumatic Heart Disease

Congenital heart disease is present in certain babies when they are born and can include one or more of the following: a hole in the wall (septum) separating sections of the heart, imperfectly formed blood vessels, valvular damage, or left ventricular imperfections. The majority of these imperfections can be corrected with surgery. Rheumatic heart disease results from a bacterial infection *(Strepto-coccus)* that has been inadequately treated and results in damage to the heart valves. Rheumatic heart disease is a downward progression from an inadequately treated strep throat, which progresses to rheumatic fever, which affects the entire body in an inflammatory process. The brain, heart, and joints can be adversely and permanently affected. In the heart, rheumatic heart disease can be seen as damage to the valves either by closing them off completely or partially. This condition may require surgery and valve replacement. The best treatment is prevention, e.g., treatment of the initial strep throat, which precludes further damage.

Angina Pectoris

Angina pectoris is chest pain resulting from an insufficient supply of blood (oxygen) to the heart muscle. The symptoms can range in severity from a mild clamping ache to a crushing pain in the chest. The impairment of blood flow can result from atherosclerosis or a spasm of a normal artery. Depending on the cause of the impairment, the pain can be relieved by medication, often nitroglycerin, which is a strong vasodilator (opening the closed blood vessel).

Peripheral Artery Disease

Peripheral artery disease is a disease of the extremities (hands, arms, but mainly in the legs and feet) in which the blood supply is diminished, and sufficient oxygen and nutrients do not reach these areas properly. Waste is not removed from these areas sufficiently either, and, as a result, a woman can experience symptoms that range from cramping and numbness to **gangrene** (tissue death), which may require amputation of the extremity. The cause of PAD is related to atherosclerosis and arteriosclerosis and is particularly associated with persons who have diabetes, who smoke, or who have hypertension.

All of these cardiovascular diseases are a result of some damage or injury to the heart or vascular system. Although some diseases are the result of congenital defects or bacterial diseases, the majority are due to atherosclerosis or arteriosclerosis, diseases that have an important antecedent in lifestyle factors such as uncontrolled high blood pressure, high blood cholesterol, cigarette smoking, lack of exercise, and uncontrolled stress.

Cardiovascular Disease and Women

Cardiovascular disease patterns show interesting gender differences. Between the ages of 25 and 35, men have three times the incidence of CHD as women. Between the ages of 36 and 49, men have 1.7 times the incidence, and the incidence does not become 1:1 until after age 75, so even though menopause decreases a woman's protection from coronary disease, she retains a biological advantage over her male counterparts until into her seventies.[13]

Epidemiology

Despite the delayed onset of disease in women, cardiovascular disease nevertheless accounts for almost half of all deaths among women. African-American women are particularly vulnerable. Up until about age 75, African-American women have higher rates of death owing to cardiovascular diseases than do white women or other women of other racial groups. The annual cost in dollars for cardiovascular diseases in women is well over $11 billion. The emotional cost to women and their families and friends is incalculable.

Of the cardiovascular diseases, CHD (primarily heart attack) and stroke are the major causes of death among adults—both women and men. CHD is the leading cause of death, killing about 500,000 people annually, about equally divided between women and men. Stroke is the third leading cause of death, killing about 150,000 people annually—about 20 percent more women than men. Although some cardiovascular diseases occur among children and adolescents, the majority of cardiovascular diseases, that is, CHD and stroke, are diseases of older individuals, usually those who are middle-aged (50 years) and beyond. The incidence (occurrence) of CHD begins to rise for men between the ages of 45 and 50 years of age and about 10 years later for women. The incidence of stroke is similar. CHD, primarily heart attack, is the number one cause of death in the United States, accounting for 765,143 deaths in 1988.[1] An estimated 250,000 of the deaths occurred suddenly, within 1 hour of the onset of symptoms, many without warning.

Cardiovascular disease imposes a large burden on the medical care system in the United States, particularly on emergency medical departments and hospitals. In 1987, an estimated $15 billion was spent for the care of persons with CHD. The biggest share of this cost can be attributed to heart attacks occurring in that year. The national economic impact of this disease is also measured in terms of lost productivity, measured by lost earnings owing to illness (morbidity) and death (mortality). Mortality costs include lost future earnings for those dying from this disease. The estimated indirect cost (indirect costs are those costs related to morbidity [lost work days] and mortality [lost future earnings]) from this disease in 1987 was $3 billion for morbidity and $25 billion for mortality. Medical costs over a 5-year period for an individual acute myocardial infarction are an estimated $51,211 in 1986 dollars.[3]

Gender Dimensions of Cardiovascular Disease

CHD (particularly heart attack) was not, and still is not, generally thought of as a woman's disease, even by the most sophisticated medical practitioners or by the woman herself. This happens in part because women do not tend to show signs and symptoms of CHD until at least 10 years later than men. Among women 25 to 64 years of age, only 10 percent suffered from CHD, whereas after age 65 approximately 90 percent of women die from CHD.[2] These later years in women present a compromised quality of life fraught with heart disease and other conditions, such as high blood pressure, high blood cholesterol, diabetes, and osteoporosis.

Although this disease can strike anyone, it is mainly a disease of the elderly, the poor, and the less educated. Among women:[14,15]

- The majority of deaths (90 percent) occur after age 65.

- Four times as many women than men are widowed.

- 32 percent live alone compared with 7 percent of men.

- 86 percent have a high school education or less compared with 79 percent of men.

- 83 percent have a family income less than $25,000 per year.

- Many have other health problems, such as high blood pressure, diabetes, cancer, and angina.

Although rates of CHD mortality are higher in men than women throughout the life span, there are almost as many CHD deaths in women as in men overall because of the larger numbers of older women who die from the disease. Under age 45, the male to female ratio is over 4:1, but that ratio decreases with age so rates are only 20 percent higher in men by age 85. Among women, the rates are higher in African-American than white women until about age 75 years.[1]

The chances of having a heart attack are not trivial. Incidence is much greater in men than women, but in women it increases steadily after menopause. Eighteen percent of heart attacks in men and 24 percent in women present with sudden death as the first and only manifestation. Often the symptoms and signs of CHD may differ substantially from those of men. Women, for example, tend to have angina pectoris as the first symptoms of heart disease as opposed to a heart attack (myocardial infarction) in men. Women may also have unspecified pain, which could lead a woman or her physician to look for other causes rather than to suspect a heart attack. Some women may not even be aware that they have had a heart attack. They may have a "silent" heart attack—a heart attack in which no signs or symptoms are seen or felt.

Women may present substantially different symptoms and signs than do men. As such, women have not been included as much as they should have been in CHD research and treatment.[4,5] The result is that both women and their physicians have been compromised in their awareness, identification, and treatment of CHD. A woman who survives a heart attack continues to face a high risk of disability, recurrence, and premature death. After surviving the acute stages, rates of recurrent attack, angina pectoris, cardiac failure, stroke, or mortality are three to seven times that of the general population.[6] Within 5 years after the initial heart attack, 13 percent of men and almost 40 percent of women develop a second infarction.[2] About two-thirds of myocardial infarction patients do not make a complete recovery.[2] Ten-year survival after an infarction is 50 percent for men and, because of women's higher early mortality, 70 percent for women.[2] In other words, once an infarction occurs, the relative immunity exhibited by women in earlier years is lost and they survive no better than men, indeed generally worse.

Racial Differences with Cardiovascular Disease

Any woman is susceptible to a stroke, but African-American women bear a disproportionate burden of stroke disability and death. Death rates from stroke start at earlier ages in African-American women and rise more sharply over time. The rate of death from heart disease is higher in African-American women than in white women (181.1 versus 144.2 per 100,000 population.)[1] Mortality from heart disease increases with age and is also higher for African-American women than for white women of all ages except for those over 85 years of age.[7] Although scientists do not completely understand why this is so, several important factors appear to contribute to these differences. African-American women in general tend to have more high blood pressure and to be, on average, more overweight or obese than white women. High blood pressure is clearly the major risk factor for stroke. **Obesity** is a major risk factor and enhancer of high blood pressure. The combination is believed to predispose a woman to stroke. Whether or not African-American women are genetically predisposed to stroke is not clear.[6]

High blood cholesterol affects all racial and ethnic groups. Although most data sources have traditionally categorized women as "black" or "white," national cholesterol screening programs have provided some rare insight into differences within ethnic groups. For example, the prevalence of high blood cholesterol levels (240 mg/dl or greater) is lower among Hispanic-American women, ranging from 17 percent of Cuban women to 23 percent of Puerto Rican women compared with 25 percent of African-American women and 28 per of white women.[1] High blood pressure is a particular problem for African-American women Indeed, the prevalence of high blood pressure (blood pressure greater than 140/90 mm Hg) among African-American women is almost twice (1.7 times) that of white women. As with high blood cholesterol, the prevalence rates for high blood pressure are lowest among Hispanic-American women, especially Cuban women. Only 14 percent of Cuban women are shown to have high blood pressure. For Native-American and Alaskan-Native women, the prevalence of high blood pressure is 22 and 23 percent.[1]

Although prevalence of high blood pressure and high blood cholesterol is lower among Hispanic-American women, the prevalence of overweight is substantially greater when compared with white women. African-American women, who have the greatest prevalence of high blood pressure also have the greatest prevalence of overweight. The two risk factors are closely associated with and contribute significantly to the higher disability and death from stroke and heart attack among African-American women. Diet also clearly plays a role in the development of these diseases and, as such, can assist in preventing and controlling them.

The prevalence of diabetes is particularly high among Hispanic-American and Native-American women, in whom obesity is also high. These factors clearly contribute significantly to earlier appearance of heart disease and stroke among these women.

Risk Factors

A risk factor for a disease is an action or a behavior that places an individual at a higher risk of developing a condition or a disease (Self-assessment 11.1). The risk factors for cardiovascular disease are summarized in Information Box 11.4. The major modifiable risk factors (those that make a major contribution to the development of the disease) for CHD are high blood pressure, high blood cholesterol, and cigarette smoking. The major modifiable risk factors for stroke are high blood pressure and cigarette smoking. In other words, these are the risk factors that are most closely associated with the development of either of these conditions in both women and men. The risk of developing heart disease in a woman who has high blood pressure, high blood cholesterol, and who smokes is eight times that of a woman who has none of those risk factors.[2]

High Blood Cholesterol

High blood levels of cholesterol (greater than 240 mg/dl) are associated with an increased risk of mortality and morbidity from CHD.[7] **Cholesterol** is a fatty substance found in all cells that is essential for the manufacture and maintenance of the cell as well as sex hormones and nerves throughout the body. Cholesterol is made in the liver and small intestine and is transported throughout the body in a **lipoprotein.** Lipoproteins are fats and protein bound together in a chemical structure that enables them to be transported in the blood. In most individuals, the body manufactures an appropriate amount of cholesterol to serve the needs of the body. In some individuals, blood cholesterol levels are excessively high, owing to genetic abnormalities. These people are at greatly increased risk for heart disease. When an excessive amount of cholesterol and saturated fat is taken in through a diet high in these ingredients, however, the body is overwhelmed, and the unused cholesterol is deposited on the inner walls of the

INFORMATION BOX 11.4

Women's Modifiable Risk Factors for Cardiovascular Diseases

High blood pressure

High blood cholesterol

Oral contraceptives (particularly with smokers)

Cigarette smoking

Obesity

Diabetes

High triglycerides

Excessive alcohol consumption

Sedentary lifestyle

Menopause

Stress

SELF-ASSESSMENT 11.1

Personal Risk Factors for Cardiovascular Disease

Age
A woman's risk of cardiovascular disease increases as she gets older, most noticeably after menopause

Genetics
A family history of cardiovascular disease increases a woman's risk

Race
Until age 75, African-American women are twice as likely to die of cardiovascular disease as white women; after age 75, white women are more likely to die of cardiovascular disease

Obesity
Being 20 percent over recommended body weight is a risk factor for cardiovascular disease

Smoking
For women, smoking is the most significant factor for cardiovascular disease

Hypertension
Elevated blood pressure is a risk factor for cardiovascular disease. A woman's blood pressure is likely to rise after menopause

Elevated cholesterol
Elevated cholesterol is a major risk factor for cardiovascular disease

Sedentary lifestyle
Failure to achieve adequate levels of physical activity predisposes an individual for cardiovascular disease

Diabetes
Diabetes is more prevalent in women and is a major risk factor for cardiovascular disease

---

arteries. Over time (usually decades), these deposits gradually accumulate, slowly narrowing the artery (Fig. 11.6). The inner walls become clogged and brittle, and pieces tear leaving jagged edges. These jagged edges stick up and catch more material as it flows by in the bloodstream, thereby adding more waste deposits to the wall. The artery is gradually closed off either by an artery closed (occluded) by fatty plaque or by a transient embolus, which may become lodged in the narrowed artery. In either case, the blood does not reach a part of the body and that part dies unless the artery is once again opened. Because the coronary (heart) arteries are so twisted and tortuous, they are particularly prone to clogging. When that happens, a heart attack occurs.

Lipoproteins are made up of the following key elements: **low-density lipoproteins** (LDL), **high-density lipoproteins** (HDL), **very-low-density lipoproteins**

(VLDL), and **triglycerides.** Everyone has each of these in varying amounts in each lipoprotein molecule. When speaking of cholesterol levels in the blood, health care professionals generally refer to the total blood cholesterol level, or to the LDL-cholesterol or HDL-cholesterol level.

LDL-cholesterol is often referred to as the "bad" cholesterol because of its affinity for sticking to the wall of the artery and lodging there. HDL-cholesterol is often referred to as the "good" cholesterol because it functions somewhat like a trash collector taking the LDL-cholesterol out of the body. A low level of HDL has been found to be a predictor of mortality from CHD in women.[8] VLDL is another lipoprotein that is associated with the transport of fats known as triglycerides. Triglycerides are associated, particularly in women, with an elevated risk of heart disease.

Women, particularly those who are fit and slender and who have not experienced menopause, tend to have slightly elevated HDL-cholesterol levels compared with men or with postmenopausal women. Elevated HDL-cholesterol levels are shown to be protective against heart disease. Indeed, after menopause, a woman's hormone levels begin to drop and so do her HDL-cholesterol levels. They can drop by as much as 10 to 20 percent. During this time, a woman's risk for heart disease continues to rise.

As discussed in Chapter 1, cholesterol levels can usually be controlled by diet. A diet low in cholesterol and saturated fat is crucial in maintaining a low overall total cholesterol level. Indeed, the "typical" American diet is far too high in cholesterol, saturated fats, and calories to be healthy. Roughly 35 to 40 percent of the typical American diet is made up of saturated fats: fats that are eaten in the form of French fries, hamburgers, potato chips, and other high-fat foods. There are three types of fats: saturated, polyunsaturated, and monounsaturated. All fats contain 9 calories per gram compared with 4 calories per gram for carbohydrates and proteins. As such, saturated fats are dense calorically and thereby provide more calories per gram of food. This can lead to excess weight gain and possibly obesity. Saturated fats eaten in food actually have a greater effect on blood cholesterol than cholesterol eaten in food. Eating saturated fats increases the total blood cholesterol, particularly the LDL-cholesterol—the "bad" cholesterol. This does not mean that a woman should not limit the amount of cholesterol she consumes; rather it means that she should be careful to limit both the dietary cholesterol and the dietary saturated fat she eats.

A diet that is low in cholesterol and saturated fat should not limit essential nutrients. In women, especially girls who are still growing, great care should be taken to include calcium-rich and iron-rich foods, such as low-fat dairy products (skim milk, low-fat yogurt, margarine, sherbet) and green leafy vegetables (spinach). Calcium is especially important for women because it is essential for bone development and growth as well as maintaining bone density as the young woman matures into an adult. Strong bones developed at an earlier age offer a hedge against the potential for osteoporosis (bone thinning), which can lead to bone fractures in later years, particularly after menopause. Iron-rich foods are important for menstruating women to assist in replacing the modest amounts of blood lost during a menstrual period.

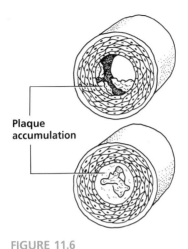

Plaque accumulation

FIGURE 11.6

Progression of athero-sclerosis—plaque deposits in artery

High Blood Pressure

In women who have not yet experienced menopause, high blood pressure has a relatively low prevalence, although women who are obese tend to have higher levels of blood pressure than do women who are more slender. After menopause, however, high blood pressure in women rises sharply with age. Control of high blood pressure depends on proper diet, salt restriction when necessary, weight maintenance appropriate for a woman's height and body type, regular exercise, and, when necessary, medication to lower elevated blood pressure. A woman with high blood pressure should be under the guidance of a health care provider. Blood pressure should be checked periodically, especially as a woman ages.

A diet that is low in cholesterol and saturated fat and calories assists a woman in maintaining a proper body weight and thereby controlling her high blood pressure. In many cases, high blood pressure can be brought under control by such a diet and weight control and maintenance. In some women, especially African-American women, salt sensitivity appears to be important in the development and control of high blood pressure. Therefore some women may have to limit the intake of salt in their diet.

Cigarettes

As discussed in Chapter 5, cigarette smoking is the greatest preventable cause of death in the United States. Not only does it increase the risk of several kinds of cancers, but also it sharply increases the risk of heart attack (especially sudden death from heart attack), stroke, and PAD. Certain elements contained in the cigarette smoke act as a **vasoconstrictor** (closes down the blood vessels). Over time in a chronic smoker, this vasoconstriction contributes to the increased fragility and brittleness of the arteries.

The threat to cardiovascular health is tremendously enhanced in a woman who smokes and has diabetes. In addition to the destructive effect on the arteries from the cigarette smoke, diabetes also exerts a powerfully destructive effect on the arteries. The combination raises the chances of a heart attack, PAD, and severe disability, possibly even death, in a woman who has both these risk factors. The good news is that when a woman stops smoking, her risk for heart disease declines, and approximately 10 years after she has stopped, her risk is about that of a person who has never smoked.

I am overweight and know that I need to lose, but how can I afford all those expensive weight loss foods in the supermarket? My kids need the fat in their diet, and I can't afford to buy and fix two separate meals.

35-YEAR-OLD MOTHER

Other Modifiable Risk Factors

Although high blood cholesterol, high blood pressure, and cigarette smoking are clearly the most important modifiable risk factors for cardiovascular disease, other factors also play a role to a lesser extent. These factors include high triglycerides, obesity, diabetes, oral contraceptives, excessive alcohol consumption, sedentary lifestyle, menopause, and stress.

Triglyceride, a fat carried in the blood, when elevated is associated with the development of diabetes and heart disease in women. Although scientists do not fully understand this effect, it is clear that women should control elevated triglyceride levels by making certain that they control the amount of alcohol and saturated fat in the diet.

Obesity is defined as being 20 percent or more over body weight as defined by the Metropolitan Life Tables. Obesity is considered a major factor in the development or the lack of progress in CHD, and high blood pressure and can lead to diabetes. Obesity, usually acquired through overeating, clogs the arteries, which in turn causes them to become more fragile. Clogged arteries place greater strain on the heart and the efficiency of the pump, which leads to heart attacks. Evidence suggests that how the fat is distributed about a woman's body may prove to be an indicator for heart disease. Truncal (body) distribution of fat (stomach and upper body) as opposed to hip and thigh fat distribution appears to place a woman at greater risk for heart disease. This distribution has been referred to as "apple" (truncal obesity) versus "pear" (hip and thigh) fat distribution.

Diabetes, sometimes called "the women's disease," is a disorder of the pancreas in which the naturally occurring insulin is not properly manufactured, and thus glucose (quick energy source from food that is stored within the cell) cannot be regulated. Several studies have shown that diabetics are at high risk for blood vessel damage and are at greatly increased risk of heart disease.[9] For reasons that are not entirely clear, women seem to be particularly vulnerable to diabetes. Diabetes appears to be a more important risk factor in women than in men, accelerating the process of atherosclerosis.[10] Obesity and high blood pressure interact negatively with diabetes and place women at even greater risk for complications of diabetes and heart disease when these factors are present. The critical factor in diabetes is keeping the disease under control through proper diet, exercise, and medication when necessary.

Sedentary lifestyle is another of the lesser but important modifiable risk factors for cardiovascular disease. Sedentary lifestyle simply means that a woman is not getting enough regular aerobic exercise—any movement that raises the heart rate significantly for an extended period of time. Whether or not this is a strong risk factor for cardiovascular diseases is not yet completely established. It is, however, a critical factor in keeping the heart and other muscles strong and in good working condition. Aerobic exercise also aids in controlling weight and in helping to raise HDL-cholesterol levels. To obtain a risk-reduction effect from aerobic exercise, a woman must exercise continuously for at least 30 minutes three times a week. Such exercise includes running, brisk walking, bicycling, swimming, cross-country skiing, and dancing. A proper aerobic workout would include a warm-up period, a vigorous exercise period, followed by a cool-down period (see Chapter 2). In a woman over 45 years of age or in a woman who has a medical problem that might be aggravated by exercise, a clinician should be consulted before starting an exercise program.

Oral contraceptive use has been found in some studies to be associated with an increase in the risk of acute myocardial infarction, particularly in smokers.[11,12] Oral contraceptives may increase the risk of cardiovascular disease by increasing blood pressure and decreasing HDL levels.[11,13] In another large study, however, women who had used oral contraceptives were not shown to be at increased

I am 60 and feel great! I exercise every day, watch my weight and diet, and am taking courses at the local college to "improve my mind." Can you beat that? Improve my mind at my age, but who cares, I feel good about myself, and my doctor says I am fine.
60-YEAR-OLD FEMALE ATTORNEY

risk for acute myocardial infarction.[16] These differences may be explained by variances in oral contraceptives. The lower doses of estrogen and progesterone in newer oral contraceptives may reduce the risk of myocardial infarction associated with their use.

Alcohol misuse is not part of a healthy lifestyle (see Chapter 3). Alcohol is essentially a poison that raises blood pressure, adds empty calories and weight, and can, in excess, be toxic to the heart muscle. In addition, it takes less alcohol to raise blood alcohol levels in women compared with men, and thus women become drunk more quickly.

Menopause is the cessation of menses in a woman either by surgical means, **hysterectomy** (removal of the uterus and ovaries), or by naturally occurring means (cessation of ovarian function) (see Chapter 13). As previously discussed, after menopause, the risk for heart disease and stroke increases significantly for women. The reason appears to be related largely to the cessation of ovarian function, e.g., the loss of production of the sex hormones, estrogen and progesterone. The loss of estrogen is believed to place a woman at increased risk for heart disease and stroke because of the effect on the arteries. Scientists believe now that after menopause women experience a decrease in HDL-cholesterol and an increase in LDL-cholesterol. Increased plaque is noted in the arteries, and heart attacks and strokes begin to occur. Evidence has shown that women who receive estrogen replacement therapy benefit by reducing the side effects of menopause ("hot flashes" and emotional irritability) and appear to be at decreased risk of developing heart disease and stroke.[17] Estrogen replacement therapy, however, is not without its risks. Studies have shown that women taking estrogen replacement therapy have an increased risk of uterine cancer and, to a lesser extent, breast cancer. The risk of uterine cancer can be countered by adding progesterones to the estrogen replacement therapy (see Chapter 13). More studies are required to understand the role of hormone replacement therapy and to determine the best treatment modalities for women.[18]

Stress is a normal part of everyday life and, in fact, essential to proper functioning. External stimulation can push a person to action: to study for a test, to sprint the final lap in a race. A kiss from a loved one can also create stress, but most would not want to do without this. Distress can create negative side effects. The extent to which these negative side effects influence a person's sense of self and well-being differs greatly. Whether women manifest stress differently from men requires additional study. What does seem clear is that women are affected by negative stress and that it can make them more susceptible to heart disease. Each woman may choose to try to relieve stress through a variety of mechanisms. More positive behaviors include exercise, meditation, and talking with a friend. Less positive behaviors include cigarette smoking, excessive alcohol consumption, and overeating. Of course, the less positive behaviors lead right back to the problems that create an increased risk for heart disease and stroke.

Cardiovascular risk factors play a crucial role in the development of cardiovascular diseases. There is a cumulative effect of multiple risk factors. A diet high in cholesterol and saturated fats leads to high blood cholesterol and depositions of fatty plaques in the arteries. That same diet, often also high in calories, leads to overweight and obesity, which strains the heart and arteries and contributes to high blood pressure and diabetes. These factors place additional strain on arteries already carrying increasing amounts of plaques. The addition of cigarette smoking compounds the problem, making the arteries fragile and more constrictive. Arteries become clogged with waste, and the supreme pump, the heart, becomes sluggish and weak, in short a scenario for disaster: heart attack, stroke, CHF, and peripheral vascular disease. These disaster events are not always fatal. If the woman survives the heart attack or stroke, she may be severely limited by a damaged heart or the effects of the stroke: impaired vision, memory, speech, or movement. Thus, even though she may be alive, the quality of her life and that of her family may be seriously impaired. Although no one can predict what will absolutely happen, this scenario can usually be prevented or controlled by establishing and maintaining good health habits early in life.

Informed Decision Making

There are several things that a woman can do to reduce her risk of cardiovascular disease. The first step is to take responsibility and develop a plan of action. The second step is prevention. The old adage says, "An ounce of prevention is worth a pound of cure." That's correct. It is so much smarter to prevent a life-threatening or disabling heart attack at 55 by never smoking, eating a prudent diet, and exercising—all behaviors that should begin in childhood. However, it's never too late to begin.

Prevention Through Lifestyle

Sensible eating is an important lifestyle variable in the prevention of cardiovascular disease. A low-cholesterol, low-saturated-fat diet aids in lowering cholesterol; limits calories; and thereby reduces the risk of overweight, obesity, heart attack, high blood pressure, and diabetes. If alcohol is consumed, it is wise to do so only in moderation. Alcohol is not part of a healthy diet or lifestyle. Cigarettes are detrimental to all aspects of a woman's health. If a woman does not smoke, she should not start, and the woman who is a smoker needs to quit as soon as possible to improve her chances of a healthy life. Maintenance of a correct body weight is also an important prevention lifestyle variable. Weight is best controlled by regular aerobic exercise, which also provides direct cardiovascular benefits. All of these lifestyle messages can perhaps be best summed up by advising women simply to take good care of themselves.

Prevention Through Health Screening

Prevention of cardiovascular disease through health screening means knowing personal numbers: blood pressure and blood cholesterol. Both levels should be checked regularly with professional health care providers. Women should also

I started having chest pains, but I thought they were just due to stress. I didn't want to make a big deal of it. My doctor didn't suspect anything either—I guess I look pretty healthy. But when they did the tests, they found that I had had a "silent heart attack." I wish I had paid closer attention to the pain, and I wish that my doctor had been more sensitive about the possibility of my having a heart attack.

60-YEAR-OLD WOMAN

I know that I shouldn't smoke cigarettes, but what the heck, it's cool and I look more sophisticated. I know that I can quit anytime I want to. Besides, a few years of smoking won't hurt.

15-YEAR-OLD STUDENT

> **INFORMATION BOX 11.5**
>
> ## *Initial Classification and Recommended Follow-up Based on Total Cholesterol Measurement in Adults 20 Years Old and Older*
>
> *CLASSIFICATION*
>
> | | |
> |---|---|
> | Less than 200 mg/dl | Desirable blood cholesterol |
> | 200–239 mg/dl | Borderline-high blood cholesterol |
> | Greater than 240 mg/dl | High blood cholesterol |
>
> *RECOMMENDED FOLLOW-UP*
>
> | | |
> |---|---|
> | Total cholesterol <200 mg/dl | Repeat check-up examination within 5 years |
> | Total cholesterol 200–239 mg/dl Without other risk factors | Provide dietary information and recheck factors annually |
> | With definite CHD or 2 other risk factors | Lipoprotein analysis; further action based on LDL-cholesterol level |
> | Total cholesterol >240 mg/dl | Lipoprotein analysis; further action based on LDL-cholesterol level |
>
> **SOURCE:** USDHHS (1993). National Cholesterol Education Program Second Report of the Expert Panel on Detection, Evaluation, and Treatment of High Blood Cholesterol in Adults (Adult Treatment Panel II), National Institutes of Health, National Heart, Lung, and Blood Institute, NIH Pub. No. 93-3096. Washington, D.C.: U.S. Government Printing Office.

have regular medical checkups to establish a personal cardiovascular health program.

Cholesterol levels are measured from a small amount of blood (about 1 teaspoonful) drawn from a vein. To obtain a total blood cholesterol measurement, the person does not have to be fasting for 12 hours before the drawing. If, however, the physician wishes to obtain an accurate measurement of the LDL-cholesterol and the HDL-cholesterol, the person must fast for 12 hours before the drawing. The measurement is shown in milligrams per deciliters (mg/dl). Similar to blood pressure measurements, there is no one "normal" level for blood cholesterol. Recommendations from the National Heart, Lung, and Blood Institute's National Cholesterol Education Program are summarized in Information Box 11.5.

Summary

Although every woman ages and her body slowly winds down, most women can live life to the fullest by taking control of factors in the environment.

A woman can control her risk factors for cardiovascular diseases by relatively simple means. The heart is a pump that must be exercised to keep it strong and healthy. The vascular system is a circular system that must be kept open and functioning. The choice is a personal responsibility to maximize cardiovascular functioning through proper personal lifestyle choices and preventive health care.

Philosophical Dimensions: Cardiovascular Disease

1. What are the social and cultural factors that must be addressed before cardiovascular disease trends will change for women and special populations of women?

2. What factors can influence younger women to adopt healthier lifestyles and reduce their risks of cardiovascular disease?

3. What actions can women take to increase the general awareness of cardiovascular problems?

4. How do political and historical factors contribute to the current problem of cardiovascular disease and women?

CURRENT EVENTS

National Institutes of Health (NIH) Launches Women's Health Initiative

Heart attacks are rare among premenopausal women. What puts a woman at risk after menopause is not exactly clear. The leading theory holds that women lose their protection against heart attacks because of a drastic reduction in estrogen levels. Because of underlying assumptions regarding heart disease and women, women who do present with symptoms are not likely to be taken as seriously as their male counterparts. Some of the medical reluctance to administer procedures and treatments to women with cardiac conditions involves age; women heart patients are generally older, and because they are older, they are more likely to have complicating conditions such as diabetes and hypertension, and they are more likely to be taking other medications. Aggravating the problem is that most major studies of cardiovascular disease have excluded female subjects.

Dr. Bernadine Healy, Director, National Institutes of Health,[1] (1991–3) announced the launch of the Women's Health Initiative. This effort is a $625 million, 14-year study of 140,000 postmenopausal women. The study will explore the effects of diet, smoking, and other factors on women's risk of developing heart disease, stroke, osteoporosis, and breast and colon cancers. The study will also evaluate the effects of hormone replacement therapy: providing women with supplemental estrogen or with estrogen plus progestin after menopause.

References

1. USDHHS (1991). *Health United States, 1990.* (DHHS Pub. No. (PHS) 91-1232.) Washington, DC: US Government Printing Office.

2. Nachtigall, L.E. (1987). Cardiovascular disease and hypertension in older women. *Obstetrics and Gynecology Clinics of North America, 14*(1), 89–105.

3. Eaker, E.D., Packard, B., Wenger, N.K., Clarkson, T.B., and Tyroler, H.A. (1987). *Coronary Heart Disease in Women. Proceedings of a NIH Workshop.* New York: Haymarket Doyma, Inc.

4. Gurwitz, J.H., Nananda, F., and Avorn, J. (1992). The exclusion of the elderly and women from clinical trials in acute myocardial infarction. *Journal of the American Medical Association, 268*(11), 1417–1422.

5. Wenger, D. (Ed.) (1992). Exclusion of the elderly and women from clinical trials. Is their quality of care compromised? *Journal of the American Medical Association, 268*(11), 1460–1461.

6. Wong, M.C.W., Giuliani, M.J., and Haley, E.C. (1990). Cerebrovascular disease and stroke in women. Cardiovascular disease in women. *Cardiology, 77,* Suppl. 2, 80–90.

7. Castelli, W.P. (1988). Cardiovascular disease in women. *American Journal of Obstetrics and Gynecology, 158,* 1553–1560, 1566–1567.

8. Kannel, W.B. (1983). High-density lipoproteins: Epidemiologic profile and risks of coronary artery disease. *American Journal of Cardiology, 52,* 9B–12B.

9. Kannel, W.B. (1985). Lipids diabetes and coronary heart disease: Insights from the Framingham Study. *American Heart Journal, 110,* 1100–1107.

10. Stokes, J., Kannel, W.B., Wolf, P.A., Cupples, L.A., D'Agostino, R.B. (1987). The relative importance of selected risk factors for various manifestations of cardiovascular disease among men and women from 35 to 64 years old; 30 years of follow-up in the Framingham study. *Circulation, 75,* 6 Pt 2, 65–73.

11. Stadel, B.V. (1981). Oral contraceptives and cardiovascular disease. *New England Journal of Medicine, 305,* 612–618, 672–677.

12. Slone, D., Shapiro, S., Kaufman, D.W., Rosenberg, L., Miettinen, O.S., and Stolley, P.D. (1981). Risk of myocardial infarction in relation to current and discontinued oral contraceptive use. *New England Journal of Medicine, 305,* 420–424.

13. Fisch, I.R., and Frank, I. (1977). Oral contraceptives and blood pressure. *Journal of the American Medical Association, 237,* 2499–2503.

14. Rogot, E., Sorlie, P.D., Johnson, N.J., Glover, C.S., and Treasure, D.W. (1988). *A Mortality Study of One Million Persons by Demographic, Social, and Economic Factors: 1978–1981 Follow-up.* U.S. National Longitudinal Mortality Study. U.S. Department Of Health and Human Services, Public Health Service. National Institutes of Health. NIH Publication No. 88-2896.

15. Kapantais, G., and Powell-Griner, E. (1989). Characteristics of Persons Dying of Diseases of Heart. *Advance Data.* 172 (August 24, 1989.)

16. Stampfer, M.J., Willett, W., Colditz, G., Speizer, F.E., and Hennekens, C.H. (1988). A prospective study of past use of oral contraceptive agents and risk of coronary heart disease. *New England Journal of Medicine, 319,* 1313–1317.

17. Colditz, G.A., Willett, W.C., Stampfer, M.J., Rosner, B., Speizer, F.E., and Hennekens, C.H. (1987). Menopause and the risk of coronary heart disease in women. *New England Journal of Medicine, 316,* 1105–1110.

18. Stampfer, M.J., Colditz, G.A., Willett, W.C., Mason, J.E., Rosner, B., Speizer, F.E., and Hennekens, C.H. (1991). Postmenopausal estrogen therapy and cardiovascular disease. Ten year follow up from the Nurses' Health Study. *New England Journal of Medicine, 325*(11), 756–762.

Resources

AMERICAN HEART ASSOCIATION

7320 Greenville Avenue
Dallas, TX 75231
214-373-6300

Local chapters also provide information and supportive services.

NATIONAL HEART, LUNG AND BLOOD INSTITUTE (NHLBI)

National Institutes of Health Information Center on Cardiovascular Disease
4733 Bethesda Avenue, Suite 530
Bethesda, MD 20814
301-951-3260

NHLBI INFORMATION CENTER

P.O. Box 30105
Bethesda, MD 20824-0105
301-251-1222

NATIONAL INSTITUTE OF NEUROLOGICAL AND COMMUNICATIVE DISORDERS AND STROKE

National Institutes of Health
9000 Rockville Pike
Bethesda, MD 20205
301-496-4000

CHAPTER 12

Cancer and Other Chronic Diseases

CHAPTER OBJECTIVES

On completion of this chapter, the student should be able to discuss:

1. The major areas of a woman's body where cancer is most likely to occur and the factors that are believed to influence carcinogenesis.

2. General trends in cancer death rates, breast cancer rates, and lung cancer rates for women: and differences in cancer incidence, survival, and death rates between minority and nonminority women.

3. Differences in chronic disease incidence rates between minority and nonminority women.

4. Common symptoms of fibrocystic breast disease.

5. Usual treatment for fibroadenomas.

6. The five levels of classifying breast cancer and their relative survival rates.

7. The major risk factors for breast cancer and the three modalities for breast cancer screening.

8. The surgical procedures associated with breast cancer and the special significance of tamoxifen as a breast cancer treatment.

9. The purpose of a Pap smear.

10. The classifications of cervical dysplasia.

11. The major risk factors for cervical cancer as well as cervical cancer screening guidelines.

12. The three primary treatment modalities for cervical dysplasia.

13. The symptoms and treatment of uterine fibroids.

14. The symptoms and treatment of endometriosis.

15. Factors that may contribute to a greater risk for endometrial cancer as well as screening guidelines for endometrial cancer.

16. Why ovarian cancer is known as "the silent cancer."

17. Possible risk factors, as well as symptoms, for ovarian cancer.

18. Risk factors for colorectal cancer and the three screening modalities for colorectal cancer.

19. Differences between melanoma and nonmelanoma skin cancers.

20. The risk factors for skin cancer.

21. The four warning signs of melanoma.

22. The four treatment modalities for skin cancer.

23. The most significant risk factor for lung cancer.

24. The two major forms of arthritis that disproportionately afflict women.

25. The risk factors for osteoporosis and treatment issues for osteoporosis.

26. The characteristics of lupus.

27. The two major forms of diabetes.

28. The major risk factors for diabetes and how pregnancy presents special risks to the diabetic mother.

29. The seven warning signs of cancer.

30. How a woman can reduce her risk of cancer through knowledge and behavior.

Introduction

Cancer is second only to cardiovascular diseases as the leading cause of death among American women of all ages, and it is the leading cause of premature morbidity for women.[1] Although cancer can occur essentially anywhere in a woman's body, most cancer deaths are accounted for by cancers of the breast, colon and rectum, and reproductive system (ovaries, cervix, and uterus).[1] This chapter provides an overview of these major cancers of concern to women and a brief review of three other chronic, disabling conditions that afflict many women.

Perspectives on Cancer and Other Chronic Diseases

Cancer is a disease characterized by uncontrolled cellular growth and reproduction. Cancer is not a new disease. The term **carcinoma,** meaning a malignant tumor, was coined by Hippocrates in the fourth century B.C. There is no one type of cancer—literally over a hundred different diseases are categorized as "cancer." Information Box 12.1 provides a summary of the major types of cancer. There are many distinctions between these types of cancer. The purpose of this chapter is to provide an overview of those cancers that present the greatest threat to women's health. Each is discussed in terms of epidemiological considerations, risk factors, screening, and treatment.

Although the language used by scientists and clinicians to describe cancer conditions is complex, a fundamental issue is the concept of benign tumors or

Types of Cancer

Adenocarcinoma: A cancer that originates from cells of the endocrine glands

Carcinoma: A cancer that is the most common of all tumors—accounting for approximately 85 percent of all cancers

Hepatoma: A cancer that originates from liver cells

Leukemia: A cancer that originates within the blood and blood-producing organs

Lymphoma: A cancer that originates from lymph tissue, which is part of the body's immune system

Melanoma: A cancer that originates within the skin cells that contain melanin

Neuroblastoma: A cancer that originates from cells in the nervous system

Sarcoma: A cancer that originates in the connective tissue, such as cartilage, tendons, and bone

malignant tumors. A cancerous growth is technically any abnormal growth of cells. Growths are generally called **tumors** or **neoplasms.** Some tumors are solid, whereas others, known as cysts, consist of a thin-walled sac filled with fluid. A **benign tumor** is one that remains localized and confined in its original growth site. It does not invade the surrounding tissue or spread to distant body sites. Examples of benign tumors include skin warts or cysts. Because benign tumors are confined and localized, they can often be surgically removed. Usually benign tumors are not life-threatening unless they are located in a surgically inaccessible location. In contrast to benign tumors, **malignant tumors** or neoplasms are capable of spreading to other tissues and organs and invading adjacent tissue. The process of cancer cell invasion and spreading is known as **metastasis.** Once metastasis has occurred, localized surgical treatment is usually impossible.

In addition to developing new, improved surgical techniques to remove tumors and biomedical modalities to treat cancer, scientists are also trying to understand how cancer happens. **Carcinogenesis** refers to the overall staging process by which normal cells become malignant. Carcinogenesis may have a hereditary factor. Increasing evidence points to an inherited link for some forms of cancer. Chemical carcinogenesis, the development of cancer as a result of chemical exposure, is another area of study. The type, dose, and time exposure of the causative chemical all play an important role in the initiation and promotion of cancer cell growth. Carcinogenesis may also be due to physical agents, such as asbestos and ultraviolet radiation. Finally, viral carcinogenesis is an important women's health cancer research area. It is now believed that certain viruses, for example, the human papillomavirus (HPV), can invade cells like the cervix and produce mutation and uncontrolled growth.

In addition to cancer and cardiovascular disease (see Chapter 11), several other chronic, disabling conditions are major causes of disability for women today. **Chronic diseases,** in contrast to **acute diseases,** are diseases or conditions that are not short-lived. They generally last longer than several weeks and often last for the remainder of a person's life. Although chronic diseases are generally thought of as afflictions of the elderly, the reality is that chronic diseases are not limited to any age group. Some chronic diseases have a greater prevalence in women. This chapter provides a brief review of arthritis, osteoporosis, lupus, and diabetes mellitus—all chronic diseases that have dramatic impact on the health of women in the world today.

Epidemiological Overview

Cancer is the second leading cause of death for women in the United States.[2] Overall for women, age-adjusted death rates from cancer have been increasing steadily, primarily owing to the rise in the death rates from breast and lung cancer (Fig. 12.1). Mortality rates for all cancer sites in women under age 55 have declined somewhat since 1973, primarily as a result of advances in early detection of cervical and uterine cancers.[1]

Breast cancer is the most prevalent of new cancer cases in women each year[1] (Fig. 12.2). Breast cancer is also responsible for nearly 50,000 deaths in women each year. Increases in breast cancer death rates have occurred for both older and younger women. The lifetime risk of breast cancer is now one in nine.[3] Some of the increase is due to improved technology, especially mammography, which has resulted in earlier identification and more reporting of breast cancer. The risk of breast cancer increases with age, particularly after age 40.[1]

Fewer new cases of lung cancer are diagnosed each year in women than breast cancer, but annual lung cancer deaths surpass breast cancer deaths in women.[1] Although the incidence (number of new cases in a given period) of lung cancer is lower now in women than in men, the death rate is steadily

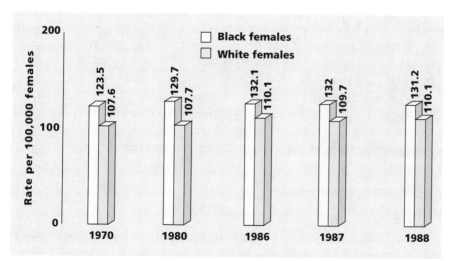

FIGURE 12.1

Death rates from malignant neoplasms, white and African-American women, 1970–88 (per 100,000 population).

SOURCE: USDHHS (1991). *Health United States, 1990.* Public Health Service, CDC. (DHHS Pub. No. (PHS) 91-1232.) Washington, DC: US Government Printing Office.

FIGURE 12.2

Comparison of new cancer cases and deaths, US women, 1993.

SOURCE: American Cancer Society (1993). *Cancer Facts and Figures— 1993*. Atlanta: American Cancer Society. Reprinted with permission.

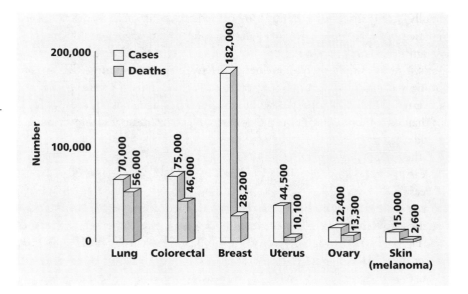

FIGURE 12.2

Comparison of new cancer cases and deaths, US women, 1993.

SOURCE: American Cancer Society (1993). *Cancer Facts and Figures— 1993*. Atlanta: American Cancer Society. Reprinted with permission.

increasing in women, while it is declining in men.[4] Five-year survival rates for lung cancer are low, and early detection is difficult because symptoms do not appear until the disease has reached advanced stages.

Other chronic conditions such as arthritis, osteoporosis, lupus, and diabetes mellitus are important health problems to women. They result in considerable impaired mobility and daily function. The epidemiological determination of prevalence for these conditions is difficult because of differences and inconsistencies in diagnostic criteria and the lack of national reporting systems. Osteoarthritis and rheumatoid arthritis are two of the most common health problems in the United States, and women are disproportionately afflicted with both conditions. A similar epidemiological picture presents with osteoporosis and lupus. Lupus, however, is even more prevalent among women than men, with women afflicted nine times more often than men.[5] Diabetes is another major chronic disease of concern to women. The prevalence of diabetes varies according to sex and race. Seven million people in the United States have been diagnosed with diabetes, and another 5 million may have the disease and not know it.[2] In general, the prevalence of diabetes increases with age.

Although these epidemiological "snapshots" of cancer and chronic disease do not provide the full picture, it is apparent that these conditions are responsible for considerable morbidity and mortality among American women.

Racial/ethnic and Socioeconomic Dimensions

The morbidity and mortality of cancer and chronic diseases are not evenly distributed across women in United States. Although cancer mortality rates have declined for younger women, rates have changed little among older and socially disadvantaged groups of women.[2] Cancer incidence rates among African Americans average 10 to 20 percent higher than among nonminorities.[6] Although racial disparity is evident in new cases of cancer for African-American and white women (Fig. 12.3), a greater racial disparity in cancer death rates among women has been a consistent epidemiological finding (see Fig. 12.1). The extent to which African-American women experience higher cancer mortality than white women is striking. Across the cancer diagnostic spectrum, not only do African Americans have higher mortality rates than nonminorities, but also the mortality rates are increasing faster. Further, mortality rates that are decreasing for whites are either still increasing for African Americans or not decreasing as fast.[7] Although overall death rates from cancer have dropped for both white and African-American women since 1973 (see Fig. 12.1), African-American women continue to experience greater overall cancer incidence rates (see Fig. 12.3), breast cancer death rates (Fig. 12.4), and similar respiratory cancer death rates (Fig. 12.5) compared with white women.

Survival rates are calculations that take normal life expectancy into account and are used as a measure of progress in detecting and treating cancer in its early stages. As with death rate data, for most cancers, the 5-year relative survival rate of African-American women is lower than that of white women (Fig. 12.6). These racial differences in breast cancer survival rates may be due to a combination of factors, including the lower likelihood of African-American women with breast cancer being diagnosed in the early disease stages and a lower survival rate in women whose disease has advanced.[7]

Because cancer risk is strongly associated with lifestyle and behavior, differences in ethnic and cultural groups can provide clues to factors involved in cancer development, such as dietary patterns, alcohol and tobacco use, and sexual and reproductive behaviors. Cultural values and belief systems can also affect attitudes about seeking medical care or following screening

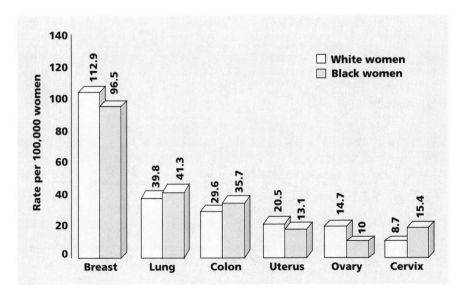

FIGURE 12.3

Age-adjusted incident cancer rates in US African-American and white women, 1988.

SOURCE: National Cancer Institute, SEER Program.

FIGURE 12.4

Death rates from breast cancer, white and African-American women, 1970–88 (per 100,000 population).

SOURCE: USDHHS (1991). *Health United States, 1990.* Public Health Service, CDC. (DHHS Pub. No. (PHS) 91-1232.) Washington, DC: US Government Printing Office.

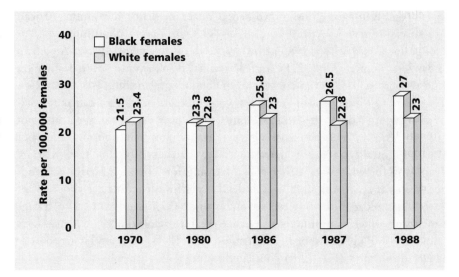

FIGURE 12.5

Death rates from respiratory cancer, white and African-American women, 1970–88 (per 100,000 population).

SOURCE: USDHHS (1991). *Health United States, 1990.* Public Health Service, CDC. (DHHS Pub. No. (PHS) 91-1232.) Washington, DC: US Government Printing Office.

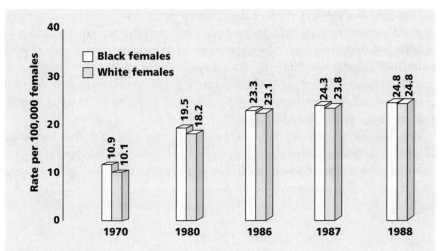

FIGURE 12.6

Age-adjusted, 5-year cancer survival rates, African-American and white women, 1981–86.

SOURCE: Adapted from National Cancer Institute (1990). *Cancer Statistics Review, 1973–87.* (NCI, NIH Pub. No. 90-2789.) Bethesda, MD: US Government Printing Office.

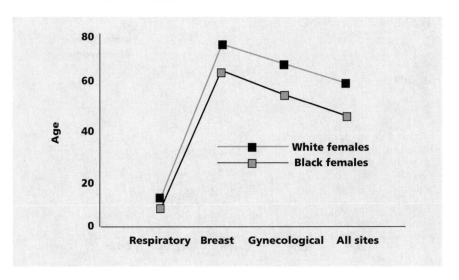

guidelines. Information Box 12.2 shows differences in health practices among white, African-American, and Hispanic-American women in the preventive health behaviors of Pap tests and mammography. Of women aged 18 and older, Hispanic-American and African-American women were more likely to have never had a Pap test while non-hispanic whites were more likely to have heard of, but never had, a mammography.

Although incidence and mortality rates for cervical cancer have declined dramatically over the last 30 years, cervical cancer remains particularly disproportionate among African-American women, who are 2½ times more likely to get cervical cancer and die from it than nonminority white women.[6] It has been estimated that 36.5 percent of deaths in African-American women from cervical cancer could be averted through appropriate screening and follow-up.[8]

Screening programs are important for early detection of cancer. Socioeconomic factors, such as the lack of health insurance, transportation, or child care, can impede women's access to care and lead to late diagnosis and poor survival. Lack of participation in and reduced access to screening have been hypothesized as the major reasons for the disproportionate cancer burden in minority women. For example, mammography use has been found to be higher among white women than among African-American women and higher among women with a higher income and more education.[9] The reasons why minority women are less likely to participate in screening programs probably relate to socioeconomic and cultural factors. Access to and use of cancer prevention services have been identified as major barriers for many minority populations. To be effective, programs must be culturally sensitive and available. Lack of respect has been identified as one of the most significant barriers to effective

INFORMATION BOX 12.2

Women's Participation in Cancer Screening Programs

| | % Women Who Never Had Test | | | |
| | Pap Smears* | | Mammography† | |
	Never Heard of Test	Heard of but Never Had Test	Never Heard of Test	Heard of but Never Had Test
All races	4.0	7.3	15.6	47.5
Whites (non-Hispanic)	2.1	6.9	12.2	48.9
Blacks (non-Hispanic)	4.1	7.8	29.4	40.9
Hispanics	15.1	9.6	31.6	42.2

*Percents are for women aged 18 and over.
†Percents are for women aged 40 and over.
SOURCE: National Health Interview Survey, National Center for Health Statistics, 1987.

prevention programs in minority populations. One study[8] found that 43 percent of African-Americans and Latinos complained that the health care system lacked respect for them as persons. It is unlikely that preventive personal health behaviors or cancer screening practice messages can be effectively sent under these conditions.

Racial differences in disease prevalence across other chronic diseases are inconsistent. No significant racial differences in the prevalence of rheumatoid arthritis have been identified, although the rate is higher among some Native-American tribes.[10] White and Asian-American women have osteoporosis more often than African-American women,[3] whereas lupus is more prevalent among African-American women than white women.[5] With diabetes, African-American women experience the highest prevalence rates.[11] In addition to the high prevalence rates among African Americans, other minority populations such as Native Americans and Hispanic Americans are at higher risk for diabetes.[12] The highest incident rates of diabetes are found among the American Indians and Alaskan Natives.[13]

Breast Conditions

More than half of all women who menstruate regularly, at one time or another, go through the frightening experience of finding a lump in a breast. In more than 90 percent of these cases, the lump is benign and may need no treatment. Being able to understand the issues and concerns about breast conditions is an important dimension of women's health.

Benign Breast Diseases

Most breast lumps are not cancer. **Fibrocystic breast disease,** also called cystic mastitis, is the most common breast disorder and the most frequent cause of a breast lump in a woman under the age of 25. The disease is most prevalent in women between the ages of 30 and 50. Common symptoms of this condition include lumpy, tender breasts, particularly during the week before menses. Several modalities have been used to treat fibrocystic breast disease, including hormonal therapy, vitamin E, and special diets, but none has emerged as a definitive treatment. Only a small subgroup of women with fibrocystic breast disease are at increased risk for breast cancer. These women have an atypical cell condition known as **hyperplasia,** which can be diagnosed by breast **biopsy,** a procedure in which a small sample of breast tissue is removed and examined under a microscope.

Another nonmalignant form of breast tumor is **fibroadenoma,** the most common breast tumor in women younger than age 25. This type of tumor produces a firm, movable, nontender lump. Fibroadenomas are usually removed both to confirm the diagnosis and to prevent further damage to breast tissue from continued localized tumor growth.

Breast Cancer

Breast cancer is a frightening condition for women. Before 1974, when First Lady Betty Ford underwent a mastectomy, breast cancer was not a public news item. Since then, news reports about breast cancer victims and breast cancer research have become more common. Women, however, still feel that the information is frightening, conflicting, and sometimes misleading. An understanding of breast cancer is important for all women. Breast cancer is one of the most treatable cancers if it is detected early.

The classification system for breast cancer consists of five levels. In situ stage breast cancer can be diagnosed by mammogram, but the tumors are usually too small to be felt. The 5-year survival rate for in situ tumors is nearly 100 percent. Stage I breast cancer remains localized to the breast and generally is smaller than 2 cm in size and has not spread to the lymph nodes. Stage II breast cancer tumors generally are larger—2 to 5 cm in size—and they also have not spread to the lymph nodes. Stage II tumors may also be smaller than 2 to 5 cm but have spread to lymph nodes. Stage III tumors are growths that are over 5 cm in size or that have grown into the chest wall, skin, or distant lymph nodes. Stage IV tumors are classified as growths that have spread to other parts of the body. Five-year breast cancer survival rates drop with the increasing size and invasiveness of the tumor.

Risk Factors

Breast cancer is the most frequent cancer in women, and several major risk factors have been identified for breast cancer (Self-Assessment 12.1). It is important to note, however, that most women with breast cancer do not have any of the known risk factors for the disease, which underscores the vital importance of regular self-examinations, clinical examinations, and screening mammography for all women. The greatest risk factor is being a woman, and the second is age. Family history plays a role in breast cancer risk. Women with mothers or sisters who had breast cancer are at greater risk themselves. Women who never had children or women who delayed their first child after the age of 30 are also at increased risk. Menstruation plays a role in risk for breast cancer. Early menarche and late menopause are associated with increased risk for breast cancer.[14] The role of estrogen as a risk factor in breast cancer has been heavily debated. Most studies have not found an association between past use of estrogen replacement therapy (ERT), including use for more than 10 years, and an increased risk of breast cancer.[15] Oral contraceptives also have not been found to be associated with an increased risk of breast cancer.[16] Other factors have been hypothesized to be associated with an elevated risk of breast cancer, such as a high-fat diet, alcohol consumption, viral infections, breast trauma, and obesity. Scientists have yet to reach consensus, however, on these factors as significant risk factors.

There is a family history of breast cancer. I am learning everything I can. I do monthly BSE, and I have regular clinical exams and mammography. There is so much research going on today. I am trying to stay informed because I know that I need to know.

32-YEAR-OLD WOMAN

*Breast Cancer Risk Factors**

Category 1: Highest Risk

Personal history of breast cancer

Mother or sister with breast cancer

Previous breast biopsy showing atypical cell changes

Previous mammogram with suspicious findings

Category 2: Lower Risk

No children or first pregnancy after age 30

Breast cancer in nonimmediate family member

Early menarche (before age 12)

History of fibrocystic breast disease

Previous cancer

Late menopause (after age 50)

Category 3: Possible Risk

Estrogen hormones

History of DES use while pregnant

Breast implants (which may reduce likelihood of breast self-examination or mammography to detect lesions)

*Most women with breast cancer do not have any of the known risk factors. This underscores the vital importance of regular self-examination, clinical examination, and screening mammography for all women.

SOURCE: National Cancer Institute.

Screening

Most of the identified risk factors for breast cancer cannot be modified by lifestyle behaviors. Early detection of breast cancer, however, can be life-saving. The prognosis for breast cancer strongly depends on early detection (Information Box 12.3). There are three basic methods for early detection of breast cancer. Breast self-examination (BSE), clinical breast examinations, and mammography are all important preventive behaviors for women to reduce their risk of breast cancer.

Breast Cancer Survival Rates

Degree of Invasion	Five-Year Survival Rate (%)
In situ (localized, no invasion)	99
Localized invasion	90
Regional spread	68
Distant metastases	18

SOURCE: American Cancer Society (1991). *Cancer Facts and Figures, 1991*. Atlanta: American Cancer Society.

BSE consists of the systematic palpation of the breast tissue of each breast while in a supine position. Most abnormalities are detected as changes or lumps in breast tissue, and most breast cancers present in the breast ducts. The American Cancer Society recommends that women over the age of 25 examine their breasts monthly after menses. For women who have reached menopause, regular BSE should be done on a scheduled monthly basis. In addition to examining for lumps, women should check for breast discharges. Figure 12.7 provides detailed guidance on the BSE procedure.

Most breast lesions are present for several years before they can be felt. Smaller breast lesions that cannot yet be felt through BSE can be detected by **mammography,** which is a low-dose x-ray of the breast tissue (Fig. 12.8). Mammography has the potential of detecting breast cancer at its earliest stages of development. Mammography involves compressing the breast between two flat disks. Two x-rays are taken of each breast, and one is taken from above the breast.

Despite the obvious appeal of mammography as a breakthrough in breast cancer diagnostics, some concerns have been raised. One concern is the potential **carcinogenic,** cancer-causing, effect of regular irradiation of breast tissue. Scientists generally agree, however, that the x-ray doses used for mammography are quite low, and the risk of developing mammography-induced breast cancers is negligible.[17] Others concerns with mammography include the cost, discomfort, and the comparatively high frequency of false-positive test results. There is some discomfort from breast compression during mammography, but surveys indicate that most women find such discomfort to be minor. Mammography costs remain high for most women, but third-party insurance payers are increas-

I had a lump in my breast, and it had been there for some time. It didn't hurt. I guess that I was hoping it was nothing and would go away. I waited too long. This has been a rough year, but I am trying to tell other women not to make the same mistake. If you feel a lump, regardless of the size, have it checked right away.

42-YEAR-OLD WOMAN

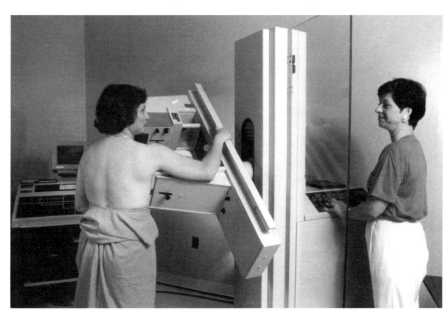

Mammography is the best breast cancer screening method currently available for detecting nonpalpable tumors.

BREAST SELF-EXAMINATION

Breast self-examination should be done once a month so you become familiar with the usual appearance and feel of your breasts. Familiarity makes it easier to notice any changes in the breast from one month to another. Early discovery of a change from what is "normal" is the main idea behind BSE. The outlook is much better if you detect cancer in an early stage.

If you menstruate, the best time to do BSE is 2 or 3 days after your period ends, when your breasts are least likely to be tender or swollen. If you no longer menstruate, pick a day such as the first day of the month, to remind yourself it is time to do BSE.

Here is one way to do BSE:

1. Stand before a mirror. Inspect both breasts for anything unusual such as any discharge from the nipples or puckering, dimpling, or scaling of the skin.

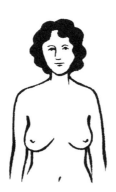

The next two steps are designed to emphasize any change in the shape or contour of your breasts. As you do them, you should be able to feel your chest muscles tighten.

2. Watching closely in the mirror, clasp your hands behind your head and press your hands forward.

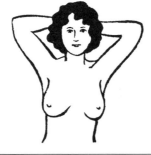

3. Next, press your hands firmly on your hips and bow slightly toward your mirror as you pull your shoulders and elbows forward.

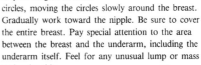

Some women do the next part of the exam in the shower because fingers glide over soapy skin, making it easy to concentrate on the texture underneath.

4. Raise your left arm. Use three or four fingers of your right hand to explore your left breast firmly, carefully, and thoroughly. Beginning at the outer edge, press the flat part of your fingers in small circles, moving the circles slowly around the breast. Gradually work toward the nipple. Be sure to cover the entire breast. Pay special attention to the area between the breast and the underarm, including the underarm itself. Feel for any unusual lump or mass under the skin.

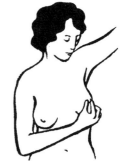

5. Gently squeeze the nipple and look for a discharge. (If you have any discharge during the month—whether or not it is during BSE—see your doctor.) Repeat steps 4 and 5 on your right breast.

6. Steps 4 and 5 should be repeated lying down. Lie flat on your back with your left arm over your head and a pillow or folded towel under your left shoulder. This position flattens the breast and makes it easier to examine. Use the same circular motion described earlier. Repeat the exam on your right breast.

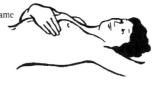

FIGURE 12.7

Breast Self-Examination (BSE). BSE should be done once a month so you become familiar with the usual appearance and feel of your breasts. Familiarity makes it easier to notice any changes in the breast from one month to another. Early discovery of a change from what is "normal" is the main idea behind BSE. If you menstruate, the best time to do BSE is 2 or 3 days after your period ends, when your breasts are least likely to be tender or swollen. If you no longer menstruate, pick a day, such as the first day of the month, to remind yourself it is time to do BSE.

SOURCE: National Cancer Institute.

ingly providing partial or total coverage for the procedures. **False-positive** (suspected breast lesions that are biopsied but that are not found to be cancerous) mammography test results are high—nearly 80 percent. The problems that arise from these false-positive results are the performance of unnecessary biopsies, expense, time, and anxiety. Nevertheless, it is generally thought that the demonstrated benefits of mammography screening for breast cancer outweigh these disadvantages. The use of mammography is recommended by several major medical and health organizations as part of an early detection program for breast cancer, in conjunction with regular physical examinations. The National Cancer Institute released a statement in 1993 noting the general consensus among experts was that routine screening every 1 to 2 years with mammography and clinical breast examination could reduce breast cancer mortality by about one third for women ages 50 and over. The Institute acknowledged that experts do not yet agree on the role of routine screening for women ages 40 to 49. To date, randomized trials have not shown a statistically significant reduction in mortality for women under the age of 50. Breast cancer screening program evaluations and clinical trials are currently being reviewed in an effort to more clearly answer questions about mammography screening.

Although a breast tumor may be suspected with an examination or mammography, the ultimate diagnosis is made by biopsy.

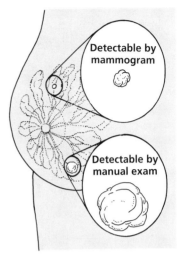

FIGURE 12.8

Finding breast lumps early. A mammogram can detect a tiny cancer (top inset) up to 2 years before it grows big enough to feel with your fingers (bottom inset).

Treatment and Reconstruction

A few years ago, a radical mastectomy was fairly standard with a diagnosis of breast cancer. A shift in recent years has been toward breast conserving surgery. Today surgery is still the primary treatment of breast cancer, but the surgery is sometimes combined with chemotherapy and hormone therapy. For early-stage localized tumors, it is often possible to remove only the tumor and some surrounding tissue, a procedure known as a lumpectomy. If the entire breast is removed, the procedure is known as a **mastectomy.** Breast cancer surgery may be performed immediately following a positive biopsy, thereby avoiding the need for a second anesthetic and procedure. Most women, however, prefer a two-step procedure in which the biopsy and the necessary surgery are separate events. The two-step process enables the woman to review her options better and make her decision carefully.

There are three major types of breast removal surgical procedures. A **radical mastectomy** is the removal of the entire affected breast, the underlying chest muscles, and the lymph nodes under the arm. A **modified radical mastectomy,** or total mastectomy, is a less extensive procedure not removing the underlying chest wall muscles. It is now the standard surgical procedure for most breast cancers. The modified mastectomy has comparable survival rates to the radical mastectomy, but it is more conducive to cosmetic reconstruction and results in greater mobility and reduced swelling. A **simple mastectomy** involves the complete removal of the breast but not the lymph nodes under the arm or the chest wall muscles.

A **segmental mastectomy** or lumpectomy involves the removal of a portion of the breast, including the cancer and a surrounding margin of breast tissue. Axillary lymph nodes are also usually removed. In women with early cancer, a lumpectomy with subsequent radiation therapy has become the primary alternative to modified radical mastectomy. Lumpectomies are usually limited to those breast tumors that are well defined and less than 1 to 2 in. in total diameter. Radiation may be used to eliminate any possible remaining cancer cells.

Adjuvant therapy, methods that enhance surgical effectiveness, include anticancer drugs, **chemotherapy,** hormone therapy, and radiation therapy. Chemotherapy and hormone therapy may also be used in the treatment of localized tumors as well as for the control of metastatic conditions. Chemoprevention of breast cancer has been a goal of medical researchers. Research has suggested that **tamoxifen,** a widely accepted chemical treatment for breast cancer, may actually prevent the disease in healthy women as well. Tamoxifen is appealing as a chemoprevention because it is far less toxic than conventional breast cancer chemotherapy. The exact mechanism by which it works is not understood, but it appears that tamoxifen inhibits the growth of tumors that have spread beyond the breast. Other studies suggest that it can reduce the number of new breast tumors. For that reason, there is scientific speculation that tamoxifen may serve as a preventive chemotherapy for women who are at risk but who have never had breast cancer. Current ongoing clinical studies will hopefully shed additional light on this important question.

After mastectomy, a woman faces the decision of whether or not to have breast reconstruction. Reconstruction of breast tissue is often an important part of breast cancer recovery. Currently approximately 30 percent of women undergoing mastectomy choose breast reconstruction.[18] The degree of difficulty with reconstruction varies with the extent of surgery. Emotional support and social support are important components of recovery. Local support groups may provide valuable information and assistance with physical and psychological breast cancer recovery issues.

Gynecological Conditions

The term, "gynecological conditions" refers to any disease process in a woman's upper or lower reproductive tract. This section provides an overview of the major gynecological conditions of the cervix, uterus, and ovaries. Malignant and nonmalignant conditions are discussed in terms of risk factors, screening, and treatment.

Cervical Cancer*

The **Pap smear** has made early detection of cervical abnormalities a reality. The Pap smear is one of the tests that is usually performed during a routine

---

AUTHORS' NOTE. The cervix is technically part of the uterus, but because the characteristics and risk factors for uterine and cervical cancer are distinctive, they are discussed separately.

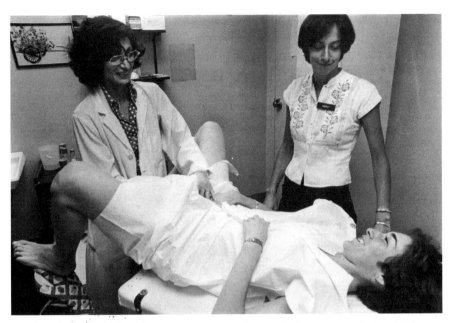

The Pap smear is a reliable screening test for cervical cancer and should be a routine part of a woman's gynecological care.

gynecological examination (see Chapter 7). A sample of cells is obtained from the cervix and then sent to a laboratory for microscopic analysis. The Pap smear is a screening test: If abnormal cells are detected, a cervical biopsy is performed to establish a firm diagnosis. Pap smears are an effective screening tool for cervical cancer because precancerous cell changes can be detected before cancer actually develops. Pap smears can also detect a portion of, although not all, endometrial cancers. Precancerous cell changes are known as **dysplasia.** Dysplasia can be classified as mild, moderate, or severe. Severe dysplasia is the type most likely to become cancerous. In its localized first stage, this form of cancer is known as **carcinoma-in-situ,** involving only the outer layer of the skin. Dysplasia and carcinoma-in-situ have nearly a 100 percent cure rate, and localized carcinoma remains curable in nearly 90 percent of cases. As with other forms of cancer, survival rates drop with invasive conditions. Regular screening for early detection is the keystone to reducing mortality from cervical cancer.

Risk Factors

The major risk factors for cervical cancer are associated with sexual practices, such as age of first intercourse and multiple sexual partners. The use of barrier methods of contraception may reduce the exposure to infectious agents and thereby reduce the risk of developing cervical cancer. Cigarette smoking also appears to be associated with increased risk for cervical cancer. Most cases of

He was a nice guy and I asked him if he had any diseases . . . he said no. But guess what? Now I have HPV and I know he gave it to me. It makes me angry at him and myself for believing him. I am adjusting to this, but the thought of cervical cancer scares me the most.

22-YEAR-OLD STUDENT

INFORMATION BOX 12.4

Major Risk Factors for Cervical Cancer*

First marriage or intercourse at an early age (teenager)

Multiple sex partners or a partner with multiple partners

History of HPV infection

More than four pregnancies

Daughter of a woman who took DES during pregnancy

*If a woman has any of these risk factors, she should have a Pap smear at least annually to screen for cervical cancer.

cervical cancer are associated with HPV (see Chapter 10), which are sexually transmitted. As many as one-third of women with HPV infections may have precancerous changes of the cervix. The major risk factors for cervical cancer are summarized in Information Box 12.4. Invasive cervical cancer rarely occurs in women who have regular gynecological examinations. When it does, however, symptoms may include bleeding between menstrual periods or spotting after intercourse.

Screening

Cervical cancer is one of the few cancers with a truly effective screening modality. Pap smears provide a reliable method of screening for very early forms of cervical cancer. Pap smear screening currently detects more than 75 percent of cervical carcinomas before they become invasive. American Cancer Society guidelines for cervical cancer screening recommend that all women who are or have been sexually active or have reached the age of 18 should have an annual Pap test and pelvic examination. After a woman has had three or more consecutive negative Pap smears, the time between screenings can be determined on an individual basis. A woman who has any of the identified risk factors for cervical cancer, however, should receive annual screening.

Treatment

Treatment following an abnormal Pap smear depends on results of a cervical biopsy. Inflammation of the cervix, known as **cervicitis,** may be associated with a vaginal infection or discharge that requires only local treatment with specific vaginal creams or suppositories. Treatment for dysplasia depends on its severity and usually consists of cryosurgery, cone biopsy, or laser cone biopsy.

Cryosurgery is a procedure that destroys tissue by a freezing process. It is most often used to treat mild or moderate dysplasia. As a procedure, cryosurgery has the advantage of producing little or no discomfort. It also presents few risks for complications, such as bleeding, further infection, or infertility from scarring. A watery vaginal discharge is common for about 2 weeks after cryosurgery. It is generally recommended that women avoid intercourse, douching, or tampons during this recovery time.

A cone biopsy or **conization** is considered to be both a diagnostic and a therapeutic procedure because it provides tissue for an accurate diagnosis while removing the abnormal tissue. Cone biopsy procedures are less common today than a few years ago because of the widespread use of **colposcopy,** an office procedure using a special microscope that permits close examination of the cervix and vagina as well as biopsy.

By the time carcinoma-in-situ has become invasive, there is likely to be an abnormal growth on the cervix. Cervical biopsy is then performed to establish the diagnosis. Treatment of cervical cancer depends on the tumor's stage when diagnosed. Carcinoma-in-situ may be treated with cone biopsy in a woman who has not completed her family. Definitive treatment of carcinoma-in-situ, however, requires **hysterectomy,** surgical removal of the uterus, because surface cancer can recur in 5 to 10 percent of the women treated with cone biopsy alone. Even after hysterectomy, a small percentage of women experience a recurrence of cancer in the vagina, so lifelong gynecological follow-up is important.

Benign Uterine Tumors

Benign tumors are not cancer. They do not spread to other parts of the body, and they seldom are life-threatening. Several types of benign tumors grow in the uterus. In some cases, there is no need for medical intervention after diagnosis; however, sometimes surgical removal of the growth is indicated.

Fibroids are benign tumors composed of muscular and fibrous tissue in the uterus. They are most often found in women older than age 35. Fibroids are the primary cause of an abnormally enlarged uterus and one of the most common reasons for hysterectomy. Although single fibroid tumors occur, multiple tumors are more common. Symptoms of fibroids depend on the size and location of the tumors and may include irregular vaginal bleeding, vaginal discharge, and frequent urination. They may increase in size under the influence of estrogen produced during pregnancy, from oral contraceptives, or from hormone replacement therapy. Fibroids often shrink and disappear with menopause. Although they are usually symptomless, large fibroids may contribute to chronic backache, pelvic pain, and heavy or prolonged menstrual periods. Fibroids are usually detected during routine pelvic examinations because they create an enlarged and irregular uterus. Surgery may be indicated for fibroids if they cause severe pain or bleeding. Surgery involves removing either the fibroid alone, **myomectomy,** or the entire uterus, hysterectomy. New drug regimens for the treatment of fibroids are currently under investigation.

Endometriosis is another benign condition of the uterus. In this condition, tissue that looks and acts like endometrial tissue begins to grow outside the uterine lining. This progressive condition is most common in women aged between 30 to 40 years. Because endometrial tissue responds to hormonal influences during the menstrual cycle, women who have this disorder often feel pain just before or during menstruation. Endometriosis also causes painful menstrual periods and abnormal vaginal bleeding. About 30 percent of women with endometriosis experience infertility. Treatment of endometriosis includes hormones to prevent ovulation. When hormonal drugs fail to relieve symptoms of pain or when the endometriosis has progressed to the point of forming large cysts, surgery may be indicated. Through operative laparoscopy, deposits of endometriosis as well as more extensive disease involving cysts and adhesions can be removed using either electrocautery, burning of tissue, or a laser. The most radical surgery as well as the only definitive cure for endometriosis involves a complete hysterectomy.

Hyperplasia is an increase in the number of normal cells lining the uterus. Although the condition is not cancer, it may develop into cancer in some women. The most common symptoms of hyperplasia are heavy menstrual periods and bleeding between periods. Treatment depends on the extent of the condition (mild, moderate, or severe) and on the age of the woman. Young women are usually treated with hormones, and the endometrial tissue is checked often. Hyperplasia in women near or after menopause may be treated with hormones if the condition is not severe. Hysterectomy is the usual treatment for severe cases.

Malignant Uterine Tumors

Uterine cancer most commonly begins in the tissue lining of the uterus, the **endometrium.** Endometrial cancer is most common in women between the ages of 55 and 70. The incidence of endometrial cancer increased rapidly in the early 1970s owing to the increased use of high-dose estrogen therapy in postmenopausal women.[19] With the decline in the use of estrogens and changes in the composition of replacement hormones used in postmenopausal women, the incidence of endometrial cancer has also declined. The higher incidence rates of endometrial cancer among white women may be related to their greater access to and use of estrogen replacement therapy during the 1970s.

Risk Factors

Endometrial cancer accounts for most uterine cancers. Risk factors for uterine cancer are believed to involve excess stimulation of endometrial cell proliferation by estrogen in the absence of progesterone. Obesity is believed to increase endometrial cancer risk, perhaps owing to fat cell estrogen production. Other risk factors for endometrial cancer include a failure to ovulate and a history of infertility. Both of these conditions may also be associated with an estrogen imbalance. Postmenopausal long-term, high-dose estrogen replacement therapy is also a risk factor for endometrial cancer. Today this risk is minimized by hormone replacement regimens of lower doses of estrogen in combination with progesterone. In addition to hormonal risk factors, cigarette smoking has been linked to an increased risk for endometrial cancer. Further research is needed to ascertain the mechanisms and roles of all these risk factors for endometrial cancer.[20]

Screening

Because endometrial cancer is inside the uterus, the tumor initially cannot be seen or felt during a pelvic examination. Unfortunately, the Pap smear is only partially effective in the diagnosis of endometrial cancer, and the disease is not usually detected until symptoms are evident. The most common symptom of endometrial cancer after menopause is vaginal bleeding. The American Cancer Society recommends that women at increased risk for endometrial cancer (history of infertility or obesity) have an endometrial biopsy at menopause. Women on estrogen replacement therapy should have endometrial biopsies repeated on a regular basis.

Treatment

Diagnosis of endometrial cancer is by biopsy or **dilation and curettage** (D&C). Both of these procedures permit the evaluation of tissue and cells lining the uterine cavity. Because uterine cancer may spread rapidly, treatment for early stages of this disease involves removal of the uterus as well as the fallopian tubes and ovaries. A combination of surgery and radiotherapy is effective in the treatment of localized disease. Regional spread of the cancer outside of the uterus is treatable by radiation. Advanced, metastatic endometrial cancer is generally treated by the administration of progesterone, which results in prolonged survival but not cure.

Ovarian Cancer

Ovarian cancer is a relatively rare but usually fatal form of cancer. It is more common in white women than African-American women,[21] and the risk increases with age. Highest rates of ovarian cancer occur in women over 60 years of age.[1] The causes of ovarian cancer are not very well defined.

Risk Factors

Because the causes of ovarian cancer are not well understood, it is difficult to define specific risk factors. The risk of ovarian cancer appears to be related to reproductive history, indicating perhaps the importance of hormonal factors. Women who have not had children have about a twofold increased risk of developing ovarian cancer, but the risk decreases to below average in women who have had several pregnancies. Oral contraceptives, which, like pregnancy, prevent ovulation, also appear to decrease the risk of ovarian cancer.[22] A history of previous cancer, particularly of the breast or endometrium, doubles a woman's risk of developing ovarian cancer.[1] A moderate direct relationship between age of menopause and ovarian cancer does appear to exist.[21] In contrast to endometrial cancer, there does not appear to be an association between estrogen replacement therapy and ovarian cancer.

Screening

Ovarian cancer, often called the "silent cancer," is usually asymptomatic until it is relatively advanced. It is not detected by Pap smears. Early detection is best accomplished through regular pelvic examinations. Ultrasound and a laboratory test for an ovarian tumor marker in the blood, called CA-125, are being evaluated as possible ovarian cancer screening methods. Early symptoms of ovarian cancer may include pelvic pressure, abdominal swelling, gas pains, indigestion, and vague abdominal discomfort. Rarely, however, are any of these symptoms attributed to ovarian cancer because they are all symptoms of other common benign conditions.

Treatment

Definitive treatment for ovarian cancer includes surgery, radiation, and chemotherapy. Surgical treatment involves removal of the uterus, fallopian tubes, and ovaries. Chemotherapy and radiation therapies are used after surgery to improve survival.

Other Cancers of Special Concern to Women

Women are susceptible to cancer anywhere in their bodies. Colorectal cancer, lung cancer, and skin cancer, however, all have special considerations in terms of women's health issues. Each of these cancers is discussed in terms of their risk factors, screening guidelines, and treatment.

Colorectal Cancer

Colorectal cancers develop in a gradual, progressive manner and may present anywhere in the colon and rectal areas. Colon cancer is about twice as common as rectal cancer. Some rarer forms of colon cancer are known to have a genetic tendency.

Risk Factors

The risk of developing colon and rectum cancers is about twice as high for individuals with an immediate family member who has had the disease as it is for the general population. A history of inflammatory bowel disease, for example, ulcerative colitis, is also associated with a high risk of developing colon cancer. An individual who has had a polyp or carcinoma is also at increased risk of developing a second carcinoma. Dietary factors are thought to be an important determinant of colon and rectal cancer risk. An increased incidence of these cancers appears to be associated with diets that are high in fat and low in fiber or other components of fruits and vegetables. The most definitive dietary risk for colorectal cancer is a high-fat diet. Warning signs for colorectal cancer include rectal bleeding, blood in the stool, or a change in bowel habits.

Screening

Similar to other forms of cancer, early detection of colorectal cancer greatly improves the likelihood of complete recovery. Three approaches to the early detection of colorectal cancer have been recommended by the American Cancer Society. These approaches include digital rectal examination, sigmoidoscopy, and fecal occult blood testing. In contrast to breast cancer and cervical cancer studies, there are fewer and more limited studies demonstrating the efficacy of these measures in terms of reducing mortality, although studies do support the efficacy of screening in terms of earlier cancer detection.

Each of these tests for colorectal screening has inherent advantages and disadvantages. Digital rectal examination is a simple part of a routine physical examination. It is, however, relatively insensitive as a screening test because very few colorectal lesions develop within the range of the examining finger. **Sigmoidoscopy** is an examination of the rectum and lower part of the colon with a thin, lighted tube. Although more tumors can be detected with this procedure, a significant disadvantage of the procedure is discomfort. Screening for tumors by fecal occult blood testing has the potential advantage over the other two methods to detect a tumor in any part of the colon. Developing tumors cause minor bleeding, which results in the presence of occult blood, small amounts of blood in the stool. Fecal occult testing is a simple procedure of smearing a small sample of stool on a slide containing a chemical that changes color in the presence of hemoglobin. Unfortunately, the testing process is still plagued by a significant number of false-positive and false-negative findings.

Despite the limitations of each method, screening for colorectal cancer is important for early detection. The American Cancer Society recommends that all individuals have yearly digital examinations starting at age 40; yearly fecal occult blood tests starting at age 50, and sigmoidoscopy every 3 to 5 years starting at age 50.

Treatment

Surgical removal of the colorectal tumor is the primary treatment modality. Surgery is sometimes combined with radiation and chemotherapy. Overall survival is about 50 percent, but this is highly dependent on the extent of tumor progression at the time of diagnosis.

Skin Cancer

Skin cancers can be classified as melanomas and nonmelanomas. Melanoma is a cancer arising from pigment-producing cells in the skin. The worldwide incidence of melanoma has been steadily increasing in recent years. The nonmelanoma skin cancers include basal and squamous cell carcinomas. They are extremely common but seldom fatal. The American Cancer Society estimates that about 90 percent of skin cancers could have been prevented by protection from the sun's rays.[1]

Risk Factors

The major risk factor for melanoma is ultraviolet radiation from sunlight. It is about 10 times more frequent among white people than African Americans. It is believed that the greater pigmentation of dark skin affords protection against radiation. In rare cases, a familial susceptibility to melanoma may be inherited. Similar to melanomas, nonmelanoma skin cancers are caused by solar ultraviolet radiation. All forms of sun tanning and sun exposure are potentially hazardous to the skin. The American Cancer Society considers the sun to be the greatest single cause of cancer in the United States. Basal cell carcinoma and squamous cell carcinoma are associated with frequent exposure to the sun over many years. Melanoma has been associated with a single, blistering sunburn early in life.

Screening

Early detection of all skin cancers is critical. Recognition of changes in skin growths or the appearance of new growths is the best way to find early skin cancer. Early detection is essential to the outcome of melanoma. Screening is best accomplished by skin examination. Melanomas may develop within a mole or as a new molelike growth. They are characterized by increasing size and changes in color. The American Cancer Society emphasizes four warnings of melanoma:

- *Asymmetry*—the shape of one-half of a lesion or mole is different from the other.
- *Border irregularities*—the edge may be uneven, ragged, or blotched.
- *Color irregularities*—there may be different colors present in the mole or lesion.
- *Size*—the mole or lesion is usually greater than 6 mm (about ¼in.) in diameter.

Treatment

There are four primary treatment modalities for skin cancer. Surgery is used in 90 percent of the cases.[1] Radiation therapy; **electrodessication,** tissue destruction by heat; or cryosurgery are also used for early forms of nonmelanoma skin cancer. Treatment for melanoma usually consists of surgical removal of the mole or lesion and sometimes regional lymph nodes. Survival rates are high for localized lesions, but metastatic disease is not responsive to therapy. Because melanomas are able to metastasize quickly, early detection is the major determinant of survival.

Lung Cancer

In 1987, more women died from lung cancer than breast cancer, and lung cancer has remained as the leading cause of cancer deaths among women.[1] Lung cancer is deadly with 5-year survival rates of only 13 percent overall for patients at all stages of diagnosis. Only 20 percent of lung cancers are detected in early stages when survival rates are higher.[1] Causes of lung cancer vary, but the commonality that exists is the persistent exposure to lung irritants, particularly those that are inhaled, such as cigarette smoke.

Risk Factors

Although exposure to radon, asbestos, radioactive materials, and some industrial compounds have been associated with lung cancer, cigarette smoking is the most significant risk factor for lung cancer. Cigarette smoking has been estimated to be responsible for 75 to 80 percent of lung cancer cases in women.[4,23] Lung cancer rates in women are expected to continue to climb. A diagnosis of cancer usually reflects the cumulative effect of many years of smoking. As the post–World War II cohort of women smokers continues to age, lung cancer rates for this group are expected to escalate. Although respiratory death rates are currently similar among African-American and white women (see Fig. 12.5), this trend is not expected to continue because minority populations today are not quitting tobacco use as fast as whites. In future years, this will be reflected in greater respiratory cancer death rates.[24]

Screening

Early detection of lung cancer is difficult because symptoms do not appear until the disease is in its advanced stages. Cough may present as a predominate symptom in lung cancer. Along with cough, common symptoms of lung cancer include weight loss, bloody sputum, recurring bronchitis or pneumonia, and chest pain. There are no specific screening techniques or guidelines for the early detection of lung cancer. A person with symptoms may have a chest x-ray and sputum tests for a more definitive diagnosis.

Treatment

Because most lung cancers are not diagnosed until they are in advanced stages, treatment options are usually limited. Treatment usually includes surgical removal of the affected regions followed by radiation and chemotherapy.

Other Chronic Diseases of Special Concern to Women

Diseases other than cancer seriously impact the quality of life and the life span of women. These diseases include but are not limited to arthritis, osteoporosis, lupus, and diabetes.

Arthritis

Recurrent joint pain in women is usually due to one of several forms of **arthritis,** an inflammation in the joint. A capsule containing lubricating fluid encases all joints, and swelling and inflammation within the joint capsule may cause stiffness, rigidity, and pain on movement. Eventually a scar between the bones may develop, resulting in joint deformity. These processes occur regardless of the cause of arthritis.

Osteoarthritis

Osteoarthritis, also called degenerative joint disease, is a common chronic health problem today. It is seen in all age groups but is most common among older adults. The weight-bearing joints such as the hip and the back are affected as are the joints in the ends of the fingers, which may become enlarged, stiff, and painful. Joint stiffness occurs at the end of the day with osteoarthritis, which is milder than rheumatoid arthritis, and other body parts are usually not affected.

Rheumatoid Arthritis

Rheumatoid arthritis is a chronic inflammatory disease with increasing prevalence among older adults. The cause of rheumatoid arthritis is not known, although there is some evidence that genetic, hormonal, and environmental factors interact to predispose disease development in certain individuals.[25] The role of hormones is particularly intriguing because pregnancy is associated with disease remission in patients and may also play a role in the prevention of the disease.[26] It is not understood why rheumatoid arthritis often gets better in pregnancy and then worsens during the postpartum period. Rheumatoid arthritis has no known deleterious effects on pregnancy, fertility, or the fetus. Oral contraceptives appear to prevent progression to severe disease but do not necessarily prevent disease development in a woman.[25] The clinical course of rheumatoid arthritis is unpredictable. Rheumatoid arthritis is regarded as the most painful and the most disabling form of arthritis in women. Symptoms often improve or worsen with and without treatment. The disease can lead to severe disability and a shortened life expectancy.

Osteoporosis

Osteoporosis is an age-related, debilitating disorder characterized by a general decrease in bone mass. It is an important cause of bone fractures in postmenopausal women and is a leading cause of frailty. The technical difficulty and expense involved in measuring bone mass has made it impractical to screen large populations. One study found that among women age 75 and older, the prevalence of osteoporosis was 89 percent.[27] The diagnosis of osteoporosis is often made when a patient is treated for a fractured bone that is the result of minimal trauma. Fractures of the wrist are the most common fractures among white women under age 75.[28] Fractures of the hip are somewhat less common, but they result in serious long-term disability. Nearly 80 percent of the hip fractures that occur in the United States occur in women.[28]

Women are at much higher risk for osteoporosis than men. It has been hypothesized that white and Asian-American women have osteoporosis more often than African-American women largely as a result of differences in bone mass and density. Slender women have less bone mass than heavy or obese women and therefore are at greater risk for osteoporotic bone fractures.[28] Other risk factors for osteoporosis include substances that may increase the likelihood of falling, such as alcohol and psychotropic drugs. Calcium deficiency is also associated with an elevated risk of osteoporosis. Most women in their young adult years do not consume adequate calcium levels to achieve peak bone mass, and in later life their inadequate calcium intake cannot prevent persistent bone loss.[28] Important throughout the life span, calcium and weight-bearing exercise may be especially helpful in slowing bone loss in older postmenopausal women.[29]

In the absence of a biomedical cure for osteoporosis, prevention is the best strategy currently available to women. Bone loss accelerates after menopause, and estrogen replacement therapy is reported to be effective in preventing osteoporosis in women by reducing bone resorption and slowing or halting postmenopausal bone loss.[29] The increased risk for endometrial cancer associated with estrogen replacement therapy can be reduced with the addition of progestin to the estrogen regimen.[30] Because sedentary lifestyle is also associated with bone loss, moderate weight-bearing exercise may help to reduce bone loss, particularly in postmenopausal women.[31]

Lupus

Lupus is a complex chronic inflammatory disorder in which the immune system forms antibodies that target healthy tissues and organs. Lupus is a mild disease in most cases, but it also may become a life-threatening condition. Although lupus may affect persons of any age, it is primarily a disease of young women of childbearing age. The prevalence of lupus is difficult to estimate owing to inconsistencies of definition, lack of reporting, and difficulties in diagnosing.

There are several types of lupus. Discoid lupus, also known as cutaneous lupus, affects the skin and causes a rash that usually appears on the face and upper body. Lupus may also be induced by certain drugs, and this form of the disease usually disappears when the drug is discontinued. Systemic lupus erythematosus (SLE) is a more severe form of the disease and can involve any organ of the body. SLE is the most common of several conditions known collectively as connective tissue or **autoimmune diseases.** SLE is characterized by unpredictable periods of disease activity and periods of symptom-free remission.

The cause of SLE is unknown, although it is hypothesized that both genetic and environmental factors play a causative role.[5] Lupus is associated with a shortened life span, and renal failure is the most common cause of death for SLE patients. Although lupus does not have a cure, several medical therapies are used to help control the disease. In the early stages of the disease, anti-inflammatory drugs and antimalarial drugs are helpful in controlling more severe joint pain or skin involvement. Corticosteroids are also used as a treatment modality, but the severe side effects require careful monitoring and cautious use.

Experimental immunosuppressive drugs are currently being tested as treatment modalities for SLE.

Diabetes Mellitus

Diabetes mellitus is a disease characterized by abnormal glucose metabolism. The body of a diabetic is unable to produce or use glucose properly. In 1988, diabetes was the seventh leading cause of death in the United States.[2] Diabetes is frequently associated with vascular changes involving many organ systems, including eyes, kidneys, peripheral nervous system, and heart. There are two clinical types of diabetes: insulin-dependent diabetes mellitus (IDDM) and noninsulin-dependent diabetes mellitus (NIDDM). IDDM is also called type I diabetes or juvenile diabetes because of its early onset. This type of diabetes is thought to have a genetic component. Persons with IDDM need daily injection doses of insulin because their pancreases are unable to produce insulin. IDDM contributes disproportionately to the excess morbidity and mortality associated with diabetes. NIDDM is also referred to as type II diabetes or adult-onset diabetes, and it is the most common type of diabetes. It usually develops after age 30. NIDDM is often controlled by diet and exercise. Sometimes oral hypoglycemia medications or insulin may be required with NIDDM. Many individuals afflicted with NIDDM are unaware that they have the disease.

Several risk factors for diabetes have been identified, including cigarette smoking, sedentary lifestyle, and hypertension. Persons with diabetes have an increased probability of a shortened life span owing to their greater likelihood of developing a variety of acute and chronic conditions. Diabetics are at increased risk for coronary heart disease, peripheral vascular disease, eye disease, and renal disease. Rates of these diabetes-related diseases are highest among African Americans and Native Americans.[13] The disproportionate burden of these diseases in these populations is among women.

Pregnancy presents special risks to diabetic women. The likelihood of a good pregnancy outcome is enhanced if the mother's diabetes is well controlled before she becomes pregnant. The risk of serious congenital malformations in babies born to mothers with diabetes is two to three times greater than in the general population.[32] Infants who are large for gestational age are common in diabetic pregnancies and increase the likelihood of cesarean delivery.

One of the hardest things I ever did was watch my mother die of lung cancer. She smoked for 40 years and she somehow thought that it wouldn't happen to her. But it did. It has really made me think about the decisions I make.

25-YEAR-OLD TEACHER

Informed Decision Making

Knowledge

Knowledge is the first step in effective health decision making. Women must increase their knowledge levels before they are able to modify their attitudes and health practices that will reduce their risk of developing cancer or improve their chances for early detection (Information Box 12.5). Knowledge is not a

---

Reduce the Risk of Cancer through Knowledge and Behavior

Eat a diet low in saturated fat and high in fiber. Add fresh fruits and vegetables and avoid red meats, high-fat dairy foods.

If alcohol is used, do so only in moderation. Alcohol is not part of a healthy lifestyle.

Shop smart. Learn products that are low in saturated fat and high in fiber. Read and understand labels. Ask questions.

Stop smoking cigarettes and don't chew tobacco. Avoid breathing other people's cigarette smoke.

Do a monthly breast self-examination and have regular Pap smears.

Know the warning signs of cancer.

Have regular medical checkups and work with your provider to establish a cancer prevention program for yourself.

Engage in sexual activities wisely and use protection for you and your partner.

Review personal risk factors carefully before using oral contraceptives or hormone replacement therapy.

Sunbathe wisely and use a sunblock.

---

static concept; every day brings new insights and information about carcinogens, dietary implications, environmental factors, hormonal influences, and preventive behaviors. Women must be alert for new information about all chronic conditions and be able to incorporate it into their lifestyle and personal decision making.

Lifestyle and Screening Behaviors

Scientists have concluded that approximately three-fourths of cancers in the United States are attributable to lifestyle factors.[23] Many of these factors were also addressed as modifiable factors for cardiovascular disease in Chapter 11. These modifiable lifestyle factors include the elimination of cigarette smoking as well as avoiding involuntary or second-hand smoke. Maintaining a desirable body weight and limiting daily intake of total dietary fats, especially saturated fats, also helps reduce the risk of cancer. The avoidance of excessive sun exposure is particularly important in the prevention of skin cancer.

It has been estimated that breast cancer death rates could be reduced by an estimated 30 percent if women received mammograms at recommended intervals.[33] A woman can maximize her possible benefits from the procedure through effective mammography consumerism (Information Box 12.6). Regular mammography is not the panacea for breast cancer, however. Unfortunately, mammography misses about 10 percent of breast cancers in women over age 50 and about half of cancers in younger women.[34] Monthly BSE must supplement mammography, and women should have a professional breast examination at

Maximizing Mammography

Schedule the procedure during menstrual period if there is any chance of pregnancy. This will avoid possible radiation exposure to a developing fetus.

Choose a facility that has "dedicated" and accredited mammography equipment. The person taking the mammogram should be a registered technician with special training in mammography. The radiologist should be specially trained to read mammograms.

Avoid any skin lotions, powders, or deodorants. This will prevent any blurring or discoloration of the film.

Remove any jewelry.

Advise the technician if you have breast implants or if you have had previous breast surgery. Implants and scar tissue may complicate the auto focusing process.

Advise the technician when and where the last mammography was done. It is often necessary to compare old films with new films to ascertain changes.

Advise the technician to note any skin moles that may cast confusing shadows or blur film images.

Cancer Warning Symptoms: C-A-U-T-I-O-N

Change in bowel or bladder habits

A sore that does not heal

Unusual bleeding or discharge

Thickening or lump in breast or elsewhere

Indigestion or difficulty in swallowing

Obvious change in a wart or mole

Nagging cough or hoarseness

SOURCE: American Cancer Society (1991). *Cancer Facts and Figures, 1991*. Atlanta: American Cancer Society. Reprinted with permission.

least once a year. Examining breasts properly requires specific techniques (see Fig. 12.7). Unusual concerns merit prompt evaluation. Any breast lump or lumps should be evaluated by a physician, especially if painless and involving only one breast. Any breast discharge should also be evaluated, especially if it is bloody or involving only one breast. Skin changes that include flaking, crusting, or weeping eruptions around the nipple should also be checked. Dimpling or retraction of the skin on any portion of the breast is another concern that merits prompt evaluation. If a woman is unsure of the BSE procedure, she should have her clinician show her how it is done when she has her annual examination.

In addition to lifestyle changes and cancer screening procedures, women should be familiar with their bodies and know the symptoms of all cancers (Information Box 12.7). Those cancers that are not detected by screening before the development of symptoms still need to be diagnosed as early as possible to maximize the advantages afforded by treatment. The cancer warning symptoms do not necessarily indicate the presence of cancer, but the symptoms should be investigated by a clinician.

Communication

Communication is an important dimension of all women's health issues. Cancer and other chronic diseases have inherent communication requirements, especially with health care providers. Discussing concerns, fears, and anxieties is usually the best strategy to alleviate them. Reporting symptoms and discussing health concerns, in fact, are two of the best preventive measures that a woman can take in the early detection of diseases.

Summary

Cancer and chronic disease issues are important dimensions of women's health. Knowledge, personal preventive practices, and lifestyle modifications are the best measures for a woman to reduce her chances of acquiring the condition, and they are the best measures to ensure early diagnosis if a disease is present.

Philosophical Dimensions: Cancer and Other Chronic Diseases

1. Data indicate that young women are initiating sexual intercourse earlier and have more lifetime sexual partners. What are the implications of this in terms of disease protection?

CURRENT EVENTS

More than Contraception: Will Doctors Prescribe the Pill to Prevent Cancer?

Family Planning World
March/April 1993, p. 14

Recent scientific evidence strongly suggests that "the pill" (oral contraceptives) may actually provide protection for women against cancer. Some medical officials are now considering prescribing low-dose pills for noncontraceptive purposes. Since several studies suggest that the pill protects against ovarian and endometrial cancer, doctors are debating what role oral contraceptives may play in future cancer studies and whether the pill should be considered preventive care for women who have increased cancer risks. Before oral contraceptives could be generally used for this purpose, however, the Food and Drug Administration (FDA) would require additional documentation and label changing. At the present time, the FDA lists cancer prevention only as a possible side effect of the pill.

The report describes a study conducted by the Alan Guttmacher Institute (AGI) that found the risk of ovarian cancer to be lowered by 30 percent for women who have used the pill for 4 years or less, compared with non pill users. Benefits appear to increase with years on the pill—among women who have used the pill for 5–11 years, the risk is decreased by 60 percent and by 80 percent after 12 years of use. Women who have used the pill were half as likely to get endometrial cancer. The relationship between the pill and breast cancer is less dramatic. AGI found that up to age 55, breast cancer occurs with equal frequency among women who have used the pill and women who have not. For women in the 30–40 year range, there is a *higher* incidence of breast cancer among long-term pill users, and among long-term pill users in the 40–50 year range, there is a *lower* incidence of breast cancer.

As more studies are conducted, there is a real possibility that oral contraceptives may be prescribed as a cancer preventive for women.

Reprinted with permission.

2. Dramatic differences present in the racial distribution of cancers and chronic diseases. What are some possible reasons for this and how can society and researchers address the problem?

3. Why is it that with so much information about lifestyle and diet do people continue to engage in behaviors that increase their risk for cancer and other chronic diseases?

4. What are some possible strategies to encourage young women to engage in preventive behaviors such as BSE, and Pap smears?

5. Prolonged involuntary smoking is a risk factor for lung cancer. How can the situation be handled when someone is being exposed to passive smoke?

6. How can academic institutions take a more active role in disease prevention for young women?

References

1. American Cancer Society (1993). *Cancer Facts and Figures, 1993.* Atlanta: American Cancer Society.

2. USDHHS (1991). *Health United States,* 1990. (DHHS Pub. No. (PHS) 91-1232.) Hyattsville, MD: US Government Printing Office.

3. USDHHS (1992). *Report of the National Institutes of Health: Opportunities for Research on Women's Health.* (PHS, NIH Pub. No. 92-3457.) Washington, DC: US Government Printing Office.

4. Centers for Disease Control (1990). Trends in lung cancer incidence and mortality, United States, 1980–1987. *Morbidity Mortality Weekly Report, 39,* 875–883.

5. Schulman, L.E. (1988). Systemic lupus erythematosus. In US Department of Health and Human Services, *Women's Health. Report of the Public Health Service Task Force on Women's Health Issues.* Vol. III. (DHHS Pub. No. (PHS) 88-50206.) Washington, DC: US Government Printing Office.

6. Garfinkel, L. (1991). The epidemiology of cancer in black Americans. *Statistical Bulletin, 72*(2), 11–17.

7. National Cancer Institute (1990), *Cancer Statistics Review, 1973–87.* (NCI, NIH Pub. No. 90-2789.) Bethesda, MD: US Government Printing Office.

8. Haynes, M.A. (1991). Making cancer prevention effective for African-Americans. *Statistical Bulletin, 72*(2), 18–22.

9. Centers for Disease Control (1990). Use of mammography, United States, 1990. *Morbidity Mortality Weekly Reports, 39*(36), 621–627.

10. del Puente, A., Knowler, W.C., Pettitt, D.J., and Bennett, P.H. (1989). High

incidence and prevalence of rheumatoid arthritis in Puma Indians. *American Journal of Epidemiology, 129,* 1170–1178.

11. Centers for Disease Control (1990). Prevalence and incidence of diabetes mellitus. *Morbidity Mortality Weekly Report, 39,* 809–812.

12. American Diabetes Association (1991). *Diabetes: 1991 Vital Statistics.* Alexandria, VA: American Diabetes Association.

13. USDHHS (1991). *Healthy People 2000: National Health Promotion and Disease Prevention Objectives.* (DHHS Pub. No. (PHS) 91-50212.) Washington, DC: US Government Printing Office.

14. American College of Obstetricians and Gynecologists (1991). Carcinoma of the breast. *ACOG Technical Bulletin.* No. 158. Washington, DC: American College of Obstetricians and Gynecologists.

15. Berkquist, L., Adami, H.O., Persson, I, Hoover, R., and Schairer, C. (1989). The risk of breast cancer after estrogen and estrogen-progestin replacement. *New England Journal of Medicine, 321,* 293–297.

16. Lipnick, R.J., Buring, J.E., Hennekens, C.H., Rosner, B., Willett, W.C., Bain, C., Stampfer, M.J., Colditz, G.A., Peto, R., and Speizer, F.E. (1986). Oral contraceptive use and breast cancer. A prospective cohort study. *Journal of the American Medical Association, 255*(1), 58–61.

17. Harris, J.R., Lippman, M.E., Veronesi, U., and Willett, W. (1992). Breast cancer (three parts). *New England Journal of Medicine, 327,* 319–328, 390–398, 473–480.

18. Phillips, L.G. (1992). Reconstructive options following mastectomy. *Journal of the American Medical Women's Association, 47*(5), 178–180.

19. Persky, V., Davis, F., Barrett, R., Ruby, E., Sailer, C., and Levy, P. (1990). Recent time trends in uterine cancer. *American Journal of Public Health, 80,* 935–939.

20. Harlan, L.C., Bernstein, A.B., and Kessler, L.G. (1991). Cervical cancer screening: Who is not screened and why? *American Journal of Public Health, 81,* 885–890.

21. Parazzini, F., Franceschi, S., LaVecchia, C., and Fasoli, M. (1991). The epidemiology of ovarian cancer. *Gynecol-Oncology, 43,* 9–23.

22. Hankinson, S.E., Colditz, G.A., Hunter, D.J., Spencer, T.L., Rosner, B., and Stampfer, M.J. (1992). A quantitative assessment of oral contraceptive use and risk of ovarian cancer. *Obstetrics and Gynecology, 80*(4), 708–714.

23. Williams, G.D. (1991). Causes and prevention of cancer. *Statistical Bulletin, 72*(2), 6–10.

24. Sullivan, L.W. (1991). Approaches for reducing cancer mortality in minorities. *Statistical Bulletin, 72*(2), 2–6.

25. Hochberg, M.C., and Spector, T.D. (1990). Epidemiology of rheumatoid arthritis: Update. *Epidemiological Review, 12,* 247–252.

26. Spector, T.D. (1990). Epidemiology of rheumatoid arthritis. *Rheumatology Disease Clinics of North America, 14,* 513–538.

27. Lawrence, R.C., Hochberg, M.C., Kelsey, J.L., McDuffie, F.C., Medsger, T.A.,

Felts, W.R., and Shulman, L.E. (1989). Estimates of the prevalence of selected arthritic and musculoskeletal diseases in the United States. *Journal of Rheumatology, 16*(4), 427–441.

28. Cummings, S.R., Kelsey, J.L., Nevitt, M.C., and O'Dowd, K.J. (1985). Epidemiology of osteoporosis and osteoporotic fractures. *Epidemiological Review, 7,* 178–208.

29. Heaney, R.P. (1990). Calcium intake and bone health throughout life. *Journal of the American Medical Women's Association, 45*(3), 80–86.

30. Peck, W.A. (1990). Estrogen therapy after menopause. *Journal of the American Medical Women's Association, 45,* 87–90.

31. Drinkwater, B.L. (1990). Physical exercise and bone health. *Journal of the American Medical Women's Association, 45*(3), 91–97.

32. Mennuti, M.T. (1985). Teratology and genetic counseling in the diabetic pregnancy. *Clinics in Obstetrics and Gynecology, 28,* 486–495.

33. Eddy, D.M. (1989). Screening for breast cancer. *Annals of Internal Medicine, 111,* 389–398.

34. Consumer Reports on Health (1991). Mammograms: Crucial but infallible. *Consumer Reports on Health, 3*(12), 89–91.

Resources

AMERICAN CANCER SOCIETY

1599 Clifton Road NE
Atlanta, GA 30329
1-800-ACS-2345

CANCER CARE, INC.

1180 Avenue of the Americas
New York, NY 10036
212-221-3300

CANDLELIGHTERS
CHILDHOOD CANCER
FOUNDATION, INC.

1901 Pennsylvania Ave NW
Washington, DC 20006
202-659-5136

ENDOMETRIOSIS
ASSOCIATION

8585 North 76th Place
Milwaukee, WI 53223
800-992-ENDO

LEUKEMIA SOCIETY OF
AMERICA, INC.

733 Third Avenue
New York, NY 10017
212-573-8484

MAKE TODAY COUNT

10½ South Union Street
Alexandria, VA 22314
703-548-9674

NATIONAL CANCER
INSTITUTE

National Institutes of Health
Bethesda, MD 20892
1-800-4-CANCER

NATIONAL COALITION FOR
CANCER SURVIVORSHIP

323 8th Street SW
Albuquerque, NM 87102
505-764-9956

NATIONAL HOSPICE
ORGANIZATION

1901 Fort Myer Drive, Suite
  901
Arlington, VA 22209
703-243-5900

CHAPTER 13

Menopause

CHAPTER OBJECTIVES

On completion of this chapter, the student should be able to discuss:

1. The basic demographic aging trends in the United States.

2. How menopause has been a basic source of confusion and misinformation for women.

3. How cultural and societal attitudes about aging have influenced attitudes about menopause.

4. How menopause can be a time of rejuvenation for women.

5. The basic biological sequence of events associated with menopause.

6. The controversy associated with hysterectomy procedures in the United States.

7. Some physical symptoms that may be associated with menopause.

8. Some psychological symptoms that may be associated with menopause.

9. How the psychological symptoms of menopause may be influenced by cultural expectations.

10. The various procedures for administering hormone replacement therapy.

11. The risks associated with unopposed estrogen therapy.

12. The cardiovascular benefits associated with hormone replacement therapy.

13. The osteoporotic benefits associated with hormone replacement therapy.

14. The cancer risks associated with hormone replacement therapy.

15. Two major national research initiatives that will help answer some important questions about menopause and hormone replacement therapy.

16. What preventive lifestyle behaviors can help prepare a woman for a healthier menopause and beyond life.

Introduction

Aging is a natural process of biological maturation. American women are aging. In 1993, there are 43 million women in **perimenopause,** a term used to describe the years immediately preceding and following the last menstrual period. In the next decade, 19 million women will be in the perimenopausal age range. The sheer numbers in this group are influencing how society addresses a fundamental, natural facet of women's aging process. By the year 2000, people over the age of 65 will compose 13 percent of the total population (Fig. 13.1). This represents a dramatic increase from 1900. The most rapid population increase over the next decade will be among those over 85 years of age.[1] This graying of the female baby boomers has created not only national demographic data changes, but also changes in how aging and menopause are viewed.

All facets of aging are important to consider from a women's health perspective. One of the most important of these facets is menopause. This chapter provides an overview of both natural and surgically induced menopause and the controversy surrounding hormone replacement therapy. Research issues and implications for informed decision making are also discussed.

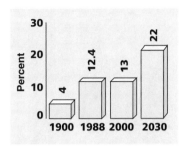

FIGURE 13.1

Percent population of the United States over the age of 65, 1900–2030.

SOURCE: Adapted from USDHHS (1991). *Healthy people 2000: national health promotion and disease prevention objectives.* (DHHS Pub. No. (PHS) 91-50212.) Washington, DC: US Government Printing Office.

Menopause

Menopause refers to the cessation of regular menstrual periods. It is also known as the **climacterium** or the "change of life." It is the end of menstruation and childbearing capability. Most women enter and complete menopause between the ages of 45 and 55. There are often variances in these ages, however. The age at which a woman has her last period is not known to be related to race, body size, or the age at which she began to menstruate. Smokers, however, generally experience menopause about 2 years earlier than nonsmoking women. Most often, menopause begins with skipped periods and a diminished menstrual flow.

Menopause has been a traditional source of confusion and misinformation for women. The myths and misinformation have been compounded, until recent years, with little coverage in lay or professional literature about menopause. It has also been badly neglected as a research area. The paucity of research and interest in menopause cannot be blamed on historical neglect because it is only since the turn of the century that women have had life expectancies that took them into and beyond the age of menopause. Today most women will live about a third of their lives postmenopausally.

Although women will live such a significant portion of their lives postmenopausally, aging has been a major phobia of twentieth-century America. In non-Western cultures, where women's status or role improves with age, aging and menopause are perceived as positive events. Today women are becoming more assertive and more informed about all aspects of their health care. Open discussions about sexuality and life issues have fostered a foundation to continue understanding facets of menopause and aging without fear, embarrassment, or stigmatization. Research has shown that the stereotypes about women are not

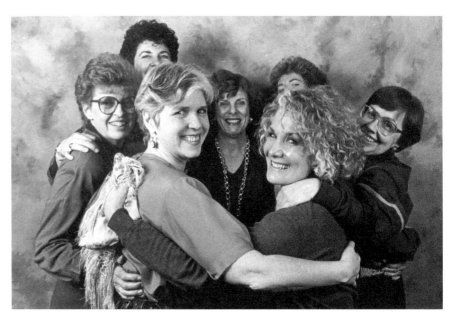

Women today are more open in their discussions about all aspects of their sexual well-being, including menopause.

I was well into my menopause before I realized what was happening. My symptoms were so minor and rather vague. I didn't understand all the hype about symptoms.

50-YEAR-OLD WOMAN

valid; for example, menopausal women do not use health care services at a higher rate than would be expected with increases in age.[2]

The confusion and misinformation about menopause have been compounded by myths, stereotypes, and "old wives tales" that have been embedded in lay and clinical "knowledge" about aging. The "change of life" has mistakenly been perceived as a difficult time for women in which they experience uncontrollable extreme moodiness, irritability, and depression. Popular stereotypes in the United States have portrayed menopause as a major life tragedy that results in hypochondria, hysteria, and irritability. The stereotype continued to imply that solace to these conditions could be found only in a physician's office with pharmacological remedies. The menopausal woman has been portrayed as a burden to herself, her family, and, if she was married, to her suffering husband. In the 1940s and 1950s, "treatment" for menopause often focused on psychiatric conditions of depression and melancholy. In subsequent decades, menopause was examined as a "disease" entity because clinical concern focused on women reporting symptoms and seeking medical intervention. When more representative samples of women were studied more recently, it became apparent that many, if not most, women experience few symptoms and life disruptions with menopause.[3,4]

Many women, in contrast to the myths, actually welcome or do not regret menopause. The cessation of menses frees women from contraception concerns, leading to increased sexual satisfaction. Others appreciate the freedom from menstrual periods, which may have been inconvenient or uncomfortable. Social and cultural influences have also influenced more positive attitudes toward menopause. Many women have delayed or postponed their careers with childbearing and child-care responsibilities. Menopause is a time of fewer obligations in these areas with increased opportunities in the work force. This combination of events is often inviting and invigorating for women who are seeking added dimensions in their personal and professional lives. The time of menopause is often more flexible in terms of leisure time and financial resources, increasing the opportunities for new forms of activity and self-expression.

Natural Menopause

The physiological mechanisms of natural menopause are not as well understood as other dimensions of a woman's reproductive health. Most descriptions of the menopausal process rely on clinical impressions (with little or no data) or on small samples of women selected from patient populations rather than from the general public.[5] Natural menopause occurs when the ovaries begin to fail to respond to the luteinizing and follicle-stimulating hormones that are produced in the anterior pituitary, which is under the control of the hypothalamus. These hormones are still being secreted into the bloodstream, but the ovaries are not producing estrogen and progesterone in response, and ovulation becomes somewhat erratic. The mechanisms for these changes are not well understood. Whatever the reasons, the woman beginning menopause will have more luteinizing and follicle-stimulating hormones present in the bloodstream and less estrogen and progesterone than she had during her regular cycling. For most women, menopause lasts from a few months to 2 to 3 years. Because ovulation may occur in sporadic intervals during this time, pregnancy is a possibility. Menopause is considered complete once monthly periods have ceased altogether.

Generally in a woman's early to mid forties—2 to 8 years before actual menopause—her menstrual cycle begins changing. These changes include the following: The level of estrogen produced by the ovaries decreases, ovulation stops or becomes irregular, and the pattern of menstrual cycling changes. Although the pattern is not consistent for all women, initially the change may be characterized by heavier, more frequent periods, which later become scantier and less frequent. Lack of ovulation may cause some light bleeding or spotting between periods. In most cases, these irregularities are normal manifestations of the transition to menopause. Sometimes if a clinician suspects that the uterine lining is not being completely shed during the flow, **progestin,** a synthetic progesterone, may be prescribed to make the cycle more regular. In cases of extremely heavy bleeding, surgery may be recommended.

After menopause, women continue to produce estrogen, but far less is manufactured in the ovaries. Most postmenopausal estrogen is produced in a process in which the adrenal gland makes precursors of estrogen, which are then converted by stored fat to estrogen. Far less estrogen, however, is produced in this manner than was produced in the ovaries before menopause.

Surgically Induced Menopause

Currently **hysterectomy,** the surgical removal of the uterus, is one of the most commonly performed inpatient surgical procedures in the United States. In

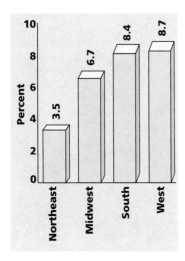

FIGURE 13.2

Rates of hysterectomies (per thousand) by geographical region, United States, women aged 15 to 44.

SOURCE: Adapted from National Center for Health Statistics, National Hospital Discharge Survey, 1987.

terms of overall frequency for surgical procedures for men and women, it is second only to cesarean sections.[6] It has been estimated that at present rates, 37 percent of all women will have undergone a hysterectomy before they reach the age of 60.[7] This high prevalence has generated significant controversy regarding the risks and benefits of the procedure. The hysterectomy controversy is further fueled, as shown in Figure 13.2, by the national geographical variance that is also present in the distribution of hysterectomy procedures.

Hysterectomy performed in conjunction with the removal of both ovaries and the fallopian tubes, known as a **total hysterectomy and bilateral salpingo-oophorectomy,** has become increasingly more common. When a woman's ovaries are surgically removed, a more abrupt and often earlier menopause results. The pituitary gland continues to produce luteinizing and follicle-stimulating hormones, but the ovaries are not present to respond with ovulation. Estrogen and progesterone are no longer produced in presurgical levels because of the absence of the ovaries. Hormones, however, are still being produced in the adrenal glands, but the levels are considerably lower without the ovarian production. It has been observed that women who have had both ovaries removed before the onset of menopause experience more severe menopausal symptoms than women who experience a natural menopause.[8]

Physical Symptoms

The endocrine changes of menopause are believed responsible for the physical symptoms of menopause. The most frequently reported physical symptom is a vascular response or instability known as **hot flashes** or hot flushes. Hot flashes may begin before a woman has stopped menstruating and may continue for a couple of years after menopause. Nearly 50 percent of menopausal women report hot flashes, but only about 10 to 20 percent of women consider them severe enough to warrant treatment.[9] Hot flashes are generally described as an uncomfortable sensation of internally generated heat beginning in the chest and moving to the neck and head or spreading throughout the body. Increased heart rate and finger temperature have been documented during hot flashes. They are often accompanied by heavy perspiration and may be followed by a chill. Hot flashes often occur at night and usually result in sleep disruption. Hot flashes are credited with much of the insomnia associated with menopause. The mechanisms of hot flashes are not completely understood but are believed to be related to decreased estrogen levels. Obese women tend to have a lower overall incidence of hot flashes, perhaps because they have higher levels of estrogen converted from stored fat.

Thinning of the vaginal lining, known as **vaginal atrophy,** is another physical symptom that occurs with some frequency following menopause. As estrogen levels decline, layers of the vaginal surface become dry and sensitive. Some women experience pain or burning during intercourse, vaginal discharge, and more frequent vaginal infections. Other physical symptoms among menopausal women are pain in muscles and joints, headaches, and increased weight.[10]

Psychological Symptoms

Psychiatric syndromes have been linked to reproductive endocrine system changes, including postpartum psychosis and depression, premenstrual syndrome, posthysterectomy depression, and menopausal psychiatric syndromes, but much of the current information with these conditions is based on myths, unwarranted assumptions, and conclusions derived from methodically flawed studies.[11] As with the physical symptoms associated with menopause, most women have few if any symptoms and feel that the psychological symptoms are manageable.[10,12] The most frequently reported psychological symptoms during menopause are feelings of irritability, depression, and anxiety. These may be due to the physical changes occurring in the body, but they may also be highly influenced by the normative traditional cultural and social expectations of a woman's worth expressed in relation to her reproductive capabilities.

Hormone Replacement Therapy

Few topics in women's medicine today are as fraught with confusion and controversy as the question of appropriate treatment for menopausal symptoms and the prevention of long-term health outcomes associated with postmenopausal women.[5] Although it can be debated whether or not menopause is a medical condition or a "deficiency disease," the reality is that today dozens of medications are currently available for treating menopause. The availability of these medications does not imply that all women should take them, however.

Replacement estrogens can be taken in a variety of different preparations, by various routes of administration, and in different dosages. Oral preparations are most often prescribed. Vaginal creams that contain estrogen help women whose only symptom is vaginal dryness. Although estrogen does enter the bloodstream with the cream, the amount is too low to provide protection against heart disease and osteoporosis. A skin patch or **transdermal therapy** is another estrogen delivery mechanism. By feeding estrogen directly into the bloodstream via the skin, the liver is bypassed. This is a plus for some women whose livers respond to supplemental oral doses of estrogen by deactivating it with enzymes that also raise triglycerides (see Chapter 11), which contribute to heart disease. For women with low levels of high-density lipoproteins (HDL), the "good" cholesterol (see Chapter 1), the oral pill form of estrogen is preferred because it increases HDL levels. Before deciding which form of estrogen therapy might be better for a woman, it is important to ascertain blood lipid levels.

Estrogen has demonstrated distinct clinical value in the treatment of postmenopausal conditions. Estrogen alleviates menopausal symptoms[13] and helps to prevent heart disease (see Chapter 11) and osteoporosis (see Chapter 12). But estrogen also increases the risk of endometrial cancer (see Chapter 12.) It is important to examine hormone replacement therapy (HRT) in greater detail for each of these conditions.

Researchers found that by adding a progestin to estrogen therapy, women could be protected against endometrial cancer by opposing the negative effects of estrogen. This led to the terms **opposed estrogen** and **unopposed estrogen.** Progestin reduces the uterine cancer risk apparently by causing shedding of the estrogen-thickened endometrium, lessening the chances of cancer development. When progestin is added to estrogen therapy, the treatment is considered to be "combined" and is often referred to as HRT or combined hormone therapy. New research suggests that it may also confer protection against osteoporosis.

Progestin is not without its side effects, however. Some studies have suggested that progestin appears to diminish estrogen's beneficial effect against heart disease,[14] whereas other longer studies have shown no adverse effects.[15] Other side effects may include menstrual-like bleeding, breast tenderness, mood swings, and bloating. The side effects of progestins vary according to the type and dosage used. Clinicians are currently experimenting with various regimens in an effort to modulate the side effects. Because of the side effects, many women prefer to take the lowest dose of estrogen and no progestin. It is unclear whether this regimen affords any protection against heart disease or osteoporosis. Until more definitive data are available, it is not possible to ascertain the long-term effects of combination replacement therapies. In general, unopposed estrogen therapy is considered acceptable as long as adequate monitoring for endometrial cancer is done with yearly biopsies.[16]

Hormone Replacement Therapy and Cardiovascular Disease

As discussed in Chapter 12, cardiovascular diseases are the leading cause of mortality in women. The incidence of cardiovascular disease in women continues to rise markedly after menopause (Fig. 13.3). Evidence clearly shows that high levels of HDL cholesterol and low levels of low-density lipoprotein (LDL) cholesterol are protective against the development of atherosclerosis (see Chapter 1). Research has also shown that natural and surgical menopause is associated with changes in serum lipid profiles, such as a decline in HDL levels and a rise in LDL levels. These serum cholesterol changes may be factors in the development of a woman's increased risk of postmenopausal cardiovascular disease.[17]

Although the mechanism of the cardioprotective effect is unclear, the evidence for the cardiovascular protective effect of estrogen is compelling. In a prospective study of nearly 50,000 women, researchers found that postmenopausal estrogen users compared with women who had never used estrogen had about half the risk of major coronary artery disease or fatal cardiovascular disease and no increased risk of stroke.[17] Studies have shown that estrogens may confer a protective effect by maintaining HDL and LDL levels at premenopausal values.[18] Although epidemiological association as demonstrated by this study does not establish cause and effect, the evidence does strongly suggest that postmenopausal estrogen has an independent, significant protective effect against cardiovascular disease.

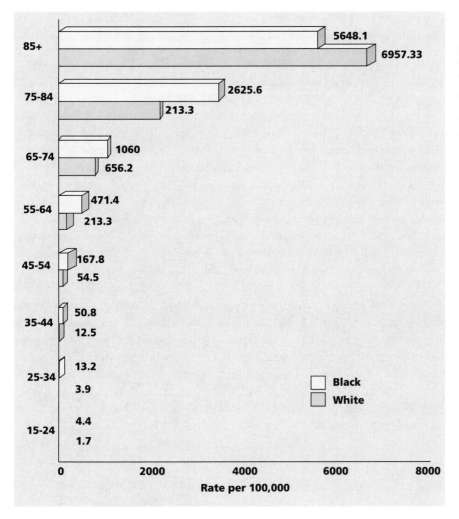

FIGURE 13.3

Death rates (per 100,000) from heart disease, according to age, white and African-American women, 1988.

SOURCE: USDHHS (1991). *Health United States, 1990.* (PHS (CDC) DHHS Pub. No. (PHS) 91-1232.) National Center for Health Statistics.

Hormone Replacement Therapy and Osteoporosis

Perhaps the most serious concern of postmenopausal women may be the development of osteoporosis (see Chapter 12), the loss of bone mass in which bones become brittle and more likely to fracture. The spine may also lose flexibility and begin to curve. Osteoporosis is a major problem for many elderly women, and falls resulting from or leading to bone fractures constitute a leading health problem. Several decades ago, researchers established the link between ovarian hormone insufficiency and increased bone loss by observing that nearly all patients with osteoporotic fractures were postmenopausal women and that women with their ovaries removed were disproportionately represented.[19] Studies have also shown that long-term use of estrogen protects against postmenopausal bone loss and osteoporosis.[20] Once estrogen replacement stops, however, bone loss resumes and at a rate faster than normal.[21] For this reason alone, some clinicians advocate long-term or lifelong estrogen therapy.

Hormone Replacement Therapy and Cancer

HRT is not without risks. Controversy exists about the risks with breast cancer, and endometrial cancer has been associated with the use of unopposed estrogen.[22] Endometrial cancer is relatively rare, but studies have found that the use of opposed estrogen at lower doses carries at least a fivefold increased risk of endometrial cancer.[23] Advocates of HRT argue that the risks of endometrial cancer are minor when compared with the associated cardiovascular and osteoporotic benefits.[17] They further argue that baseline endometrial biopsies and annual biopsies afford a clinical opportunity to detect early cancer development and treat with hysterectomy if endometrial cancer should present.

The link between breast cancer and HRT is more controversial. It is generally accepted that naturally occurring estrogens, known as **endogenous estrogens,** play an important role in the causation of breast cancer,[24] but a recent meta-analysis has suggested that lower doses of estrogens do not pose an increased risk for breast cancer.[25] Comparison of existing studies is difficult owing to biases from methodological issues, definitions, complex and confounding biological and pharmacological factors, and heterogeneous study populations. A carefully designed large-scale study is needed to address this and many other questions regarding HRT.

Research Issues

The millions of American women in their perimenopausal years are generally surprised and somewhat angry that so little is known about menopause as a normal and universal aging dimension of women's health. The few available studies that have examined menopausal issues provide some insight, but many of these studies are flawed. Past studies of menopausal symptoms, for example, have mistakenly combined women who experience a natural menopause with women who have had surgically induced menopause. This error may be responsible for some of the overstatements associated with menopause symptoms.[5]

Two new major research efforts have been launched by the National Institutes of Health (NIH) to answer some of the many questions associated with menopause. The first large-scale clinical trial of HRT is underway, and it is hoped that it will provide a more definitive basis for hormone replacement decision making. The study, called PEPI (Postmenopausal Estrogen/Progestin Interventions), is following nearly 1,000 women randomly placed in five groups, each with a different treatment. The groups are estrogen alone, estrogen and progestin in three different combinations or doses, and a placebo. The study is measuring the effects of the drugs on cholesterol, blood pressure, and bone density as

I am so frustrated by the lack of definitive information about menopause and hormone replacement therapies. I feel like my generation of women has been shortchanged by the research community. How can it be that so little is known about such a basic and universal phenomenon?

45-YEAR-OLD LAWYER

well as cancer of the breast and uterus. Hormone use is also being correlated with personal matters, such as sexual satisfaction, mood, and general outlook on life.

Another major NIH effort is the Women's Health Initiative, a 14-year clinical trial that will track, among other things, the incidence of heart disease, osteoporosis, and breast and uterine cancer in 55,000 postmenopausal women taking either estrogen or a combination therapy. Together these two major studies should provide some insight and answers into the myriad of questions that women are asking about menopause and replacement therapies.

Informed Decision Making

Although it is commonly believed that health problems in old age are inevitable, many in fact can actually be prevented or controlled. Clearly it is best to have a full lifetime of healthy behaviors, but changing unhealthy behaviors, even in later years, can improve quality and quantity of life. Health promoting behaviors include cessation of cigarette smoking (it is best to never start), maintenance of good nutrition, losing excess weight, and regular physical exercise. For some women, menopause is a time of reflection and renewed determination to engage in healthier living. Waiting until one is older is not the time to start preventive health care: Protecting the body from heart disease and osteoporosis means not smoking, exercising throughout the life span, eating a healthy diet, and knowing one's body.

Perspectives on menopause require personal and societal reevaluation: It is no longer seen as the beginning of the end of life but rather as the beginning of a second life, no longer confined or defined by procreative abilities. The phobia about aging and the myths and misconceptions about the aging process need to be replaced with knowledge and insight into the myriad opportunities that exist in the second half of a woman's life. Menopause is also not a disease. It is a transition period and an opportunity for reevaluation.

The decision whether or not to use HRT is a personal one that must be individualized. No two women respond exactly the same way. Dosages, products, and regimens may require readjusting more than once to find an appropriate balance. Women with difficult menopause symptoms, those who have thin bones as measured by a bone density test, and those at high risk of heart disease are possible candidates for HRT. Women with a history of liver disease or who are prone to blood clots and women who have had breast cancer are generally considered to be at too high a risk for HRT. As stated recently by the Office of Technology Assessment, "The debate over hormone therapy—in particular unopposed estrogen—focuses on whether it should be used to treat menopausal symptoms for a short period of time, thereby reducing any risks associated with long-term treatment, or whether it should also be used to prevent future disease, thereby requiring longer treatment that could increase the risk of cancer."[2] As with any form of medication, treatment, or procedure, the benefits must be carefully weighed and considered against the spectrum of associated risks before

I couldn't believe the intensity of my hot flashes. They would come out of the blue and I felt like I was on fire. I couldn't sleep at night. I realize that my symptoms were extraordinary. Fortunately, my doctor was understanding, and she helped me work through various combinations of replacement hormone therapies until we found the best one for me. It was important that I could talk to her about what I was feeling—not just the physical symptoms but the psychological symptoms as well.
49-YEAR-OLD PRODUCER

a decision is made. In future years, it is hoped that women will have access to more information to help them better make these important health decisions.

As in any acute, chronic, or infectious condition, prevention is the best strategy. Prevention of cardiovascular disease and osteoporosis by lifestyle modification is the best option available to women of all ages. Regardless of her age, quitting cigarettes (or better yet, never starting), eating a diet low in fat and with adequate levels of calcium, and regular physical exercise are a woman's most proactive healthy behaviors.

Philosophical Dimensions: Menopause

1. Why has medical research been slower to understand the physiological dimensions of menopause than other reproductive health matters?

2. What can be done to change societal images of menopause, aging, and older women?

3. Should menopause be viewed as a "disease of deficiency"? If not, how should it be viewed?

4. What can a woman do to maximize the effectiveness of her decision making about hormone replacement therapy?

References

1. USDHHS (1991). *Healthy People 2000: National Health Promotion and Disease Prevention Objectives.* (DHHS Pub. No. (PHS) 91-50212.) Washington, DC: US Government Printing Office.

2. Avis, N.E., and McKinlay, S.M. (1991). A longitudinal analysis of women's attitudes toward the menopause: Results from the Massachusetts Women's Health Study. *Maturitas, 13,* 65–79.

3. Goodman, M. (1980). Toward a biology of menopause. *Journal of Women in Culture and Society, 5,* 739–753.

4. Baruch, G., Barnett, R., and Rivera, C. (1983). *Life Prints: New Patterns of Love and Work for Today's Women.* New York: New American Library.

5. Office of Technology Assessment (1992). *The Menopause, Hormone Therapy, and Women's Health—Background Paper.* (S/N 052-003-01284-7.) Washington, DC: US Government Printing Office.

6. Pokras, R. (1989). Hysterectomy: Past, present, and future. *Statistical Bulletin, 70*(4), 12–21.

7. Bachmann, G.A. (1990). Hysterectomy: A critical review. *Journal of Reproductive Medicine, 35*(9), 862.

8. Weinstein, L. (1990). Hormonal therapy in the patient with surgical menopause. *Obstetrics and Gynecology, 75,* 4 Suppl., 47–50S.

9. McKinlay, S.M., Brambrilla, D.J., and McKinlay, J.B. (1991). Women's experience of the menopause. *Current Obstetrics and Gynecology, 1,* 3–7.

10. Anderson, E., Hamburger, S., Liu, J.H. and Rebar, R.W. (1987). Characteristics of menopausal women seeking assistance. *American Journal of Obstetrics and Gynecology, 156*(2), 428–433.

11. Gitlin, M.J., and Pasnau, R.O. (1989). Psychiatric syndromes linked to reproductive function in women: A review of current knowledge. *American Journal of Psychiatry, 146*(11), 1413–1422.

12. Hunter, M.S. (1990). Emotional well-being, sexual behaviour, and hormone replacement therapy. *Maturitas, 12*(3), 299–314.

13. Brenner, P.F. (1988). The menopausal syndrome. *Obstetrics and Gynecology, 72,* 6–10S.

14. Whitehead, M.I., Hillard, T.C., and Crook, D. (1990). The role and use of progestogens. *Obstetrics and Gynecology, 75,* 4 Suppl., 69S–76S.

15. Gambrell, R.D., and Teran, A.Z. (1991). Changes in lipids and lipoproteins with long-term estrogen deficiency and hormone replacement therapy. *American Journal of Obstetrics and Gynecology, 165,* 307.

16. American College of Obstetricians and Gynecologists (1990). Estrogen replacement therapy and endometrial cancer. *ACOG Committee Opinion,* No. 80. Washington, DC: American College of Obstetricians and Gynecologists.

17. Stampfer, M.J., Colditz, G.A., Willett, W.C., Manson, J.E., Rosner, B., Speizer, F.E., and Hennekens, C.H. (1991). Postmenopausal estrogen therapy and cardiovascular disease: Ten year followup from the Nurses' Health Study. *New England Journal of Medicine, 325,* 756.

18. Egeland, G.M., Kuller, L.H., Matthews, K.A., Kelsey, S.F., Cauley, S.F., Cauley, J. and Guzick, D. (1990). Hormone replacement therapy and lipoprotein changes during early menopause. *Obstetrics and Gynecology, 76,* 776–782.

19. Albright, F., Bloomberg, F., and Smith, P.H. (1940). Postmenopausal osteoporosis. *Transactions of the Association of American Physicians, 55,* 298–305.

20. Genant, H.K., Baylink, D.J., and Gallagher, J.C. (1989). Estrogens in the prevention of osteoporosis in postmenopausal women. *American Journal of Obstetrics and Gynecology, 161,* 6, Pt. 2, 1842–1846.

21. Lindsay, R., and Tohme, J.F. (1990). Estrogen treatment of patients with established postmenopausal osteoporosis. *Obstetrics and Gynecology, 76*(2), 290–295.

22. Ernster, V.L., Bush, T.L., Huggins, G.R., Hulka, B.S., Kelsey, J.L. and Schottenfeld, D. (1988). Benefits and risks of menopausal estrogen and/or progestin hormone use. *Preventive Medicine, 17*(2), 201–223.

23. Barrett-Connor, E. (1987). The risks and benefits of long-term estrogen replacement therapy. *Public Health Reports,* Suppl. Sept/Oct, 62–65.

24. Kelsey, J.L., and Berkowitz, G.S. (1988). Breast cancer epidemiology. *Cancer Research, 48,* 5615–5623.

25. Steinberg, K.K., Thacker, S.B., and Smith, J. (1991). A meta-analysis of the effect of estrogen replacement therapy on the risk of breast cancer. *Journal of the American Medical Association, 265*(15), 1985–1990.

Resources

NATIONAL INSTITUTE OF
AGING INFORMATION
CENTER
2209 Distribution Center
Silver Springs, MD 20910
301-495-3455

NATIONAL OSTEOPOROSIS
FOUNDATION
2100 M Street NW, Suite
  602
Washington, DC 20037
202-223-2226

NATIONAL WOMEN'S
HEALTH RESOURCE CENTER
2440 M Street NW
Washington, DC 20037
202-293-6045

Glossary

Abortion   The spontaneous or induced expulsion of an embryo or fetus before it is viable or can survive on its own.

Abruptio placenta   A complication of pregnancy in which the placenta separates prematurely from the wall of the uterus.

Abstinence   No penis-in-vagina intercourse. Couples may substitute oral sex or mutual masturbation without fear of pregnancy.

Active neglect   The intentional failure or refusal to acknowledge an obligation to care for an elder.

Acute diseases   Diseases that are characterized by being severe and of relatively short duration.

Addiction   Psychological or physiological dependence upon a substance with a tendency towards increased use of the substance.

Additive   A combined effect of drugs that is equal to the sum of the individual effects.

Adenocarcinoma   A cancer that originates from cells of the endocrine glands.

Adjuvant therapy   Methods such as chemotherapy and radiation therapy that enhance surgical effectiveness in cancer treatment.

Aerobic bacteria   Bacteria that are oxygen dependent.

Aerobic exercise   Any activity in which the amount of oxygen taken into the body is slightly more than, or equal to, the amount of oxygen used by the body.

Aerobic training   The process of increasing the body's ability to utilize oxygen and improve endurance.

Afterbirth   The placenta and amniotic sac that are expelled after the infant is delivered.

Afterburn   The elevated metabolic rate of the body for an extended period following exercise.

Agility   Ability to coordinate such movements and change directions quickly and safely.

AIDS-Related Complex   also known as ARC—a general term used in the earlier years of the AIDS epidemic to identify an intermediate phase of HIV infection between no symptoms and full-blown AIDS. It was generally diagnosed when an HIV infected individual had swollen lymph nodes, fever, night sweats, fatigue, diarrhea and weight loss that persisted for at least 3 months.

Alcohol dehydrogenase   An enzyme that metabolizes alcohol into aldehyde.

Alcoholic   A person whose experiences interfere with normal life activities due to regular and continuous drinking of alcohol.

Alcoholism   Pattern of alcohol use characterized by emotional and physical dependence as well as a general loss of control over the use of alcohol.

Alpha-fetoprotein screening   A prenatal screening test which measures a substance produced by the baby's kidneys between the 13th and 20th week of pregnancy.

Amniocentesis   Procedure to detect fetal defects in which the amniotic sac is punctured with a needle and syringe and amniotic fluid is obtained for analysis.

Amnion   The innermost membrane of the sac enclosing the embryo or fetus.

Amniotic fluid   Watery fluid that surrounds a developing embryo and fetus in the uterus.

Anabolic steroids   Synthetic derivatives of the male hormone testosterone usually taken to increase muscle mass, that often result in serious physiological and psychological side effects.

Analgesic   Medication that relieves pain without inducing loss of consciousness.

Androgyny   A blending of typical male and female behaviors in an individual.

Anerobic bacteria   Bacteria that are intolerant of oxygen.

Angina pectoris   Chest pain resulting from insufficient supply of blood (oxygen) to the heart muscle.

Anorexia nervosa   An eating disorder characterized by self-starvation and excessive weight loss.

Antagonistic   Opposing or counteracting.

Antihistamine   A medication used to treat allergic reactions and cold symptoms that inactivates histamine, a substance found in body tissues that plays a role in allergic reactions.

Anus   Outlet of the rectum between the fold of the buttocks.

Aorta   The great artery arising from the left ventricle; largest artery.

Aortic valve   Valve located between the left ventricle and the aorta.

Arrhythmias   Erratic heartbeats.

Arterioles   Small arteries.

Arteriosclerosis   The thickening and loss of elasticity of the arterial walls, slowing the flow of blood.

Arthritis   Chronic disease characterized by joint inflammation.

Atherosclerosis   Condition characterized by impaired constriction of blood vessels.

Athletic amenorrhea   The cessation of regular menstrual periods due to excessive exercising.

Autoimmune diseases   Diseases caused by autoantibodies or lymphocytes that attack molecules, cells, or tissues of the organism producing them.

Autoinoculation   Spreading infection from one area of self to another area.

B

Barbiturate   A class of sedative medicines that have a depressant effect on the central nervous system.

Bartholin's glands   Two small glands slightly inside the vaginal opening that secrete a few drops of fluid during sexual arousal.

Basal Metabolic Rate (BMR)   The amount of energy expended, usually expressed in terms of calories, per unit of time under resting conditions.

Battering   Repeatedly subjecting a woman to forceful physical, social, and psychological behavior in order to coerce her, without regard to her rights.

Benign tumor   A non-cancerous growth that does not spread to other parts of the body.

Beta-carotene   A substance found in yellow-orange fruits and vegetables which is believed to provide some level of protection against cancer by mopping up free radicals.

Bicuspid valve   Valve that separates the left atrium and the left ventricle of the heart.

Bingeing   Characteristic of bulimia nervosa—eating large amounts of food.

Biopsy   The removal and microscopic examination of a tissue sample to see if cancer cells are present.

Birth control   Umbrella term that refers to procedures that prevent the birth of a baby, including all contraceptive measures, sterilization and abortion procedures.

Birth canal   Passage through which the fetus travels during childbirth.

Bisexual   A person who feels sexual attraction or who has sexual contact with members of both sexes.

Blackout   The loss of memory or consciousness while drinking.

Blastocyst   Mass of cells that result from repeated divisions of the zygote.

Blood   Liquid medium of the circulatory system.

Blood Alcohol Concentration (BAC) or BAL (blood alcohol level)   A measure of the amount of alcohol present in the total blood of an individual, presented as a percentage of the total blood volume.

Blood pressure   The pressure exerted against the walls of the arteries when the heart pumps, specifically when the left ventricle contracts.

Body mass index   Weight (in kilograms) divided by height squared (in meters). A value of 25 or greater shows obesity-related health risks.

Braxton-Hicks contractions   The contraction of the uterus at irregular intervals throughout pregnancy. These contractions are not like "real" labor contractions in that they do not gradually increase in frequency, intensity or duration.

Breech   Birth presentation in which the fetus' buttocks present before the head.

Bulimia nervosa   An eating disorder characterized by a secretive cycle of bingeing and purging.

C

Calorie   The amount of heat required to raise the temperature of 1 gram of water by 1 degree Celsius.

Cancer   A general term for more than 100 diseases that are characterized by uncontrolled, abnormal growth of cells. Cancer cells can spread through the bloodstream and lymphatic system to other parts of the body.

Capacitation   Process of biochemical changes in the sperm cells that permit the sperm to penetrate the egg.

Capillaries   Minute, hairlike vessels connecting arterioles and venules.

Carbohydrate   An organic compound such as starch, sugar, or glycogen—composed of carbon, hydrogen, and oxygen: a source of bodily energy.

Carcinogenesis   The overall staging process by which normal cells become malignant; may be induced by chemical, physical, or viral agents.

Carcinogenic   Cancer causing.

Carcinoma-in-situ   Cancer that involves only the top layer of the organ without invading deeper tissues.

Carcinoma   A cancer that is the most common of all tumors—accounting for approximately 85 percent of all cancers; generally refers to cancer that begins in the tissues that line or cover an organ.

Cardiovascular accident (stroke)   Condition in which blood vessel damage occurs in the brain.

Cardiovascular fitness   The ability of the heart to pump blood through the body efficiently.

Cardiovascular system   The heart, arteries, veins, and capillaries.

Cauterization   The use of heat to destroy abnormal cells.

Cephalopelvic disproportion   A complication of pregnancy in which the size of the baby's head is deemed too large for the mother's pelvis; an indication for Cesarean delivery.

Cerebral aneurysm   Abnormal outpouching of an artery, which, due to the stress of blood rushing through it, may weaken and rupture.

Cervical cap   Contraceptive device made of plastic and individually fitted to fit snugly over the cervix.

Cervicitis   An inflammation of the cervix.

Cervix   The small end of the uterus, located at the back and extending into the vagina.

Cesarean delivery   The surgical procedure in which an infant is delivered through an incision made in the abdominal wall and uterus.

Chemotherapy   The treatment of disease with anticancer drugs or chemicals.

Child abuse and neglect   Physical or mental injury, sexual abuse or exploitation, negligent treatment, or maltreatment of a child by a person who is responsible for the child's welfare, under circumstances which indicate that the child's health or welfare is harmed or threatened.

Chloasma   Darkening of skin pigment on the upper lip, under the eyes, and on the forehead—occasionally a consequence of taking oral contraceptives,

Cholesterol   One of the steroids or fatlike chemical substances manufactured by the body and also consumed in foods of animal origin. It is essential for the manufacture and maintenance of the cell as well as sex hormones and nerves throughout the body.

Chorion   Outer membrane that forms outer wall of the blastocyst.

Chorionic villi sampling (CVS)   Procedure to detect fetal abnormalities in which the chorionic villi are examined.

Chromosomes   The structures in the nucleus of each cell composed of DNA and protein that contain the genes which provide information for the transmission of inherited characteristics.

Chronic bronchitis   A persistent inflammation of the bronchi due to irritation by air pollutants and tobacco smoke.

Chronic diseases   Diseases which are not of a short or acute nature; may be lifelong conditions and usually result in some sort of impairment or disability.

Chronic obstructive lung disease (COLD)   Any one of several lung diseases characterized by breathing obstruction. Includes COPD (Chronic Obstructive Pulmonary Disease) and emphysema.

Circuit training   A fitness routine that seeks to raise the heart rate by lifting moderate amounts of weight quickly and skipping the rest period between exercises.

Circumcision   Surgical removal of the foreskin of the penis.

Cirrhosis A chronic liver disease, characterized by a degeneration of cells and excessive scarring.

Climacteric Physiological changes that occur during the transition period from fertility to infertility in both sexes.

Climacterium Another term for menopause.

Clitoridectomy The removal of the clitoris; also known as female circumcision.

Clitoris A highly sensitive structure of the female external genitalia, the only purpose of which is sexual pleasure.

Co-dependent A person in a continuing relationship with a chemically dependent person and whose actions enable the addiction to continue.

Cohort A group of individuals who share a common condition or characteristic.

Coitus Technical term for penile-vaginal intercourse.

Colposcope A magnifying instrument used to examine the vagina and cervix.

Complex carbohydrate A starch found in cereals, fruits, and vegetables.

Conceptus The products of conception or fertilization.

Conditioning To develop the state of physical fitness.

Condom A protective sheath that fits over the penis to prevent sperm from entering the vagina and as a protection against sexually transmitted diseases.

Condyloma Wartlike growth(s).

Congenital heart disease A heart condition present when a baby is born and includes a variety of conditions, most of which can be surgically corrected.

Congestive heart failure (CHF) Condition in which the heart loses its ability to contract properly or sufficiently to meet the demands placed upon it.

Conization The surgical removal of a cone shaped piece of tissue from the cervix and cervical canal; may be used to diagnose or to treat a cervical condition. Also called cone biopsy.

Consensual   In terms of an extramarital sexual relationship—a sexual and/or emotional relationship that occurs outside the marriage with the consent of one's spouse.

Contraception   Measures that prevent fertilization of an ovum.

Contraceptive film   Spermicide that is contained in a small thin sheet of glycerine. It is placed over the cervix prior to intercourse. Its effect is similar to that of contraceptive suppositories in that as the sheet dissolves, the spermicide is released.

Contraceptive foam   Spermicide that is contained in a foam format.

Contraceptive sponge   Contraceptive device that acts both as a cervical barrier and a source of spermicide and the sponge absorbs the ejaculated semen. It is available without fitting or prescription.

Contraceptive suppositories   Spermicide that is available as vaginal suppositories. As the suppository dissolves, the spermicide is released.

Contraindication   A medical condition that renders a course of treatment inadvisable or unsafe that might otherwise be recommended.

Cool-down   The gradual slowing of an intense exercise period; prevents an abrupt drop in blood pressure.

Coordination   The ability to organize physical activities involving all parts of the body in a skillful manner.

Corpus luteum   A yellowish body that forms on the ovary at the site of the ruptured graafian follicle and secretes progesterone.

Crack   A highly addictive smokeable form of cocaine; also known as "rock."

Criminal violence   Includes robbery, burglary, aggravated assault, forcible rape, and homicide.

Cross-addiction   A state of physical dependence in which psychological need for one psychoactive substance leads to the dependence on similar substances.

Cross-tolerance   The capacity to endure the effects of psychoactive substances similar to one for which a tolerance has developed.

Crude fiber   Primarily cellulose and lignin; what remains of dietary fiber after acid and alkaline treatment.

Crura   The innermost tips of the cavernous bodies that connect to the pubic bones.

Cryosurgery   Procedure that freezes and destroys abnormal tissues

Cryotherapy   Surgical freezing of an infected area.

Cumulative   The increase in effects upon successive additions of the same drug or another substance.

Cunnilingus   Oral stimulation of the vulva.

Cystitis   Bladder infection.

D

Date rape   Also known as "acquaintance rape," is defined as rape in which the victim and the rapist were previously known to each other and may have interacted in some socially appropriate manner.

Delirium tremens (DT)   A condition induced by alcohol withdrawal and characterized by excessive trembling, sweating, anxiety, and hallucinations.

Dependency   State in which there is a compulsion to take a drug in order to experience its effects or to avoid the discomfort of the absence.

Depressant   A drug that relaxes the central nervous system.

Designer drug   An illegally manufactured psychoactive drug that has dangerous effects.

Diabetes   A disorder of the pancreas in which naturally occurring insulin is not properly manufactured and thus glucose cannot be regulated.

Diaphragm   Rubber, dome-shaped cap inserted over the cervix to prevent conception.

Diastolic   The second reading of blood pressure which represents the amount of pressure the blood exerts against the wall of the artery when the heart rests between beats.

Dietary fiber   Substances in plant foods that are not digested in by the processes present in the stomach and small intestine.

Differentiation   The process by which an individual develops distinct physical characteristics.

Dilation and curettage   A minor operation in which the cervix is expanded enough (dilated) to permit the cervical canal and uterine lining to be scraped with a spoon-shaped instrument called a curette; also called D & C.

Dilation   The opening of the uterus before delivery.

Disulfram   A drug that causes an aversive reaction when taken with alcohol; used to treat alcoholism; also known as antabuse.

Diuretic   Drug that expedites the elimination of fluid from the body.

Deoxyribonucleic acid (DNA)   A complex protein found in all living cells; carries the organism's genetic information.

Dorsal lithotomy position   A position for a gynecological examination; the woman lies on her back with her bottom at the very end of the examining table and her legs are supported in foot stirrups.

Down's syndrome   Congenital condition of various degrees of mental retardation and abnormal development caused by extra chromosome, usually number 21 or 22.

Drug abuse   The excessive use of a drug that has dangerous side effects.

Drug misuse   The use of a drug for a purpose other than its original intent.

Drug   Any substance other than food that, when taken, affects body processes.

Duration   The length of the exercise activity period.

Dysmenorrhea   Pain or discomfort before or during menstruation.

Dyspareunia   Pain or discomfort during intercourse.

Dysplasia   Abnormal cells that are not cancer; classified as mild, moderate or severe.

E

Ectopic pregnancy   Result of implantation of a fertilized egg outside the uterus.

Edema   An abnormal accumulation of fluid in body parts or tissues that results in swelling.

Effacement   The thinning of the cervix before delivery.

Elder abuse The injury, maltreatment, or neglect of an older person from a physical, psychological, or material perspective.

Electrocardiogram (ECG) The record produced by electrocardiography.

Electrocautery Electrical burning of an infected area.

Electrodessication Tissue destruction by heat.

Emboli A clot circulating in the blood stream.

Embryo transfer A fertility procedure in which the sperm of the infertile woman's partner are placed in another woman's uterus during ovulation. The fertilized egg is removed a few days later and transferred to the uterus of the infertile woman.

Embryo An organism in its early stage of development in humans; the embryonic periods lasts from 2nd–8th week of pregnancy.

Emetine A drug that induces vomiting.

Emphysema A condition caused by overdistention of the pulmonary alveoli or by the abnormal presence of air or gas in the body's tissues.

Endogenous estrogens Naturally occurring estrogens.

Endometriosis A benign condition in which tissue that looks like endometrial tissue grows in abnormal places in the abdomen.

Endometrium The tissue that lines the inside of the uterine walls.

Enzyme Linked Immunosorbent Assay test (ELISA) If HIV antibodies are found with this test, it is repeated. If antibodies are found on a second ELISA test, a Western Blot test is performed.

Episiotomy An incision in the mother's perineum that provides more room for the infant during delivery and helps prevent tearing of the vaginal tissues.

Estrogen A class of hormones that produce female secondary sex characteristics and affect the menstrual cycle.

Ethyl alcohol (ethanol) The intoxicating agent in alcoholic beverages.

Ever-smoker A person who has smoked as least 100 cigarettes during her lifetime.

Excision   Removal by cutting.

Excitement phase   Term used by Masters and Johnson to describe the first phase of the sexual response cycle, in which engorgement of sexual organs and an increase in muscle tension, heart rate, and blood pressure occur.

Extramarital relationship   Sexual interaction by a married person with someone other than his or her spouse.

F

Failure rate   A determination of the number of pregnancies that can be expected in a contraceptive method with normal use. A failure rate of 2 percent means 2 pregnancies per 100 women per year studied.

Fallopian tubes   Two tubes in which the egg and sperm travel, extending from the sides of the uterus.

False-positives   Test results which are initially thought to be positive but are later determined to be negative.

Fat-soluble vitamins   A vitamin absorbed with the aid of fats in the diet or bile from the liver, through the intestinal membrane and stored in the body.

Fat   A lipid with one, two, or three fatty acids, responsible for multiple body functions.

Fellatio   Oral stimulation of the penis or scrotum.

Feminine   Those behaviors believed to be appropriate for females.

Feminization of poverty   Referral to the fact that women and children are overwhelmingly the victims of poverty.

Fertilization   The union of an ovum and a sperm.

Fetal Alcohol Effect (FAE)   A term used to describe less serious cases of Fetal Alcohol Syndrome.

Fetal alcohol syndrome (FAS)   Alcohol-related defects among infants due to prenatal maternal alcohol consumption. They are usually characterized by growth retardation, facial malformations, and central nervous system dysfunctions including mental retardation.

Fetus   The unborn baby in the uterus from the 8th week of gestation to birth.

Fiber   Plant parts which cannot be digested in the human digestive tract: high fiber diets have been shown to protect against certain cancers and heart disease.

Fibroadenoma   A non-malignant form of breast tumor.

Fibrocystic breast disease   Also known as cystic mastitis; the most common breast disorder in women resulting in tender and lumpy breast tissues.

Fibroid   A benign uterine tumor composed of muscular and fibrous tissue.

Fimbriae   Fingerlike projections that form fringe around the fallopian tubes.

Flexibility   The range of motion permitted by joints.

Follicle Stimulating Hormone (FSH)   A pituitary hormone secreted by a female during the secretory phase of the menstrual cycle. It stimulates the development of ovarian follicles.

Forceps   Instruments for extracting a baby from the birth canal during delivery.

Forcible rape   An event that occurs without a woman's consent and involves the use of force or threat of force, and involves sexual penetration of the victim's vagina, mouth or rectum.

Foreskin   A covering of skin over the penile or clitoral glans.

Former smoker   A person who does not now smoke cigarettes, but who once did.

Fortification   The addition of any nutrient to a food.

Free radical   Toxic substances which are short-lived forms of compounds that exist with an unpaired electron in their outer shell. This causes it to have an electron-seeking nature, which can be very destructive to electron-dense areas of a cell, such as DNA and cell membranes.

Frequency   The regularity of an exercise program.

Fundus   The upper, rounded portion of the uterus.

G

Gamete intrafallopian transfer (GIFT)   A procedure for infertility which involves placing sperm and egg cells into fallopian tubes.

Gangrene   Localized tissue death due to inadequate cellular nutrition.

Gastritis   Inflammation of the stomach lining.

Gay   A homosexual, particularly, a homosexual man.

Gender dysphoria   A transsexual; a person whose psychological gender identity is opposite to his or her biological sex.

Gender identity   How one psychologically perceives oneself as either male or female.

Gender role   Also known as sex role—a collection of attitudes and behaviors that are considered normal and appropriate in a specific culture for people of a particular sex.

General sexual dysfunction   Formerly defined as "frigidity" this term refers to a condition where little or no erotic pleasure is experienced from sexual stimulation.

Glans   The head of the penis or clitoris, richly endowed with nerve endings.

Gonadotropins   Pituitary hormones that stimulate activity in the testes or ovaries.

Gonadotropin-Releasing Hormone (GRH)   Hormone responsible for reproductive hormone control.

H

Hallucinogen   A drug that causes hallucinations.

Heart attack   Death of a certain portion of the heart.

Heavy smoker   A person who smokes 25 or more cigarettes a day.

Hemoglobin   The iron-containing protein in the red blood cell that carries oxygen to the cells and carbon dioxide away from the cells; also responsible for the red color of blood.

Hemoglobin   The oxygen-carrying protein of red blood cells.

Hepatitis   Inflammation and destruction of liver cells.

Hepatoma   A cancer that originates from liver cells.

Herpes Simplex Virus (HSV)   Virus that causes skin eruptions.

Heterosexual   A person whose primary social, emotional, and sexual orientation is towards members of the opposite sex.

High density lipoprotein (HDL)   A type of lipoprotein—HDL-cholesterol is often referred to as the "good" cholesterol because it functions somewhat like a trash collector taking the LDL-cholesterol out of the body and lubricating the inner lining of the arteries.

Homeostatic   A constant environment.

Homologous   Refers to the "same" parts—the external genitals, gonads, and some of the internal structures of males and females originate from the same embryonic tissue.

Homophobia   Irrational fears of homosexuality, the fear of the possibility of homosexuality in oneself, or self-loathing towards one's own homosexuality.

Homosexual   A person whose primary erotic, psychological, emotional and social orientation is toward members of the same sex.

Host uterus   Procedure in which the sperm from a man and the egg from a woman are combined in a laboratory. The fertilized egg is then implanted into the uterus of a second woman who agrees to bear the child which is not genetically related to her.

Hot flashes   An uncomfortable sensation of menopause consisting of internally generated heat beginning in the chest and moving to the neck and head or spreading throughout the body.

Human chorionic gonadotropin (HCG)   A hormone produced by the chorionic villi.

Human Immunodeficiency Virus (HIV)   The virus that causes AIDS.

Human Papilloma Virus (HPV)   Viral infections that cause genital warts. In women, some strains are known to cause cervical cancer.

Hymen   Tissue that partially covers the vaginal opening.

Hyperplasia   A precancerous condition in which there is an increase in the number of normal cells.

Hypertension   Also known as high blood pressure—a blood pressure that remains elevated above what is considered a safe level.

Hypnotic   Drug that induces sleep or a trancelike state.

Hysterectomy   The surgical removal of the uterus; results in surgically induced menopause.

I

Immune system   The body's natural defense system, which works to eliminate pathogens.

Implantation   The embedding of the fertilized ovum in the uterine lining six to seven days after fertilization.

Incubation period   The period of time between the entrance of a pathogen into the body and the development of symptoms.

Inferior vena cava   The largest vein in the body and the venous trunk for the lower viscera.

Infertility   The inability to conceive a child.

Inhalant   A substance that produces vapors and has psychoactive effects when sniffed.

Inhibited sexual desire (ISD)   A sexual difficulty involving lack of interest in sexual fantasy and activity.

Insoluble fiber   Fiber that, for the most part, is not dissolved in water or by bacteria in the large intestine.

Intensity   Work per unit of time, usually measured by target heart rate.

Interferon   An antiviral substance secreted by infected cells that helps protect uninfected cells.

Intima   Inner portion of an artery.

Intimate violence   Includes child abuse, incest, courtship violence, date rape, battering, marital rape, and elder abuse.

Intoxication   Condition produced by excessive use of alcohol.

Intramuscular (IM)   The process of injecting drugs directly into muscle tissue.

Intrauterine growth retardation   Poor fetal growth for a given duration of pregnancy.

Intravenous (IV)   The process of injecting drugs directly into a vein.

Introitus   The opening to the vagina.

Invitro fertilization (IVF)   A procedure for infertility which involves removing the ova from a woman's ovary. The ova and sperm (from the woman's partner) are placed in a medium and, if development occurs, the conceptus is returned to the woman's uterus.

Involution   The returning of the uterus to its nonpregnant shape and size after delivery.

J

Jaundice   A condition in which accumulation of pigments in the blood produces a yellowing of the skin.

K

Korsakoff's psychosis   Nervous system disease associated with chronic alcoholism.

L

Labia majora   The outer lips of the vagina.

Labia minora   The inner lips of the vulva, one on each side of the vaginal opening.

Laparoscopy   Surgical procedure into a woman's abdomen which permits the surgeon to view the oviducts and other structures.

Laparoscope   An instrument consisting of an illuminated tube with an optical system that is inserted into the abdomen for diagnostic or therapeutic purposes (such as tubal ligation).

Lean body weight   The result of total body weight minus body fat.

Left atrium   One of the two upper chambers of the heart. It collects blood.

Left ventricle   One of the two lower chambers of the heart. It pumps blood from the heart.

Lesbian   A female homosexual.

Lesion   An anatomical change or disruption of part of the body.

Leukemia   A cancer that originates within the blood and blood-producing organs.

Leutinizing Hormone (LH)   The hormone secreted by the pituitary gland that stimulates ovulation in the female.

Lipoprotein   A compound found in the bloodstream containing a core of lipids with a shell of protein, phospholipid, and cholesterol.

Low-density lipoprotein (LDL)   A type of cholesterol that is considered harmful because it promotes fatty deposits on the inner lining of arteries.

Lupus   Chronic inflammatory disorder in which the immune system forms antibodies that target healthy tissues and organs; forms of the disease include discoid lupus and systemic lupus erythematosus.

Lymphoma   A cancer that originates from lymph tissue which is part of the body's immune system.

M

Macromineral   One of the six major minerals—calcium, chloride, magnesium, phosphorus, potassium, and sodium.

Mainstream smoke   The smoke directly inhaled by the smoker.

Malignant   A term used to describe a tumor that is capable of spreading to other tissues and invading adjacent areas.

Mammography   Procedure which results in a low dose x-ray of the breast to detect tumors.

Masculine   Those behaviors believed to be appropriate for males.

Mastectomy   Removal of entire breast tissue and underarm lymph nodes.

Masturbation   Stimulation of one's own genitals to create sexual pleasure.

Material elder abuse   The abuse or exploitation by the misuse or misappropriation of financial resources of an older person.

Melanoma   A cancer which originates within the skin cells that contain melanin.

Menarche   The initial onset of menstrual periods in a young woman.

Menopause   The cessation of regular menstrual periods by surgical or natural means. It is also known as the climacterium or the "change of life."

Menstrual phase   The phase of the menstrual cycle when menstruation occurs.

Metastasis   The spread of cancer from one part of the body to another. Cells in the metastatic tumor (the second tumor) are like those in the original tumor.

Mineral   A naturally occurring inorganic substance; a small amount is essential to life.

Minipills   Newest birth control pills. They are estrogen-free and provide a continuous, low-dose of progestin. Minipills are slightly less effective than the phasic pills and often cause irregular menstrual patterns. Minipills do not totally suppress hormone production.

Miscarriage   A pregnancy that terminates before the 20th week of gestation.

Modified radical mastectomy   Also known as total mastectomy; a less extensive procedure than radical mastectomy because underlying chest wall muscles are not removed.

Monounsaturated   A fatty acid containing one $C=C$ double bond that has been shown to lower only LDL.

Mons veneris   A triangular mound over the pubic bone above the vulva.

Mucosa   Collective term for the mucous membranes which are the moist tissues that line certain body areas such as the vagina and the mouth.

Multiple orgasms   More than one orgasmic experience within a short time period.

Muscular endurance   The ability to withstand the stress of physical exertion.

Muscular strength   Physical power such as the amount of weight one can lift, push or press in a single effort.

Myocardial infarction   Heart attack.

Myomectomy   Surgical removal of a uterine fibroid.

Myometrium   The smooth muscle layer of the uterine wall.

N

Narcotic   Derived from opium, a drug that relieves pain and induces sleep.

Neoplasm   A type of tumor that is a new growth of tissue serving no physiological function.

Neuroblastoma   A cancer which originates from cells in the nervous system.

Never-smoker   A person who has never smoked as many as 100 cigarettes (5 packs) in her lifetime.

Node   Specialized heart tissue that sends electrical stimulation for heartbeats.

Nonconsensual   In terms of an extramarital sexual relationship—a sexual and/or emotional relationship that occurs outside the marriage without the consent of one's spouse.

Nutrient   A food element essential to life and that the body cannot produce on its own.

Nutrition   The science studying the need for and the effects of food on an organism.

O

Obesity   The excessive accumulation of fat in the body; a condition of being 20 percent or more above ideal weight.

Opiate   A drug derived from opium.

Opportunistic infections   Infections that seldom cause disease in people with normal immune function but "take the opportunity" to cause disease in people with AIDS.

Opposed estrogen   Estrogen replacement therapy that is taken with the opposing effects of progestin.

Oral contraceptives   Birth control pills that cause the woman's own reproductive hormone cycle to be suppressed by the synthetic estrogen and progestin. Without the natural signals, the ovary egg follicle cannot mature and ovulation does not occur.

Orgasm   A series of muscular contractions of the pelvic floor muscles occurring at the peak of sexual arousal.

Orgasmic dysfunction   An inability to experience the orgasmic component of the sexual response cycle.

Orgasmic phase   Term used by Masters and Johnson to describe the third phase of the sexual response cycle in which the rhythmic muscular contractions of the pelvic floor occur.

Os   The opening of the cervix which connects the vagina to the uterine cavity.

Osteoarthritis   Degenerative joint disease.

Osteoporosis   Debilitating disorder characterized by a general decrease in bone mass.

OTC drugs   Over-the-counter drugs—those available without a prescription.

Ova   Female reproductive cells that are released in single units from the ovary.

Ovaries   Female gonads that produce ova and sex hormones.

Overuse syndrome   Injuries that occur to the body affecting the muscles, tendons, ligaments, joints, or skin, when the body is exercised beyond its biological limit.

Ovulation   The release of a mature ovum from the graafian follicle of the ovary.

Ovum   The female reproductive cell.

P

Pap smear   Gynecological procedure in which a sample of cervical cells are examined for the presence of precancerous or cancerous cells.

Passive neglect   Intentional failure to fulfill an obligation to care for an elder person.

Passive smoking   Breathing the smoke from others who are smoking. Occurs when a nonsmoker lives or works with smokers.

Pelvic floor   The muscles which provide the basis of support for a woman's uterus, bladder, and rectum.

Perimetrium   The thin membrane covering the outside of the uterus.

Perineum   The area between the vagina and the anus of a female.

Peripheral artery disease   Disease of the extremities in which the blood supply is diminished and sufficient oxygen and nutrients do not reach the areas properly.

Petting   Physical contact which includes kissing, touching, and manual or oral genital stimulation but excluding coitus.

Phenylketonuria (PKU)   A genetic disorder in which a crucial liver enzyme is absent, resulting in severe mental retardation if not treated.

Physical dependence   The physiological attachment to, and need for, a drug.

Physical elder abuse   Any activity which causes pain or injury to an older person.

Physical fitness   The ability to meet routine physical demands with a reserve to meet sudden challenges.

Physical violence   Includes slapping, choking, punching, kicking, pushing, and the use of objects as weapons.

Placenta previa   A complication of pregnancy in which the birth canal is obstructed by the placenta.

Placenta   An organ that develops after implantation and to which the embryo attaches, via the umbilical cord, for nourishment and waste removal.

Plaque   Fatty deposits on the lining of arteries.

Plateau phase   Term used by Masters and Johnson to describe the second phase of the sexual response cycle, in which muscle tension, heart rate, blood pressure, and vasocongestion increase.

Platelets   Disk-shaped structures in the blood for blood coagulation.

***Pneumocystis carinii* Pneumonia (PCP)**   The most common AIDS-related opportunistic infection in the U.S. HIV infected men.

Polyabuse   The use of more than one drug.

Polypharmacy   The dual use of alcohol and prescription drugs.

Polyunsaturated   A fatty acid containing two or more $C = C$ bonds which lowers both LDL and HDL.

Pornography   Sexually arousing images in film, print, or electronic media.

Post-pill amennorrhea   A delay in the return of normal menstrual cycles after taking oral contraceptives

Potentiating   The process of making more effective or powerful.

Premenstrual syndrome   A group of cyclic symptoms that occur in some women about a week before menstruation including breast tenderness, abdominal bloating, fatigue, fluctuating emotions and depression.

Premature labor   Labor that begins before the completed 9th month of fetal gestation.

Prepuce   The foreskin or fold of skin over the glans penis or clitoris.

Prodrome   Period of infectiousness before the first signs of infection are present.

Progestational phase   Second half of the endometrial cycle. Also known as the secretory phase.

Progesterone   The hormone produced by the corpus luteum of the ovary that causes the uterine lining to thicken.

Progestin   A synthetic progesterone used in conjunction with estrogen in hormone replacement therapy.

Progressive Resistance Training   The gradual and incremental increase, usually in the form of weights, to normal body motion.

Prolapsed cord   A complication of pregnancy in which the umbilical cord comes through the pelvis before the baby and can result in a disrupted flow of oxygen to the baby due to a compressed cord.

Proliferation phase   The phase in the menstrual cycle in which the ovarian follicles mature.

Prostaglandins   A family of hormones present in many body tissues. The release of prostaglandins as uterine living cells shed is believed to be the cause of menstrual cramping.

Protein   A substance that is basically a compound of amino acids; one of the essential nutrients.

Psychedelic   A drug that produces a heightened sense of reality with visual hallucinations and sometimes, psychoticlike behaviors.

Psychoactive   Affecting mood and/or behavior.

Psychological and social violence   Threats of harm, physical isolation of a woman, extreme jealousy, mental degradation, and threats of harm to children.

Psychological dependence   The emotional or mental attachment to the use of a drug.

Psychological elder abuse   The infliction of mental anguish upon an older person.

Puberty   The stage of life between childhood and adulthood during which the reproductive organs mature.

Pulmonary arteries   Vessels from the right ventricle to the lungs—carries blood for oxgenation.

Pulmonary veins   Vessels from the lungs to the left atrium.

Purging   Characteristic of bulimia nervosa—use of vomiting, laxatives, or diuretics after a bingeing episode.

Pus   Result of an infection process. Pus is composed of dead bacteria, dead white blood cells, and fluid.

R

Radiation therapy   Treatment with high-energy radiation from x-rays or other sources.

Radical mastectomy   Removal of entire affected breast, underlying chest muscles and underarm lymph nodes.

Red blood cells   One of the formed elements in peripheral blood—contains hemoglobin and transports oxygen

Relationship violence   Domestic violence between individuals in a significant relationship; formerly known as "wife abuse," or "spouse abuse."

Resolution phase   Term used by Masters and Johnson to describe the fourth phase of the sexual response cycle in which the sexual systems return to their nonexcited state.

Rheumatic heart disease   A heart condition resulting from a bacterial infection (Streptococcus) that has been inadequately treated and results in damage to the heart valves.

Rheumatoid arthritis   Chronic inflammatory disease of the joints.

Right atrium   One of the two upper chambers of the heart. It collects blood.

Right ventricle   One of the two lower chambers of the heart. It pumps blood from the heart.

Rubella   An infectious disease often causing birth defects in pregnant women; also called German measles.

Rugae   The folds of tissue in the vagina.

S

Sarcoma   A cancer which originates in the connective tissue, such as cartilage, tendons, and bone.

Saturated fat   Fats which come primarily from animal sources.

Secondary sex characteristics   The physical characteristics other than genitals that indicate sexual maturity, such as breasts and body hair.

Secretory phase   The phase of the menstrual cycle in which the corpus luteum develops and secretes progesterone.

Sedative   Drug that depresses the central nervous system resulting in a sleep or a trancelike state.

Segmental mastectomy   Lumpectomy, or the removal of a breast lump and minimal surrounding tissue.

Septum   A dividing wall between the right and left sides of the heart.

Sex role   Also known as gender role—a collection of attitudes and behaviors that are considered normal and appropriate in a specific culture for people of a particular sex.

Sexual dysfunction   The inability of an individual to function adequately in terms of sexual arousal, orgasm, or in coital situations.

Sexual harassment   Any unsolicited nonreciprocal male behavior that asserts a woman's sex role over her function as a worker. It can include staring, commenting, touching, requests for sexual favors, repeated requests for dates or sexual intercourse, or rape.

Sexual violence   Forced sexual activity in any form.

Shaft   The length of the clitoris or penis between the glans and the body.

Sickle-cell anemia   A debilitating genetic disorder of the blood characterized by sickle-shaped red blood cells, primarily affecting blacks.

Sidestream smoke   The smoke indirectly inhaled by a nonsmoker.

Sigmoidoscopy   Procedure that uses a thin lighted tube to examine the rectum and lower colon.

Simple carbohydrate   A sugar; provides the body with glucose.

Simple mastectomy   Complete removal of breast but not lymph nodes under the arm or chest muscles.

Sitz bath   A tub in which one bathes in a sitting position with hips under water and legs out.

Socialization   The process whereby a society conveys behavioral expectations to the individual.

Soluble fiber   Fiber that either dissolves or swells in the presence of water or is metabolized by bacteria in the large intestine.

Spontaneous abortion   Miscarriage.

Staging   The process of learning whether cancer has spread from its original site to another part of the body.

Stereotype   A generalized notion of what a person is like that is based only on that person's sex, race, religion, ethnic background, or similar criterion.

Sterilization   Any process that removes the organs of reproduction or makes them incapable of functioning effectively.

Sternum   The breast bone.

Stimulant   A drug that excites the central nervous system.

Strength training   The process of enhancing the size and strength of particular muscles and body regions.

Stress urinary incontinence   The involuntary release or leaking of small amounts of urine; usually associated with sudden exertion.

Stroke (cerebrovascular accident)   Condition in which blood vessel damage occurs in the brain.

Subcutaneous   The process of injecting drugs under the skin.

Superior vena cava   The venous trunk draining blood from the head, neck, upper limbs, and thorax.

Surrogacy   Procedure for infertility in which a woman is artificially inseminated with the sperm of an infertile's woman's partner. She then carries the pregnancy to term for the infertile couple.

Synergistic   Characterized by a combined effect that is greater than the sum of the individual effects.

Sphygmomanometer   Cuff device connected to a hose and measuring device to ascertain blood pressure.

Systolic   First reading of blood pressure which represents the amount of pressure the blood exerts against the wall of the artery when the heart contracts.

T

T-cell   A cell that governs the immune system and assists the B-lymphocyte in producing antibodies; T-cells are reduced in a person with AIDS.

Tamoxifen   A chemical treatment for breast cancer; may also inhibit breast tumor growth.

Target heart rate   A rate 60 to 90 percent of the maximum heart rate; the rate at which the maximum benefit is derived from exercise.

Tay-Sachs disease   A genetic disorder resulting in death by age 5 or 6; occurs almost exclusively among Jews of Eastern European ancestry.

Teratogens   Drugs which cause defects in developing embryos.

Tetrahydrocannabinol (TCH)   The primary psychoactive ingredient in marijuana and hashish.

Thrombus   A blood clot that blocks an artery.

Tolerance   The condition of requiring increasing levels of a drug in order to produce a constant level of effect.

Total hysterectomy and bilateral salpingo-oophorectomy   Hysterectomy performed in conjunction with the removal of both ovaries and the fallopian tubes.

Toxemia   A complication of pregnancy in which fluid is retained and toxic substances end up in the blood.

Toxicity   Level at which a drug becomes poisonous to the body, causing either temporary or permanent minor or major damage.

Transdermal therapy   A skin patch for estrogen replacement therapy. By feeding estrogen directly into the blood stream via the skin, the liver is bypassed.

Transient ischemic attack (TIA)   An event in which an artery may close momentarily in a spasm and result in a brief memory lapse or garbled speech.

Transsexual   A person whose psychological gender identity is opposite to his or her biological sex.

Transverse lie   A fetal position in which the baby lies horizontal to the birth canal; an indication for a Cesarean delivery.

Triglycerides   A type of lipoprotein—triglycerides that are associated, particularly in women, with an elevated risk of heart disease.

Tricuspid valve   Heart valve which has three points or cusps; situated between the right atrium and the right ventricle.

Tumor   An abnormal mass of tissue that results from excessive cell division. They may be benign or malignant.

U

Ultrasound   A procedure which uses high-frequency sound waves to project an image of the fetus.

Unopposed estrogen   Estrogen replacement therapy that is taken without the opposing effects of progestin.

Unsaturated fat   Fats which come from plants and include most vegetable oils.

Urethra   The tube through which urine passes from the bladder to outside the body.

Urethritis   Inflammation of the urinary opening.

V

Vaginal atrophy   A condition often associated with menopause that refers to the thinning of the vaginal lining.

Vaginismus   A sexual difficulty in which a woman experiences involuntary spasmodic contractions of the muscles of the outer third of the vagina.

Vasocongestion   The engorgement of blood vessels in particular body parts in response to sexual arousal.

Vasoconstrictor   A compound that results in closing down—narrowing—of blood vessels.

Vertex   Fetal presentation at delivery with the head delivered before the buttocks.

Very low density lipoprotein (VLDL)   A type of lipoprotein—VLDL-cholesterol is another lipoprotein which is associated with the breakdown of fats known as triglycerides which are taken in through food.

Vestibular bulbs   Part of the vast networks of bulbs and vessels that engorge with blood during sexual arousal. They cause the vagina to increase in length and the vulvar area to become swollen.

Vestibule   The area of the vulva inside of the labia minora.

Villi   Short vascular projections attaching the fetus to the uterine wall.

Violence   The unjust use of force and power.

Viruses   Small pathogens incapable of independent metabolism; can only reproduce inside living cells.

Vitamin   An organic substance needed by the body in a very small amount; carries out a variety of functions in metabolism and nutrition.

Vulva   The external genitals of a female, including the mons veneris, labia majora, labia minora, clitoris, and urinary and vaginal openings.

Vulvitis   Inflammation of the vulva.

W

Warm-up   A pre-exercise series of light activity that gradually raises the heart flow and increases the blood flow; decreases the chance of an injury.

Water-soluble vitamins   A vitamin used up or excreted in urine and sweat; must be replaced daily.

Wernicke's syndrome   A manifestation of malnutrition and alcoholism characterized by neurological symptoms.

Western Blot Test   Test for HIV antibodies—performed after two positive ELISA tests.

White blood cells   Elements in peripheral blood—protects the body against pathogenic microorganisms.

Withdrawal   Adverse physiological reactions exhibited when a drug-dependent person stops using that drug.

Withdrawal   Also known as coitus interruptus. It involves interrupting intercourse before the male ejaculates.

Y

Yo-yo dieting   The practice of losing weight and then regaining it, only to lose it and regain again. This practice makes it more difficult to succeed in future attempts to lose weight because thyroid hormone levels may drop very low in subsequent dieting, thereby significantly slowing basal metabolism.

Z

Zygote   A fertilized egg.

Index